369 0163705

D1778088

NEUROSCIENCE RESEARCH PROGRESS

MENINGITIS: CAUSES, DIAGNOSIS AND TREATMENT

GRIGORIS HOULLIS
AND MAGDALINI KARACHALIOS
EDITORS

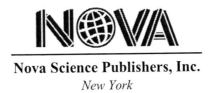

Nova Science Publishers, Inc.
New York

NOTICE TO THE READER

The Publisher has taken reasonable care in the preparation of this book, but makes no expressed or implied warranty of any kind and assumes no responsibility for any errors or omissions. No liability is assumed for incidental or consequential damages in connection with or arising out of information contained in this book. The Publisher shall not be liable for any special, consequential, or exemplary damages resulting, in whole or in part, from the readers' use of, or reliance upon, this material. Any parts of this book based on government reports are so indicated and copyright is claimed for those parts to the extent applicable to compilations of such works.

Independent verification should be sought for any data, advice or recommendations contained in this book. In addition, no responsibility is assumed by the publisher for any injury and/or damage to persons or property arising from any methods, products, instructions, ideas or otherwise contained in this publication.

This publication is designed to provide accurate and authoritative information with regard to the subject matter covered herein. It is sold with the clear understanding that the Publisher is not engaged in rendering legal or any other professional services. If legal or any other expert assistance is required, the services of a competent person should be sought. FROM A DECLARATION OF PARTICIPANTS JOINTLY ADOPTED BY A COMMITTEE OF THE AMERICAN BAR ASSOCIATION AND A COMMITTEE OF PUBLISHERS.

Additional color graphics may be available in the e-book version of this book.

LIBRARY OF CONGRESS CATALOGING-IN-PUBLICATION DATA

Meningitis : causes, diagnosis, and treatment / editors, Grigoris Houllis and Magdalini Karachalios.
  p. ; cm.
Includes bibliographical references and index.
ISBN 978-1-62100-833-0 (hardcover)
I. Houllis, Grigoris. II. Karachalios, Magdalini.
[DNLM: 1. Meningitis--etiology. 2. Meningitis--diagnosis. 3. Meningitis--therapy. WL 200]
616.82--dc23
                  2011039204

Published by Nova Science Publishers, Inc. ✛ *New York*

NEUROSCIENCE RESEARCH PROGRESS

Additional books in this series can be found on Nova's website
under the Series tab.

Additional E-books in this series can be found on Nova's website
under the E-book tab.

NEUROLOGY - LABORATORY AND CLINICAL RESEARCH DEVELOPMENTS

Additional books in this series can be found on Nova's website
under the Series tab.

Additional E-books in this series can be found on Nova's website
under the E-book tab.

NEUROSCIENCE RESEARCH PROGRESS

MENINGITIS: CAUSES, DIAGNOSIS AND TREATMENT

CONTENTS

Contents

countries.Patients present to clinics with at least two of the following symptoms; headache, fever, neck stiffness and altered mental status.Proper and swift diagnosis is pivotal to attain a proper treatment and a successful outcome.Prior to the development of molecular diagnosis, traditional culture methods were used for the identification and confirmation of the etiologic agent. For example, bacterial meningitis was detected by culturing bacteria on specific media. Such methods needed several days to identify and confirm presence of the agent.In the last two decades, the development and use of molecular diagnostic techniques for the early detection of meningitis has revolutionized the management of the disease and has remarkably contributed to positive treatment outcomes which has resulted in a vast decrease in mortality and morbidity among cases. Nucleic acid based methods primarily polymerase chain reaction (PCR) targeting specific genes in the suspected agents have been used extensively for diagnosis of meningitis.PCR-based systems especially multiplex PCR enabled the detection of multiple etiologic agents from clinical samples with a degree of certainty and speed. In addition, PCR techniques are pivotal to diagnosis of fastidious and unculturable meningitis agents or detecting very low numbers which otherwise will not be detected by traditional methods.PCR diagnosis coupled with DNA sequencing is frequently used for confirmation of the etiologic agent or when there is ambiguity in the differential diagnosis of closely related agents.This review will give a comprehensive considerationof the major bacterial agents-causing meningitis with their diagnosis using molecular methods currently in practice.

Chapter 3 - Tuberculous meningitis (TBM) is the most severe form of tuberculosis. It is an important cause of death and disease among both children and adults throughout the world, especially in developing countries.

The prognosis is worse in patients with HIV, in patients with severe neurological impairment, in chronic cases, and in patients with a resistance to drugs. The disease's pathogenesis has not as yet been sufficiently understood. Despite progress achieved over the past decades, a diagnosis of TBM is difficult to reach in many cases, because there is not as yet any diagnostic test sufficiently sensitive, targeted and timely. The percentage of patients where a definitive diagnosis of TBM can be established is low. TBM diagnosis and treatment are a challenge for neurologists. There is no characteristic medical profile, which makes it difficult to reach a diagnosis. Systemic symptoms of infection by Mycobacterium tuberculosis (MT), along with meningeal signs, may be suggestive of tuberculous meningitis. HIV infection does not change how tuberculous meningitis is presented.

In 80% of patients with TBM, symptoms appear at least one week before diagnosis. The time profile for the onset of TBM symptoms could be used to differentiate tuberculous meningitis from bacterial meningitis. The percentage of patients diagnosed as having tuberculous meningitis might increase if a molecular diagnostic test were applied. Hydrocephalus, pre-contrast hyperdensity-hyperintensity, basal leptomeningeal enhancement, obliteration of the basal cisterns, infarcts and tuberculomas are highly frequent findingson CT and MRI studies. The diagnostic approach is based on clinical criteria, laboratory test results, and image findings.

TBM prognosis depends on the presence of HIV, resistance to drugs, abnormal CT or MRI, substantial rise of proteins in CSF and onset of antituberculosis treatment three days after admission to hospital. The need to reach a diagnosis and administer early antituberculosis treatment is very important to reduce death and improve the prognosis. Recently, a consensus in terms of clinical diagnostic, laboratory and imaging criteria have been defined and recommended for tuberculous meningitis to be used in future clinical research.

Chapter 4 - Autoimmune diseases can be organ-specific or systemic, with the latter type affecting many different organs. As a neurological complication particularly of systemic autoimmune diseases such as systemic lupus erythematosus and Behçet disease, meningitis can occur at any stage of the disease and can be a main symptom as well as a prognostic factor. Mechanisms of meningitis associated with autoimmune diseases are still unclear, although disease-specific autoantibodies and cytokines are considered to play critical roles in the pathogenesis.

In meningitis associated with autoimmune disease, the main symptoms are fever, headache, nausea, and neck stiffness, which are similar to those presenting in infectious, malignant, or other forms of meningitis. The clinical course is also varied and can be acute, chronic, or recurrent, and thus is not that helpful in differential diagnosis. It is extremely difficult to prove that comorbid autoimmune disease is a direct cause of meningitis, but the exclusion of other etiologies is essential for accurate diagnosis. Such diagnosis is made from a full set of physical and laboratory data and imaging findings. Furthermore, in patients with autoimmune diseases treated with immunosuppressive or immunomodulating agents, it is often difficult to differentiate meningitis associated with autoimmune disease from infectious or drug-induced meningitis.

Treatment options for meningitis related to autoimmune diseases are targeted to suppress activated autoimmunity, and immunosuppressive agents such as pulsed cyclophosphamide and steroids are often recommended for acute relapse or severe forms of the disease. Recently, new agents such as monoclonal antibodies have been tested in cases involving the central nervous system; however, their efficacy remains unclear.

In this chapter, we discuss autoimmune diseases with which meningitis can occur, and review the clinical features, diagnosis, and treatments for meningitis associated with autoimmune diseases.

Chapter 5 - Meningitis is a bacterial, viral and fungal infection causing inflammation of the protective membrane covering the brain and spinal cord (meninges). Viral and other forms of meningitis are mild and get cured automatically within one or two week. Whereas, bacterial meningitis is life threatening disease if not being diagnosed or treated in time. Meningitis is contagious infection and can spread from one person to another by coughing, sneezing and through close contact.The diagnosis of the disease is carried out from CSF and blood of patients mostly by culture, latex agglutination, biochemical tests, PCR, MALDI, microarray and nucleic acid sensors. The treatment, prevention and therapy of especially bacterial meningitis are discussed in this chapter.

Chapter 6 - Bacterial meningitis is an infection of arachnoid membrane, subarachnoid space, and cerebrospinal fluid caused by bacteria. It is an infectious disease ranked among the top ten infectious causes of death [1]. A small number of pathogens such as Escherichia coli, group B Streptococcus (a.k.a. Streprococcus agalactiae), S. pneumoniae, Haemophilus influenzae type b (Hib), Neisseria meningitidis, and Listeria monocytogenes can cause meningitis in neonates, children, and adults with pathogenetic mechanisms elusive to scientists several years ago. The major pathogens of bacterial meningitis are Streptococcus pneumoniae and Neisseria meningitidis, accounting for 80% of the cases observed in community-acquired, bacterial meningitis in adults [2]. Nowadays, pneumococci are the most important cause of bacterial meningitis in children and adults worldwide. Haemophilus influenzae has disappeared in developed countries due to the wide employment of programs of successful vaccination. The incidence of the disease ranges from 1.1 to 2 per 100,000 population in USA [3-5] and Western Europe [6]. However, in Africa the incidence rises to 12 cases per 100,000 population per year [7]. The risk of disease is highest in individuals younger than 5 years and older than 60 years. In the adult subgroup (patients older than 16 years of age) the annual incidence of bacterial meningitis is 4 to 6 cases per 100,000 people [2]. Predisposing factors such as a previous splenectomy, malnutrition, or sickle cell disease have been identified [1, 8-10]. Bacterial meningitis can also be identified as a complication in 0.8 to 1.5% of patients undergoing craniotomy, and in 4 to 17% of patients with internal ventricular catheters. The incidence of meningitis after moderate or severe head trauma is up to 1.4% [11]. Leakage of cerebrospinal fluid (CSF) is the major risk factor for the development of meningitis, although most that occur after trauma remain undetected.

Besides classical meningitis, meningococci frequently cause systemic disease including fulminant gram-negative sepsis, and disseminated intravascular coagulopathy. The World Health Organization estimates that least 500,000 new symptomatic infections per year occur worldwide, leading to at least 50,000 deaths [12].

Bacterial meningitis remains a significant cause of morbidity and mortality throughout the world, despite the progress of antimicrobial therapy, especially in developing countries because of lack of preventive medical services, such as vaccination programs. Mortality rates are up to 34% [2, 13-15], while more than 50% of the survivors suffer from long-term neurological sequelae [3, 15-17]. The evolution of the disease can frequently result into a medical emergency with devastating consequences whenever inappropriate treatment is administered. However, mortality and morbidity vary by age and geographical location of the patient as well as the underlying pathogen. Patients at risk for high mortality and morbidity include newborns, those living in low-socioeconomical status, and those infected with Gram-negative bacilli and Streptococcus pneumoniae. Severity of illness on presentation (e.g. low Glasgow Coma Scale score), infection with resistant organisms, and incomplete knowledge of the pathogenesis of meningitis are additional factors contributing to increase mortality and morbidity. Age at infection is a crucial epidemiological factor. Different bacteria are the causative organisms of bacterial meningitis at different ages. Group B haemolytic Streptococcus, gram negative rods, Streptococcus pneumoniae, and Listeria monocytogenes are the main causes of neonatal and early childhood bacterial meningitis, and their presence is attributed to the acquisition through an infected maternal genital canal [18]. Streptococcus pneumoniae, Neisseria meningitis and Haemophilus influenzae type b appear usually responsible for meningitis occurring among patients with ages ranging between 6 months to 6 years [19, 20]. Epidemiology changes again between 6 years and 60 years, when Neisseria meningitis and Streptococcus pneumoniae predominate. In addition to this unacceptable mortality, there is a high rate of neurologic sequelae in children and adults who survive after episodes of bacterial meningitis.

High morbidity imposes the need to study the pathogenesis and pathophysiology of bacterial meningitis in an attempt to improve the response to conventional antimicrobial therapy. Many researchers have tried to analyze the pathogenesis of bacterial meningitis in an effort to develop new treatment approaches. Bacterial meningitis is an infectious disease that requires

PREFACE

Meningitis is an inflammation of the three thin membranes covering the brain and the spinal cord which are collectively called the meninges. It is a serious and sometimes fatal infection affecting the central nervous system and is caused by different bacterial and viral etiologic agents. In this book, the authors present topical research in the study of the causes, diagnosis and treatment of meningitis. Topics include the molecular diagnosis and epidemiological typing of bacterial meningitis; novel dissemination and invasion routes of bacterial meningitis; contemporary management of nosocomial bacterial meningitis in neurosurgical practice; meningitis associated with autoimmune diseases and Mollaret's meningitis syndrome.

Chapter 1 - Meningitis per se is a pathological process confined to the lepto-meninges without grossly affecting the brain, spinal cord. However, in complicated meningitis, there is involvement of the brain, spinal cord and or nerve roots also.

The pathological process is an inflammatory and or allergic response of the meninges to a wide variety of etiological factors.

The etiological spectrum of the meningitis has changed recently due to emergence of immuno-compromising diseases.

The causative factors are mainly categorized in following groups: 1.Infections and infestations (viruses, bacteria, fungi, parasites); 2.Cancer cells 3.Foreign materials including blood, chemicals, drugs etc.4.Other causes i.e., serum sickness, systemic lupus erythematosus, vasculitis, Behcet's disease, sarcoidosis, iatrogenic, etc.

The pathogenesis of the meningitis is better understood now due to increasing research activities: host factors, characteristics & virulence of the infective microorganism, level of innoculum, etc.

Irrespective of the type of etiological factor involved, the clinical features of meningism are more or less same: headaches, neck stiffness, vomiting and fever. However depending on the nature of the etiological factor, there may be prodromal symptoms, systemic symptoms, as well as the features of neurological involvement. Ideally, brain imaging (CT head) is carried out prior to the lumbar puncture to exclude the cerebral mass lesion and raised ICP.

The diagnosis mainly depends upon the detailed analysis of the cerebrospinal fluid (CSF). CSF, blood, urine, stool and throat swabs may be sent, where indicated, for culture and antimicrobial sensitivity. This may be supported by hematological, biochemical and microbiological studies, neuro-imaging, radiological studies of the other organ systems, etc. CSF, blood, urine, stool and throat swabs may be sent for culture, serological testing and antimicrobial sensitivity. Recently developed molecular technologies help in precise diagnosis.

The management is mainly focused on the treatment of the causative factors for meningitis along with the symptomatic supportive care. It is also pertinent to exclude more serious causes with certainty at that time. Inpatient care with anti-microbial drugs, bed rest, analgesics, anti-emetics, anti-cancer therapy, steroids and supportive measures are important steps in the overall management.

Efficacy of the treatment must be reviewed as per the practices of the evidence based medicine.

Though, in great majority of cases, the diagnosis is reached quickly and appropriate treatment started in time with a good outcome as compared to before. But, in some cases, this may not be possible. Occasionally, the differentiation of infective from non-infective etiologies may be perplexing and rarely there may be more than one causative factor for meningitis.

Meningitis, in general, carries higher risks of morbidities and mortality and therefore needs precise diagnosis and appropriate management strategies in time to optimize the outcome.

Unfortunately, despite much scientific advancement in diagnostics and therapeutics, there is still considerable morbidity and mortality. In future, we need to focus on the preventive measures (public educational activities, immuno-prophylaxis and chemo-prophylaxis), modern diagnostics and appropriate treatment strategies to achieve optimum results.

Chapter 2 - Meningitis, an inflammation of the meninges is a medical emergency that requires prompt treatment to minimize or eliminate its devastating outcome. Its incidence is estimated at 0.6-4 cases per 100,000 adults in developed countries and might be far more than that in developing multidisciplinary and specialized medical treatment. Better understanding of the infection route, concerning the cascade of events that spread the disease from the primary infection site of the nasopharynx or the middle ear, would aid in the development of more effective treatment strategies [1, 9].

Chapter 7 - Nosocomial meningitis are rare but potentially serious and life-threatening complications of both cranial and spinal surgeries as well as head injuries. In a postoperative neurosurgical context, an important issue consists in differentiating accurately bacterial meningitis from aseptic meningitis. This latter is mainly related to the release of blood products in the cerebrospinal fluid (CSF) and the use of dural substitutes or haemostatic substances. Clinical presentation and CSF characteristics are identical between both entities while aseptic meningitis' outcome is usually benign under corticosteroids. Prompt and aggressive antibiotic treatment is mandatory in the first hours of postoperative meningitis after accurate CSF and blood samplings and adequate cultures. Only the absence of bacterial culture growth in the CSF at the 72nd hour justifies the interruption of antibiotherapy in the postoperative course. This review details the epidemiology and the risk factors of postoperative meningitis, pathophysiology of central nervous system infection, pathogenesis of chemical or aseptic meningitis, paraclinical exams and treatment modalities according to meningitis type. Short term and long term complications including hydrocephalus, ventriculitis and/or vasculitis, may occur depending upon precocity of treatment, accuracy of antibiotic choice and bacteriological diagnosis

Chapter 8 - Mollaret's meningitis is defined as benign recurrent aseptic meningitis characterized by recurrent episodes of fever and signs of meningeal irritation, lasting between 2 and 5 days and is associated with spontaneous recovery. Mollaret's meningitis is seldom seen in clinical practice.

The syndrome was named after Pierre Mollaret, a French neurologist, that in 1944 described recurrent episodes of aseptic meningitis in three patients during a 15 year period. The cerebrospinal fluid (CSF) taken from these patients, 24 hours after the onset of these recurrences, revealed leukocytosis containing many large mononuclear cells, thought to be of endothelial origin (Mollaret cells). After a few days, these cells disappeared. Later immunocytological examination of CSF cells revealed that the so-called Mollaret cells are actually monocytes .

The clinical presentation is indistinguishable from meningitis of other aetiologies, including fever, headache, neck and back pain, myalgias, and neck stiffness. Transient neurologic abnormalities such as epileptic seizures, facial palsy, disequilibrium, speech impairment, syncope and extensor plantar response may be present in 50% of the patients. There is a female to male predominance, approximately 26:15. In general, the episodes tend to reoccur in a period of days to years and the syndrome usually resolves automatically after 3 to 5 years according to some studies.

The aetiology of the syndrome remained obscure for many years. Steel et al. in 1981 were the first to isolate Herpes Simplex Virus type 1 (HSV-1) in the CSF of a patient with diagnosed Mollaret's meningitis, suggesting a viral aetiology of the syndrome. Some researchers followed Steel's hypothesis associating different viruses, such as Herpes Simplex Virus type 2 (HSV-2) or EBV, to the syndrome . However, it was not until the development and the use of the polymerase chain reaction (PCR) technique that the Mollaret's meningitis aetiology became clearer. Since 1991, 69 patients diagnosed with Mollaret's meningitis had their CSF tested with PCR for HSV and were reported in the literature. Remarkably, 56 were positive for HSV-2. Five cases tested negative for HSV. Among them, one was finally attributed to SLE, another to herpesvirus type 6 and only three remained idiopathic.

It has been proposed that the term Mollaret's meningitis should be reserved for recurrent aseptic meningitis where no cause is identified. However, with the existing evidence, recurrent herpetic meningitis is presumably the benign condition that was previously identified as Mollaret's meningitis.

Due to the rarity and the benign course of the disease, there is no definitive treatment recommendation. Intravenous acyclovir may be of value because it has shown to resolve symptoms within 72 h and the majority of patients remain symptom free for many years. However, intermittent or continuous prophylaxis may be considered for frequent episodes.

In: Meningitis: Causes, Diagnosis and Treatment   ISBN 978-1-62100-833-0
Editors: G. Houllis et al. pp. 1-82   ©2012 Nova Science Publishers, Inc.

Chapter 1

CURRENT CONCEPTS OF MENINGITIS: ITS ETIOLOGICAL FACTORS, MANAGEMENT OPTIONS AND PROGNOSIS*

Rewati Raman Sharma, Apollina Sharma and Sameer Raniga
First page affiliation
First page affiliation

ABSTRACT

Meningitis per se is a pathological process confined to the lepto-meninges without grossly affecting the brain, spinal cord. However, in complicated meningitis, there is involvement of the brain, spinal cord and or nerve roots also.

The pathological process is an inflammatory and or allergic response of the meninges to a wide variety of etiological factors.

The etiological spectrum of the meningitis has changed recently due to emergence of immuno-compromising diseases.

The causative factors are mainly categorized in following groups: 1.Infections and infestations (viruses, bacteria, fungi, parasites); 2.Cancer cells 3.Foreign materials including blood, chemicals, drugs etc.4.Other

---

* Credentials: Dr. Sameer Raniga [FRCR, MD, DNB- Radiology] Consultant Radiologist [Senior Specialist in Radiology], Khoula Hospital, Muscat, Oman.

causes i.e., serum sickness, systemic lupus erythematosus, vasculitis, Behcet's disease, sarcoidosis, iatrogenic, etc.

The pathogenesis of the meningitis is better understood now due to increasing research activities: host factors, characteristics & virulence of the infective microorganism, level of innoculum, etc.

Irrespective of the type of etiological factor involved, the clinical features of meningism are more or less same: headaches, neck stiffness, vomiting and fever. However depending on the nature of the etiological factor, there may be prodromal symptoms, systemic symptoms, as well as the features of neurological involvement. Ideally, brain imaging (CT head) is carried out prior to the lumbar puncture to exclude the cerebral mass lesion and raised ICP.

The diagnosis mainly depends upon the detailed analysis of the cerebrospinal fluid (CSF). CSF, blood, urine, stool and throat swabs may be sent, where indicated, for culture and antimicrobial sensitivity. This may be supported by hematological, biochemical and microbiological studies, neuro-imaging, radiological studies of the other organ systems, etc. CSF, blood, urine, stool and throat swabs may be sent for culture, serological testing and antimicrobial sensitivity. Recently developed molecular technologies help in precise diagnosis.

The management is mainly focused on the treatment of the causative factors for meningitis along with the symptomatic supportive care. It is also pertinent to exclude more serious causes with certainty at that time. Inpatient care with anti-microbial drugs, bed rest, analgesics, anti-emetics, anti-cancer therapy, steroids and supportive measures are important steps in the overall management.

Efficacy of the treatment must be reviewed as per the practices of the evidence based medicine.

Though, in great majority of cases, the diagnosis is reached quickly and appropriate treatment started in time with a good outcome as compared to before. But, in some cases, this may not be possible. Occasionally, the differentiation of infective from non-infective etiologies may be perplexing and rarely there may be more than one causative factor for meningitis.

Meningitis, in general, carries higher risks of morbidities and mortality and therefore needs precise diagnosis and appropriate management strategies in time to optimize the outcome.

Unfortunately, despite much scientific advancement in diagnostics and therapeutics, there is still considerable morbidity and mortality. In future, we need to focus on the preventive measures (public educational activities, immuno-prophylaxis and chemo-prophylaxis), modern diagnostics and appropriate treatment strategies to achieve optimum results.

CURRENT PERSPECTIVE

General Background

In general, the majority of significant infective disorders of the internal organs in humans are commonly aggressive, clinically expressive and lending themselves for their management. In order of their occurrences, respiratory infections (including upper respiratory infections) are far more common followed by the gastrointestinal and urinary tract infections. Infections of the bones & joints and the cardiovascular system (including the blood) are next in the list. Comparatively, the central nervous system (CNS) infections are least common. These are usually more serious, and may be devastating and catastrophic with higher morbidities and mortality despite their aggressive management. Even after achieving their effective clinical control, these CNS infections leave short term, long term or permanent sequalae in significant number of cases with perplexing concerns, consequences and disabilities.

The current understanding of the incidence, epidemiology, clinical spectrum, diagnostic requirements and management plans of the infective disorders of the central nervous system is still far from complete. Recent advances have definitely improved our knowledge in these areas and have presented hope for the better results in future.

Infections of the nervous system present with protean clinical manifestations, difficult diagnostic dilemma and special therapeutic challenges. Currently, the main causes of the CNS infections are viral (commonest), bacterial (common), parasitic-protozoal (less common) and fungal (uncommon or rare) organisms. [1]

Definitions

The brain and the spinal cord within the cranio-spinal region are well protected by the meningeal coverings {dura mater –(pachy meningeal layer) peripherally adherent to the protective craniospinal bony structures} and two leptomeninges { an outer, arachnoid membrane potentially adherent to the internal surface of the dura mater and an inner, pia mater completely conformably blending and making the outer surface of the brain as well as the spinal cord and a protective cushion of the cerebrospinal fluid along with blood vessels and cranio-spinal nerves in the webbed sub arachnoid spaces between these two leptomeninges}.

The spectrum of CNS infections is broad and therefore a wide variety of clinical manifestations /presentations encounter in CNS infections.

Inflammation of the dura mater is denoted as pachymeningitis. Lepto-meningeal inflammation is called lepto-meningitis or simply meningitis. The chronic form of lepto-meningitis is usually termed as arachnoiditis.

Irritation of the meninges (pia mater and arachnoid mater) due to any cause i.e., blood, etc is referred as meningism. Significant inflammation of the meninges due to non-infective causes is called aseptic meningitis, whereas meningeal inflammation due to micro-organisms is referred as infective meningitis.

Among the cases of CNS infection, many patients solely present with meningitis per se but in a significant number of cases, meningeal inflammation is a concurrent part of the wide variety of CNS infections such as encephalitis (inflammation of the cerebral tissue per se), myelitis (inflammation of the spinal cord tissue), radiculitis (inflammation of the cranio-spinal nerve roots) and neuritis (inflammation of the peripheral nerves), etc.

Many a times there is combination of these disease entities as per the spread and extension of the inflammatory process in the parts of the nervous system (focal/ localized, multifocal or diffuse process),i.e.; cerebritis, ventriculitis, vasculitis, cranial neuritis, meningo-encephalitis, encephalo-myelitis, etc.

When the infective etiological factor is clearly defined then the suffix –itis – is used i.e.; meningitis, meningoencephalitis, meningo-encephalo-myelitis etc. However, when no causative factor is either identified or the cause is metabolically then the suffix-pithy is used commonly used i.e.; meningo-encephalopathy, myelopathy, radiculopathy, neuropathy.

Infective process causing meningitis may also lead to ischemia, infarction, hemorrhage, epidural /subdural hygromas/ empyema/ abscesses, as well as cerebritis, cerebral abscesses and ventriculitis.

Clinical presentation therefore may be protean in a significant number of patients depending upon the extent of the neural tissue involvement.

Classification

According to the causative factors, we can classify meningitis in following broad groups:-

1.   Viral meningitis

2. Bacterial meningitis
3. Fungal meningitis
4. Parasitic meningitis
5. Chemical meningitis
6. Carcinomatous meningitis

Meningitis is an inflammation of the cerebrospinal membranes covering the brain and spinal cord (meninges) due to the aforementioned causative factors, singly or in various combinations.

1. Viral Meningitis [2-11]

The viral meningitis per se is the pathological process of viral etiology involving mainly the lepto-meninges without affecting the brain or spinal cord. However, it is usually associated with involvement of one or more parts of the nervous system. Practically, viral meningitis (more common) and encephalitis(less common) may occur concurrently as a part of same infectious process (meningo-encephalitis), right from the onset of the illness.

Viral meningitis runs commonly a benign course and is also non-specifically called as aseptic lymphocytic meningitis, but in general, there are many other causes of aseptic meningitis.

Epidemiology [3-11]

The viral meningitis is relatively common, uncommonly serious but rarely fatal illness with multiple viral etiologies. It is ubiquitous with world wide distribution. The actual incidence is difficult to ascertain because many cases of viral meningitis are treated symptomatically by the general practitioners with good clinical outcome without establishing a proper clinico-pathological diagnosis as well as lack of reporting of such cases. This situation often complicates the clinical picture in some patients. However, the approximate estimate is reported as close as to 11-20 individuals per 100,000 people in USA, 05-20 cases per 100,000 in UK and about 25-35 individuals per 100,000 populations internationally in general. Japanese-B encephalitis Virus is being the commonest to infect in Asian countries and is responsible for causing meningitis in many more folds of population. In Finland, it is reported as 200 cases per 100,000 infants. Mumps is one of the leading causes in places where vaccines are not available. There is an increase in the incidence of viral meningitis in summers due the seasonal increase in the entero-viruses. History of vaccination, sex and travel should always be taken.

There is no bar to age and sex. However, younger the age more is the incidence of viral infection and being highest during the neonatal period and infancy. There are some age preferences such as St.Louis encephalitis virus infects infants and old aged people predilection, California virus affects young children where as Japanese-B virus contracts all age groups. However, more vulnerable group includes patients with recurrent upper respiratory infections, immuno-compromised patients, health care professionals, children in day care setups. In some generalization, infants are infected more with entero-viruses; young children with arboviruses; school going children with polio virus, measles and mumps; teenagers and college going subjects with mumps and measles; adults and middle aged people with herpes virus family and old aged persons with enteroviruses. Males are more commonly affected with mumps and enteroviruses as compared to the females.

Etio –pathogenesis: Some classes of viruses have a worldwide distribution whilst others are more localized to particular areas.

Viral meningitis is commonly (80-85%) caused by the enteroviruses (Coxsackie viruses A & B; Echoviruses); less commonly (10-15%) by the Arboviruses, Herpes viruses and mumps; and rarely (5% or less) by the measles, lymphocytic choriomeningitis viruses, HIV and adenoviruses. [2-4]

It is often not possible to precisely identify the causative virus. [3] However, in general, Entero-viruses (a group of the picornaviruses) are more commonly responsible for viral meningitis in majority of cases where as arbo-viruses (arthropod borne viruses by tics and mosquitoes) cause meningitis in a small percentage of patients. More than the 80% cases of viral meningitis are caused by the entero-viruses especially Coxsackie viruses A & B and echoviruses, polio viruses, and Enterovirus-71. In fact, in neonatal and early pediatric meningitis cases, Coxsackie virus-B remains accountable for more than 60-70 % cases. Enter viruses have more affinity towards meninges whereas arboviruses towards parenchymal tissues. Both infections occur in the warmer whether such as in summer and early fall. The population of blood sucking vectors, mosquitoes and tics, is much higher in such whether conditions.

More frequently involved viral families from the arboviruses group (more than 450 members) are as follows: 1.*Alpha-viruses* (Eastern, Western as well as Venezuelan equine encephalitic viruses); 2. *Bunya-viruses* (California encephalitic viruses and Jamestown Canyon viruses); 3.*Flavi-viruses*(Japanese B encephalitis virus, Colorado tick fever virus, West Nile virus, St. Louis encephalitis virus, Murray valley viruses), etc. The two most common viruses from this list are St. Louis encephalitis virus and Japanese B encephalitis virus for the majority of cases in the USA and worldwide. Arbo-viruses are mainly transmitted by an insect vector causing meningo-encephalitis in a small number of people bitten.

Among these arboviruses, St. Louis encephalitic virus infect more commonly -the neonates, infants and elderly; California virus -young children ,West Nile virus- adults and Japanese B virus infect all age groups-world wide. Recent appearance of West Nile virus in the United States has resulted in significantly higher incidence of cases with viral encephalitis.

The other less common cause of viral meningitis is the infection with the Herpes family viruses which are collectively responsible for about less than 5% of cases of viral meningitis but Herpes simplex virus-2 remain the most common cause of meningitis as well as meningo-encephalitis in this group of viruses. [5-8] These are ubiquitous, spread world wide and can cause infection during any time of the year. Many of these viruses are known to remain latent within the central and peripheral nervous systems. In this family, following members are more clinically significant—Herpes simplex viruses (HSV-1 & HSV-2), Varicella-zoster virus(usually causing chickenpox and shingles), Human herpes virus-6, Epstein-Barr virus (EBV) and cytomegalovirus(CMV).

In this family Cytomegalovirus causes congenital fetal intracranial infections with long term disabilities. Herpes simplex viral (HSV-2) meningitis in neonates occurs due to viral infection of the new born contracted from the mother during the vaginal delivery. In adults, HSV meningitis is associated with primary genital infection and HIV infection; however, this is usually self limiting in immuno-competent individuals. In the initial phase it is difficult to differentiate between meningitis, encephalitis or meningo-encephalitis. Complicated Varicella-zoster virus, uncommon but serious chicken pox, infection causing meningitis and meningo-encephalitis is rare. Rabies virus infection is although extremely rare but invariably fatal encephalitis. Aforementioned members of the Herpes family viruses may cause Mollaret meningitis. Interestingly this form of meningitis is benign, self limiting but may be recurrent. In these cases, Mollaret cells are detected in the cerebrospinal fluid during the early stage of infection. These are monocytes with large bilobed nuclei and amorphous cytoplasm.

Paramyxoviruses such as mumps and measles are uncommon cause of viral meningitis. [5] These infections were very common before immunization era; but now with universal immunization policy (measles, mumps and rubella {MMR} vaccination program), fortunately, these are uncommon or rare causes of meningitis. In the Europe and Japan, the incidence of mumps meningitis was much higher even after the vaccinations—so called vaccine derived(few strains identified and then taken care of) mumps meningitis. Due to the vaccination programs, the incidences of these infections are definitely low elsewhere in the range of less than one per 100 thousand populations in USA although much more common in the developing countries. Parotitis in mumps and maculo-papular rashes in measles during the winter seasons in young people help in the diagnosis.

There are many rare causes of viral meningitis including influenza virus which can be looked up elsewhere and are beyond the scope of this write up; however, some rare causes such as *lympphocytic choriomeningitis virus (LCMV), adenovirus and retroviruses* need mentioning. [6] Adenoviruses, especially Ad 3 and Ad 7, are rare cause of meningitis in the immuno-competent subjects; but a major cause of meningitis in AIDS cases, patients with severe combined immunodeficiency (SCID) and immunocompromised hosts as well as in bone marrow transplant recipients. Lymphocytic choriomeningitis is a rodent (mice, rats, hamster)borne especially in high risk people such as pet owners, laboratory workers or people living in rodent infestated areas.

Retroviruses usually, Human Immunodeficiency virus (HIV) and Human T cell lympho-trophic virus (HTLV), may cause atypical meningitis—initially at the time of sero-conversion in about 4-10 % of HIV infections and in few cases the condition becomes chronic and in rare cases it has been recurrent. Some cases it may even progress to raised ICP with increased CSF pressure. Usually these patients develop sub acute encephalitis either early or after some delay following the meningitis. AIDS patients are well known to develop other viral infections (LCMV) concomitantly.

Viral transmission occurs via various routes. Entero-viruses are transmitted mainly via oro-fecal route. Entero-viruses are commonly spread by direct contact with the fecal matter, hand-to-mouth contact and from aerosols during sneezing and coughing, hence common in young children. Adenovirus, mumps and measles are contracted in the same ways in the schools. Arbo-viruses are injected through the skin by the biting from tics or mosquito vectors. Infection due to arboviruses is, therefore, arthropod borne disease and is spread mainly by the blood sucking arthropods. Herpes family viruses are mainly communicable through the personal contact. Unlike others, Herpes family viruses(HSV-1,HSV-2,VZV-B) and rabies virus get to CNS from muco-cutaneous regions by retrograde extension up the peripheral nerves (olfactory, trigeminal and spinal nerves) and then via the cranial or spinal ganglia to the CNS. Reactivated Herpes simplex virus (HSV) type-1 is the most frequently travels up the olfactory nerves to the temporal lobes causing necrotizing-hemorrhagic encephalitis and HSV-2 is mainly causing meningitis. LCMV is contracted from the rodent's fresh urine, saliva, droppings, nesting materials, etc. Retroviruses are well known to spread by direct physical contact. Potentially, the viral infection is also caused by the infected blood transfusion and infected donor organs. The incubation period for enteroviral meningitis is about 2 days and it is different for other viral meningitis.

Fortunately, a smaller number/ percentage of systemic viral infections progress to meningitis, encephalitis or meningo-encephalitis. The occurrence of meningitis depends on many factors such as the virulence of the specific virus, inoculum's level, the immunological status of the human host (local and systemic immune status, muco-cutaneous barriers, blood brain barrier, etc) and the tropism of the virus for specific CNS cell types, such as Herpes simplex virus-1 has predilection for the temporal lobes and rabies viruses for the limbic system.

Initial viral infection and rapid replication occurs in the primary focus outside the central nervous system in the gastrointestinal system, respiratory system, muco-cutaneous regions, genitourinary system, etc. *This results in the local extension and primary viremia* causing hematogenous spread to the reticulo-endothelial system (lymph nodes, spleen and liver).If viral replication is unchecked, *the secondary viremia causes CNS seeding.* Infective viruses reach CNS either via hematogenous spread from the primary focus or by direct neuronal penetration and retrograde transportation/migration along the neural extensions from the brain and the spinal cord or nerve roots from the adjacent structures like nasal mucosa, cutaneous tissues and spinal ganglia, capillary endothelial defects in BBB/ areas lacking BBB such as area postrema, locus ceruleus, choroid plexes, etc.

There is an inflammatory response within 24-48 hours following the viral inoculum. Initial response is polymorphonuclear leukocytosis, followed later by progressively increasing monocytosis and T-lymphocytosis. The CSF study will confirm active meningitic process. If the infective process involves the cerebral or spinal cord parenchyma then there will be parenchymal edema, vasculitis, leucocytic /lymphocytic penetration of the brain /spinal cord tissues, glial cells proliferation and neuronal degenerations depending on the type of the virus , its virulence and penetration with spread which will increase morbidity and mortality in such cases. Therefore, the prompt attention to details for the diagnosis and management is mandatory.

Clinical Presentation and Differential Diagnoses [2-11]

The initial presentation is commonly with *non-specific prodromal symptoms* such as fever, chills and rigors, general malaise, lethargy, muscle pains, tiredness as well as *extra-neural symptoms* such as sore throat, upper respiratory infection, skin rashes, joint pains, nausea, vomiting and abdominal pains as well as focal or generalized lymphadenopathy.

Once the meningeal inflammation well establishes, the aforementioned symptoms are then followed by neck stiffness, headaches, and photophobia. Then either the toxic-metabolic effects of the infective process or the build up of raised intracranial pressure or the direct involvement of the brain parenchyma result in various degrees of confusion, disorientation, irritability, agitation, drowsiness, seizures, focal neurological deficits or coma may be observed.

Acute meningitis is sudden in appearance with clinical features suggestive of upper respiratory infection or constitutional symptoms, meningeal irritation and mental changes. Whereas, sub acute or chronic meningitis such as in tuberculosis or mycoses, may present with features of raised intracranial pressure (headaches, vomiting, papilledema, visual obscuration and drowsiness) and disturbances of higher mental faculties (forgetfulness, confusion, disorientation, changes in personality, etc).

The clinical features of meningeal irritation per se are headaches, nausea-vomiting, photophobia, irritability, neck & low back pains with stiffness as well as restriction of the movements. There is increasing resistance to the passive flexion of the neck (Brudzinski' sign) as well as inability to extend the knee when the hip (thigh) is flexed at 90 degrees with the trunk (Kernig's sign). Immune compromised and geriatric subjects may not present with classical features of meningitis and therefore may present a diagnostic challenge. Careful evaluation may reveal fever, neck stiffness and mental changes in these patients. One should look for muco-cutaneous vesicles in Coxsackie viruses ,Herpes family viruses as well as rashes in HIV sero-conversion.

Therefore, uncomplicated viral meningitis is often self-limiting with appreciable recovery in about fortnight in majority of cases; however when the meningitis is complicated with the spread of the inflammatory process in the cerebro-spinal parenchymal tissues and manifesting as encephalitis and myelitis then the clinical course is more likely to be protracted. Seizures, altered sensorium, focal and general neurological deficits in the face, limbs and body, and the features of raised ICP should be carefully assessed.

Adenoviruses, especially Ad 3 and Ad 7, are rare cause of meningitis in the immuno-competent subjects; but a major cause of meningitis in AIDS cases, patients with severe combined immunodeficiency (SCID) and immunocompromised hosts as well as bone marrow transplant recipients.

Asymptomatic or mildly symptomatic cases of LCM are fairly common; however, in general there is a biphasic clinical course: the initial febrile systemic extra-neural phase lasting for about one week is mainly marked with pro-dromal and constitutional general symptoms such as fever, malaise, myalgia, loss of appetite ,nausea, vomiting and headaches along with upper respiratory symptoms such as sore throat, cough and chest pains; poly-arthritic pains as well as glandular pains-parotid and testicular pains. This is usually followed with recovery and then the appearance of the second phase in some cases commonly with the symptomatology of meningitis, less commonly with encephalitis and raised intracranial pressure and hydrocephalus may need CSF diversion; and rarely, the occurrence of myelitis especially sacral radiculo-myelitis in HSV-2 meningitis. There may be recurrent enteroviral meningitis in some cases.

Differential diagnosis of meningitis, meningo-encephalitis and simply meningism will mainly include to differentiate viral meningitis and meningoencephalitis from other infective causes(bacterial including tuberculosis, fungal, parasitic and rickettsial infections), post vaccinal causes (especially in cases of measles and rubella vaccines), vascular causes (intracranial subarachnoid hemorrhage, migraine), neoplastic causes (carcinomatosis), drugs(NSAIDs, allopurinol, azathioprine etc), systemic disorders(vasculitis, sarcoidosis), trauma, etc.

Investigations [3, 7-11]
Three pronged investigations may be required:

1. *Laboratory confirmation of virus identification using serological tests or isolation techniques.* Whenever possible, identification of the viral agent is important to diagnose the case appropriately and this may be commenced by taking samples from the muco-cutaneous vesicles, throat washings, stool, blood or CSF and then performing tissue cultures or animal inoculation. Virus culture is the standard method of detection for entero-viruses but this is time consuming. Nowadays, molecular techniques such as PCR (for the identification of the viral nucleic acids) and typing based on genome sequences are performed

as the serotype-specific PCR primers are available for majority of viruses.

Mandatory test to diagnose the meningitis per se is the lumbar puncture and CSF analysis. If in doubt of raised ICP, one can do a CT scan of the head prior to lumbar puncture to rule out other potentially dangerous causes producing / mimicking meningeal irritation—intracranial tumor or bleed. The CSF analysis usually shows viral meningitis pattern : mild lymphocytic pleocytosis, with normal sugar and moderately raised proteins as well as no bacterial organisms seen on microscopy or in CSF cultures and more over, no bacterial antigen detected in the CSF analysis. The CSF is sent for virological studies especially viral culture and PCR (polymerase chain reaction) studies for the detection of the type of the virus, e.g., enteroviruses, and herpes family viruses, etc. These tests are rarely undertaken in the routine practice. Anti body tests in the CSF and Serum are done to ascertain arthropod borne meningitis or encephalitis.

2. *Tests to assess the general status of the patient*-hematological, biochemical, coagulation screen, systemic infective screen including the blood cultures and assessment of intake and output. These are usually normal.

3. *Tests to assess neuronal spread / progression of viral meningitis in the CNS and its attendant complications.* The CT brain scan is performed which usually shows normal findings until unless there is an acute hydrocephalus or the meningitis became complicated with progression to the encephalitis and or myelitis stages. In these cases periodic CT scans as well as MRI scans will be needed to monitor and treat the patients.

Management [2-4, 8-11]

The management of viral meningitis is mainly supportive. The clinical presentation of viral meningitis may be similar to the bacterial meningitis; but both need to be differentiated with the help of CSF analysis. However, the caution must be exercised so as to not to miss the bacterial meningitis where the delay in diagnosis may be life threatening and may be associated with high morbidity in the survivors. If meningitis is suspected, the patients, especially pregnant women, infants and elderly people, immune-compromised individuals etc, must be referred to the hospital for prompt further evaluation and management. In majority of cases, the viral infection is basically destroyed by the patient's own immune system and the medically derived treatment is a symptomatic adjuvant help in time to create a suitable environment for it. When patient's immune system can not overcome it, then the medical help is essential to counteract the infection.

The main pillars of the management are as follows—

I.   *Symptomatic treatment of the patient with uncomplicated viral meningitis: Supportive therapy*
   1.   An adequate rest in a quiet mildly lighted or dark room, away from the noises and having least interaction with the people
   2.   An adequate re-hydration with nutritional support
   3.   An adequate control of the fever (antipyretics such as acetaminophen) as well as relief in the concomitant headaches and body aches with acetaminophen as needed but within the prescribed limits. When the adult patients are having intolerable headaches then long acting NSAIDs, Tramadol or opiate analgesia may be required. Aspirin is avoided especially in children.

II   *Anti-microbial therapy*
   1.   Majority of the cases with uncomplicated viral meningitis is mild and may show recovery with symptomatic treatment whilst being investigated.
   2.   Significant symptoms warrant Lumbar puncture and CSF analysis.
   3.   Viral meningitis is treated with antiviral therapy wherever indicated. Immunological status of the patient must be checked and if there is hypo-gamma-globulinemia then the needed immuno-globulins must be instituted. In cases of HSV-1 encephalitis and HSV-2 meningitis, a full course of intravenous acyclovir must be started immediately for a period of 5-7 days. Similarly, Ganciclovir should be given in cases of CMV infections or AIDS related infection. The toxicities of the Ganciclovir should be monitored and controlled. Enteroviruses are usually self limiting and need no specific antiviral therapy. For the prevention of the meningitis due to the mumps, measles, varicella, polio virus, influenza virus, Japanese-B encephalitis virus etc, the vaccinations are given.

4. Anti-bacterial antibiotic medications are usually not indicated except when the bacterial meningitis is suspected, or when the diagnosis is not clear and bacterial meningitis has not been ruled out, or patient's clinical symptomatology being severe, or there is superadded bacterial infection at the primary system and/or in the CNS. Periodic CSF analysis is the key to the diagnosis in majority of cases. However, one simple rule is that if you are in doubt, it is better to start broad spectrum intravenous antibiotics and which is continued till the definitive exclusion of the bacterial meningitis from the diagnosis..

5. *Intensive Care Management* of the complicated meningitis and meningo-encephalitis with recurrent seizures, altered state of consciousness, unstable vital parameters, neurological deficits, raised intracranial pressure, cerebral edema, intracranial hemorrhage or cerebral infarction, etc. The periodic neuro-imaging studies are mandatory and close ICP monitoring is done where indicated. Here, the patient may need anti-cerebral edema medications (mannitol, 3% hyper tonic saline); anticonvulsant drugs; ventilation support; CSF diversion procedure depending on the state of the ICP, ventricular dilation and degree of CSF infection. These patients require periodic corrections of hematological values, biochemical changes, coagulation derangements if any, ventilatory-respiratory parameters and maintenance of adequate intake and out put charts. These are done whilst keeping an eye on the infection screen, antimicrobial medications, findings of periodic CSF analysis and periodic neuro-imaging studies to monitor and modify the day to day appropriate management options. These are done to control and treat severity of infection, cerebral edema, raised intracranial pressure. Cerebral edema and raised ICP can cause extensive brain damage and even death if unchecked.

III *Precautions to prevent the spread and recurrence* whilst receiving the treatment by using frequent hand washing, use of barriers (tissues) whilst coughing and sneezing, barrier nursing and universal methods of care by the health care professionals. Family members and friends should be evaluated for obvious reasons.

Prognosis: Complications with Long Term Effects

The overall prognosis in viral meningitis is better than the other infective causes except in infants and young children. Usually there is complete recovery within 2-4 weeks. However, the complicated viral meningitis / meningo-encephalitis are the fifth leading cause of mortality and a host of long term morbidities especially in the infants. In other age groups, it accounts for only about 1 % of mortality and less than 5 % of morbidity. In acute phase meningitis may progressed to encephalitis and myelitis to cause, seizures, cerebral edema, intracranial hemorrhages, coma, hydrocephalus, weakness of limbs with short term and long term squeal. This stage needs intensive care managements so as to reduce mortality and morbidities.

Majority of patients with viral meningitis and meningo-encephalitis recover almost completely with in 4-6 weeks period. However, a small but significant number of cases do suffer long term effects where cerebro-spinal parenchymal tissues are involved in meningo-encephalitis and meningo-myelitis especially in infancy and early childhood. The brain , spinal cord and nerve damage remain a possible complication of viral meningitis. Meningitis per se may give rise to communicating hydrocephalus(may need CSF diversion procedures) and meningo-encephalitis may result in cerebral atrophy with ex-vacuo ventricular dilatation, higher mental function disorders including impaired memory and intelligence, behavioral problems, speech disorders, learning disabilities, seizure disorders, syndrome of inappropriate (more) ADH secretion, neuromuscular disabilities with weakness of limbs or various forms of inco-ordinations in the eye movements, use of limbs and balancing of the trunk muscles. Cranio-spinal nerves are involved with variable loss of their functions in many cases especially optic nerves (blindness), abducent nerve (diplopia), trigeminal nerve (neuralgia), facial nerve(facial palsy) , vestibulo-cochlear nerve(dizziness, sensory neural hearing loss), lower cranial nerves(swallowing and speech disturbances) & the thoracic spinal nerves(neuralgic pains), etc.

Due to the aforementioned effects, the prognosis of CNS viral infection in infancy is poor; whereas in other groups, it is variable. However, in the great majority of cases, the overall prognosis remains excellent following an appropriate management. Prompt recognition and treatment will reduce symptomatology, lessen morbidity and reduce mortality.

Prevention is certainly better than the cure. Therefore, preventive measures such as the strict hand washing to avoid entero-viruses, protection against mosquitoes and tics to avoid arbo-viruses (insect eradicating sprays, netting, use of insecticides at the breeding sites), avoidance of exposure to rodents to avoid LCMV, use of barriers during sex to avoid herpes family viruses as well as HIV and strict Vaccination programs to ward off mumps, measles, polio, varicella viruses. Pregnant women should take extra-care in the aforementioned measures.

2. Bacterial Meningitis [11-14]

Bacterial meningitis in its terminology is simply the inflammation of the cerebrospinal meninges (mostly lepto-meninges, uncommonly pachy-meninges and rarely, both, meningeal groups involved) due to the bacterial infection. Among the causes of CNS infection, it is one of the most life-threatening illnesses with considerable higher rates of mortality and morbidities even in the present antibiotic era. Interestingly, quiet contrary to the viral infections, the bacterial infections in general, although not always, initially involve a principle / particular anatomical location such as either skull bones, meninges , ventricle or brain parenchyma and if not checked and controlled then the infection spread at the site of seeding, extend locally and progress to the other parts of the CNS.

Commonly used defined terminologies in the bacterial infections of the CNS. The terminologies commonly used in the bacterial infections of the CNS in particular are derived from the following factors: anatomical location; place/event from where the infection acquired; type of bacterial family involved in infection; degree of the infectivity of the bacteria; age of the patient; rapidity of the symptoms; products of inflammation; duration of illness; positive and negative responses to the antibiotic and general treatment; effects on the vital parameters and level of consciousness of the patients, focal neurological deficits, etc. These terminologies are also similarly used in fungal, parasitic and other forms of infections.

Following terminologies are commonly used—

1. Anatomical location: meningitis (primarily meningeal infection), encephalitis (primarily brain matter/ parenchymal infection), & vasculitis (infection of the blood vessels);
2. Meningeal involvement: pacchymeningitis (infection primarily of the dura mater), lepto-meningitis (infection of the pia-arachnoid membranes and contained CSF);
3. Type of meningeal inflammatory response—Pyogenic (polymorphonuclear response as in acute bacterial meningitis), lymphocytic (predominantly lymphocytic response as in partially treated bacterial meningitis, chronic bacterial meningitis or viral

meningitis), granulomatous (monocyte-macrophages response to chronic infection such as in tuberculosis infection);

4. Complicated meningitis: Meningitis may evolve into other conditions in the intracranial cavity--- subdural empyema (an infective collection in the subdural space), cerebritis (an initial stage of focal brain infection with parenchymal necrosis), cerebral abscess(Later stage of the focal brain infection with parenchymal necrosis, liquefaction and pus collection as a space occupying lesion), granuloma (granulomatous lesion of the meninges or parenchyma of the brain), ventriculitis (infection of the ventricular/ ependymal lining), hydrocephalus (collection of the CSF in the ventricular system under increased pressure).

5. Different Types of the organisms involved: Pneumococcal meningitis (S pneumoniae), Hib meningitis (H. influenzae-B), Meningococcal meningitis (N. meningitidis),tubercular meningitis (Mycobacterium tuberculosis), etc;

6. The age of the patient: Congenital (infection during fetal development), neonatal (infection within first 6 weeks of life), infantile (infection from 7th week of life to one year), Children (pediatric meningitis), adult meningitis and the meningitis in the elderly group;

7. Presentation at the onset: Fatal (acute onset of infection with rapid progression to death), Fulminant (acute onset with rapid progression to extreme severity), Severe (advanced meningeal infection), and acute (sudden onset of meningitis— 1-3 days), sub acute (onset, progression and persistence for 2-3 weeks after infection), chronic meningitis (more than 3-4 weeks of meningeal infection);

8. Place from where the infection is acquired: community or hospital (nosocomial);

9. Antibiotic effect: antibiotic responsive meningitis or single / multiple drugs resistant meningitis

10. Degree of the virulence of the bacteria: mild, moderate, severe, fatal, etc.

Epidemiology [11, 12, 15]

Bacterial meningitis is ubiquitous with worldwide distribution and is the second most leading cause of CNS infections in general and meningitis in particular. It is slightly more common in males as compared to the females in the ratio of 5::4 and more so in the neonates in the ratio of 3 males to one female baby. It is also more common in the blacks as compared to others. In USA, bacterial meningitis is in the range of 0.5-4.0 cases per 100,000 adult populations and about 0.25 -1 case per 1,000 live births, being 10 times more in premature then the term neonates. Meningococcal meningitis had resulted in outbreaks in 1805 in Switzerland but the causative organism was identified only in 1887 and then many serious outbreaks occurred such as in World War I & II, outbreak in Sub-Saharan African region (African meningitis belt from Ethiopia to Senegal) during 1950s, periodic outbreaks in Norwegian regions in 20th century, and out break in East Mediterranean region in 1988, etc. Vaccination programs gave much relief from such outbreaks. However, in USA before 1990s, H. influenzae was the leading cause of meningitis in the range of 2.8 to 3.0 cases per 100,000 population, but after the introduction of new conjugate vaccine to H. influenzae type–B (HIB), the incidence has significantly reduced to 0.7 per 100,1000 population. Currently in the USA, S. pneumoniae is the leading cause of meningitis followed by the N. meningitidis and then H. influenzae.

Recent developments such as the world wide impact of the HIV infection and widespread use of available vaccines have changed the epidemiology of the bacterial meningitis: much less number of meningitis cases in children (especially of the HIB related); where as the tuberculosis and other opportunistic infections have increased in the adult populations due to the HIV infection. Tuberculosis remains the 7th leading cause of death and disability in the world. In the early age group there is no male to female difference; however, in the adult population, the males are affected twice the number of the females and is highest in Asians and Pacific Islanders. The incidence of the tuberculosis has declined in the developed countries due to preventive measures (vaccination) and newer antibiotics; but, it is still a huge problem in the developing world especially in the infants and early childhood period (the age group less than five years)as well as in adults where it is resulting in significant morbidity and remains one of the leading causes of mortality. In the western society it is more common in the immigrants. There is a high risk of active TBM in patient with co-existing tuberculosis and HIV and the causative organism may be M. avium intracellulare with poor prognosis.

The wide spread use, of the conjugate vaccines against 7 serotypes of S pneumoniae, Serogroup-C meningococcal conjugate vaccine and HIB vaccines, has significantly reduced the incidence of meningitis due to these organisms and changing the epidemiological distribution of the meningitis cases.

Etio-Pathogenesis [14-20]

Community acquired bacterial meningitis: In adults, three principle causes of community acquired bacterial meningitis are Neisseria meningitidis, [20-25] Streptococcus pneumoniae (encapsulated bacteria) [24-26] and Hemophilus influenzae type-B or HIB (NHS-in increasing order of incidence). [21-23] These three organisms (NHS) cause meningitis rarely in neonates and infrequently in infants. In the neonates, E coli, Streptococcus agalactiae (group B streptococci) and Listeria monocytogenes are the main causative bacteria as these are present in the maternal vaginal cavity, perineum and her colonized gut. These are acquired by the new born during the delivery or hospital stay (nosocomial infection). Also during early infancy (between 5-12 weeks of age), these organisms predominate; however, three aforementioned organisms causing meningitis in adults also causing infection in infants. In this age group, S. pneumoniae and Neisseria meningitidis account for about 10 cases per 100,000 population but meningitis due to HIB has declined due to the use of effective vaccines. In elderly and aged group of people as well as immune-compromised patients, the L. monocytogenes and aerobic gram-negative bacilli join the group of the organisms (except H.influenzae, also a Gram negative bacilli) causing meningitis in adults.

S pneumoniae [27] is a lancet- shaped Gram positive diplo-cocci and N meningitidis Gram negative intracellularly placed Kidney bean shaped cocci; whereas H.influenzae type B is a Gram negative pleomorphic (shape changes from coccobacilli to a long curved rod) bacilli. These infections can be transmitted from the person to person and their incubation period, approximately, ranges from 4-7 days.

Neisseria meningitidis, Gram negative cocci, has three Sero-groups A, B & C; the Serogroup-A usually causes meningitis in adults and other two primarily result in systemic infections. In endemic form, sporadic cases occur in general population. Where as in epidemic form, there are outbreaks of meningococcal meningitis on wider scales. Patients and asymptomatic carriers harbor Neisseria meningitides & S. pneumoniae in their naso-pharynx and H. influenzae in their paranasal sinuses.

Nosocomial bacterial meningitis: [11-26] In post-operative neurosurgical cases (including the craniotomies, shunt surgeries, external ventricular drains, lumbar punctures, intrathecal medication infusions, spinal anesthesia as well as in the cases of post traumatic compound fractures of the calvaria), the cutaneous organisms over the calvaria of the skull or hospital acquired nosocomial organisms such as Gram positive cocci (Staphylococcus aureus, staphylococcus epidermidis and other coagulase-negative staphylococci), aerobic Gram negative bacilli (Pseudomonas aeruginosa) as well as Propionibacterium acnes are predominantly responsible for the infections. In cases where the continuity of the skull base is breached due to the surgery or fractures then the organisms residing at the skull base regions such as H. influenzae (nasal cavities), S pneumoniae (nasopharynx) and Group A streptococci (oro pharynx) are mainly responsible. Majority of infection manifest in the first month following surgery (90-95%).Craniotomy is associated with 1-3% rate of nosocomial infection whereas the internal shunts about 5-10% ,external ventricular drains 10%, lumbar punctures/ invasive techniques approximately 1-2%. The best preventive measures are use of antibiotics at the time of anesthesia, undivided attention to the details of the aseptic techniques and to the procedural details, and prevention of the CSF leakage intracranial hemorrhage. Once it is diagnosed, it must be promptly treated to have a good outcome.

In the chronic cases of meningitis, micobacterium tuberculosis, brucella, Treponema pallidum etc are commonly thought over and these are worldwide distribution. For tuberculosis and spirochete infections, the humans are main reservoir. The mycobacterium tuberculosis is an aerobic gram positive acid fast bacillus. The CNS tuberculosis is usually secondary to primary focus in the lungs, and less commonly in the gastrointestinal, genitourinary or the musculo-skeletal system. Hematogenous dissemination results in CNS tuberculosis. Initially, Bacilli seed to the meninges and the brain parenchyma to form subpial and subependymal tiny caseous lesions known as Roch foci. These sub pial foci usually enlarge and rupture in the subarachnoid spaces but parenchymal Roch foci extremely rarely rupture in the ventricular system and more commonly grow to form tuberculomas and or abscesses. Gelatinous exudate is the byproduct of the tuberculous infection, which fills the subarachnoid space and infiltrate the blood vessels in it Meningeal, vascular and parenchymal inflammation result in fibrous adhesions in basal cisterns(subsequently resulting in communication hydrocephalus needing treatment), obliterative vasculitis (progressive inflammation, vascular obstruction and focal cerebral infarction resulting in dysfunctions of the mental faculties and cranial nerves including vascular brain stem syndromes needing symptomatic treatment) and encephalitis/ myelitis (abscess or granuloma formation needing medical and or surgical treatment).

The predisposing risk factors are naso-oro-pharyngeal and respiratory infections, middle ear and mastoid infections, contaminated objects, compound head injuries, other bodily infections such as HIV, immune compromised states etc. Human migration, HIV infection, malnutrition, alcoholism, drug abuse, diabetes mellitus, corticosteroid use etc are important risk factors for the tuberculous meningitis.

The common mode of transfer of bacterial infections is via person to person contacts and spread of the respiratory droplets during coughing, sneezing, kissing and using the shared objects. Use of contaminated milk and cheese (L. monocytogenes) can also meningitis. Initially, the bacteria multiply & form colonies and adhere to the nasal mucosa and then infect nearby tissues and gain access to the blood stream to spread systemically including CNS through the BBB. The bacteria may spread from blood vessels to the meninges, parenchyma, choroid plexuses and ventricles.

Bacteria gain access to the sub-arachnoid spaces via hematogenous routes from systemic infections, direct route from the infections in the skull base region such as para-meningeal, para-nasal and temporo-mastoid structures, as well as direct implantation of the bacteria during the head injury or neurosurgical procedures. Fetal infections may occur insidiously due to transplacental spread of the maternal bacteria such as enteric Gram negative bacilli, Listeria monocytogenes and B-streptococci with serious consequences. Early neonatal infections occur due to the bacteria colonize the maternal genital tract (mainly Gram negative enteric flora and Group B streptococci called S. agalactiae) as well as from the surroundings (staphyloccocus epidermidis, L monocytogenes, etc). Rare neonatal infections such as citrobacter diversus, citrobacter koseri, and Salmonella species are also reported with higher morbidities. In immuno-compromised patients, Diphtheria, Serratia, Pseudomonas and Proteus can cause meningitis with serious consequences.

Bacteria reaching the CSF multiply rapidly due to high sugar contents in the CSF and produce intense inflammation of the lepto-meninges (pia-arachnoid).This results in immediate poly-morphonuclear response, high protein and low sugar contents with presence of bacteria and pleocytosis. As the host defenses destroy the bacteria and in turn, the products of the bacterial cell wall destruction excite cytokine activation.Interleukin-1 (IL-1) and tumor necrosis factors (TNF) as well as increased production of nitric acid are implicated in further enhanced inflammatory responses in the meninges. The local inflammatory responses in the meninges mediated by the IL-1 and TNF generally result initially in the production of platelet activating factors in arachidonic acid pathway and then later on these factors (prostaglandins, thromboxanes and leukotrienes) promoting activation of the leukocyte adhesion promoting receptors on the endothelial cells. Leukocyte adhesions and destruction with release of proteolytic enzymes results in BBB permeability: activation of coagulation cascade, cerebral edema, multi-focal infarction, hemorrhages and brain swelling. These patho-physiological changes are translated in the clinical state of the patients which we can evaluate on periodic basis.

In the CSF, whenever, the antibacterial antibodies and the compliment activities are of low titers and then these are unable to combat such bacterial infections successfully and result in immediate widespread of the infections to the vessels, brain and spinal cord.

As a matter of fact, all the cerebrospinal blood vessels are present in the sub-arachnoid spaces prior to entering the brain and spinal cord parenchyma. Only the penetrating small vessels enter parenchyma with a sleeve / cuff of the pia mater with CSF called Virchow-Robin spaces. These penetrating vessels are called cortical vessels with their end territories. The direct bacterial attack as well as the effects of the inflammatory responses on the cortical blood vessels usually results in the swelling of their walls and narrowing of the lumen with proliferation of the endothelial cells. As explained above, there are mural thrombi and obstruction to the vascular blood flow with resultant multi-focal ischemia, cerebral edema, infarctions (neuronal injury and apoptosis) and loss of functions with clinical deterioration. In a considerable number of patients with meningitis, the syndrome of inappropriate (increased) antidiuretic hormone secretion (SIADH) results in the accumulation of free water in the body which further adds to the cerebral swelling and thereby, the cellular injury. This may lead to the phase of severe cerebral edema-swelling, recurrent seizures, sub-dural effusions, hydrocephalus, raised ICP (Cushing's triad: bradypnea, bradycardia and secondary hypertension), brain shifts and brain herniations (sub-falcine, trans-tentorial and trans-foraminal herniations), coma and this may be followed by death even after instituting the highly advanced intensive care management. In such situations, the severity of the meningitic process fails to come under control due to its biological unresponsiveness and in fact refractoriness even to the advanced therapeutic measures.

Clinical Presentation and Differential Diagnoses [11-27]
The clinical presentation of the meningitis vary according to the age of the patients , severity, duration of illness, type of pathogen involved, intracranial effects etc.

In immuno-competent adults, the initial presentation of an acute (onset less than 72 hours) bacterial meningitis is initially with high grade fever, general muscle pains especially in the back, neck stiffness, headaches, photophobia, anorexia, nausea and vomiting and then later with various degrees of confusion, disorientation, irritability, agitation, drowsiness, seizures, focal neurological deficits or coma may be observed. *In the elderly patients*, it may present with disturbances of higher mental faculties (forgetfulness, confusion, disorientation, changes in personality, etc). *Chronic meningitis* (onset more than 3 weeks) may present with features of raised intracranial pressure (headaches, vomiting, papilledema, visual obscuration and drowsiness) and disturbances of higher mental faculties. Usually, there is fever in these cases; even if it is very mild.

Attention to details must be paid on the primary sources of infection such as upper respiratory infection (pharyngitis), paranasal sinusitis and ear infections, orbital cellulitis, bacterial endocarditis, infected implants, congenital dermal sinus, exposure to the patients with systemic infection (N. meningitidis or H.influenzae),etc.

The clinical signs of meningeal irritation in adults are as follows: photophobia, a positive Brudzinski' sign and a positive Kernig's sign. Initially the CNS examination may otherwise be normal. About 10-15 % patients then develop cranial nerve signs (second, sixth and eight cranial nerves more frequently than others). The presence of papilledema suggest raised ICP which may be due to hydrocephalus, subdural effusion/ empyema ,venous thrombosis, cerebral abscess ,etc. Deterioration in mental faculties and the level of consciousness as well as the fresh appearance of the focal neurological deficits herald the progression of meningitis to a complicated stage. In complicated meningitis, clinical features will depend on the extent of meningitis process, severity and involvement of the vital areas of the brain along with the raised ICP. Periodic neuro-imaging studies (CT or MRI scans) will be of great importance in the clinical management at this stage.

Clinical symptomatology of meningitis in the neonatal period is non-specifically different than that in adults. [28-30]The neonates are assessed as per their limited basic bodily functions such as the maintenance of vital parameters (look for hypothermia or mild fever, shock, and apnea), feeding habit (look for poor feeding), sound production (look for shrill cry), bodily status and limb activities (look for hypotonia, lethargy, listlessness and paucity of movements), social activities (apathy and lack of smile), signs of cerebral irritation and increase ICP (irritability, seizures and bulging fontanelle) and features of systemic derangements (pallor, jaundice, hypoglycemia and metabolic acidosis),etc. There is hardly any nuchal rigidity in neonates. *Whereas the infants may present with the some features of meningism :* fever, photophobia, and nuchal rigidity with opisthotonus posture), constitutional symptoms (lethargy, anorexia, nausea and vomiting) and signs of cerebral irritation (irritability, excessive crying, seizures and bulging fontanelle). *Young children may even complain* of headaches, neck pains, photophobia, tiredness and bodily pains and there may be papilledema. In meningococcal meningitis, there may be petechial purpuric rashes, endotoxic shock and intravascular coagulopathy with poor prognosis. [31-36]

Gram negative meningitis [11-20] caused by the Gram negative bacteria is much more serious than the gram positive meningitis and is far more common in the infants than in adults. [36] The main pathogenic Gram negative bacteria are acineto-bacter baumannii, Escherichia coli, Enterobacter aerogenes, Klebsiella pneumoniae, Pseudomonas aeroginosa, etc. The predisposing factors commonly seen are premature infants, immune compromise states, urogenital abnormalities, urinary tract infections, spinal meningo-myeloceles, shunt surgery, etc. These infants show rapid clinical deterioration in their level of consciousness, with irritability, agitation and seizures. Recurrent vomiting and fever with toxic look may be present. The feeding is poor with tachycardia, tachypnea and bulging fontanelles. These infants may have abnormal postures such as decerebrate, decorticate and opisthotonos. Obviously there may be neck stiffness. The CT Brain scan and then the LP for the CSF studies which will clinch the diagnosis are now mandatory to know the correct initial intracranial status and the type of meningitis. Obviously, the blood, CSF, urine and throat swab cultures are done along with the antibiotic sensitivity. These cases are treated on emergency basis in the intensive care units with full supportive therapies and removal of the infected shunt if any. The initial antibiotic of choice are third or fourth generation cephalosporins such as Ceftazidime or Cefepime till the results of the culture and sensitivity testings are available. Their is very high mortality(3-4 patient out of five) in these cases despite intensive management. The short and long term mobidities in the survivors depend on the virulence and extent and the severity of the illness as well as effectiveness of the treatment. Encephalomalacia as an aftermath of the cerebritis, sub-dural effusions, hydrocephalus, physical and mental mal-development, recurrent seizures, and cranial nerve palsies, etc.

*Staphylococcal meningitis [11-21]*results due to hematogenous spread of the staphylococcus bacteria from the skin contamination and implantation of the bacteria during the surgery. Staphylococcus aureus and Staphylococcus epidermidis are main culprits especially after the neurosurgical procedures (craniotomy and shunt surgery), cranio-spinal trauma, and heart valve replacement surgery. These patients initially present with typical features of meningitis, namely, severe headaches, fever, neck stiffness, photophobia, nausea and vomiting. Later, it progresses to confusion, agitation, recurrent seizures, and decreased level of consciousness. Especially, in the infants, it will manifest with tachycardia, tachypnea, poor feeding, bulging fontanelles and abnormal posturing such as opisthotonus. These patients are investigated with the CT head (to see the current status of the intracranial structures, to inspect surgical site and to rule out acute hydrocephalus, hemorrhage and features of raised ICP), CSF studies (lumbar puncture) and blood cultures (to rule out septicemia). Depending on the results of the bacterial cultures and antibiotic sensitivity testing, the appropriate antibiotics (cephalosporin-ceftriaxone, Nafcillin, vancomycin, etc) are started along with the supportive therapy and removal of the causative factor. The prognosis is much better with early removal of the cause and institution of the appropriate antibiotics. However, in 5-10% cases, severe morbidities (physical and mental retardation, sub-dural effusion, hydrocephalus, cranial nerve palsies, recurrent seizures and mortality result despite all efforts.

Immune compromised and geriatric subjects may not present with classical features of meningitis and therefore may present a diagnostic challenge. Careful evaluation may reveal mild fever, subtle neck stiffness and mental changes in these patients. One should look for rashes in meningococcal meningitis (70-80% cases).

Uncomplicated bacterial meningitis responds well to the medical treatment with appreciable recovery in a short period of time; however when the meningitis is complicated with the spread of the inflammatory process in the cerebro-spinal parenchymal tissues and manifesting as cerebritis, ventriculitis, cortical infarctions with ischemic changes and hydrocephalus, cerebral abscess etc, then the clinical course is more likely to be protracted. Seizures, altered sensorium, focal and general neurological deficits, raised ICP etc must be carefully assessed and managed as needed.

This is usually followed with recovery and then the appearance of the second phase in some cases commonly with the symptomatology of meningitis, less commonly with raised intracranial pressure and hydrocephalus which may need CSF diversion; and rarely, the occurrence of myelitis especially sacral radiculo-myelitis. Complicated meningitis may be associated with septicemia with high fever, hypotension, seizures and coma with high fatality and morbidity despite appropriate intensive care treatment.

In tubercular meningitis, [37-38] the symptomatology depends on the severity of the illness. In acute stage, due to widespread inflammatory process in the basal cisterns, the typical features of the meningitis are noted with raised proteins & reduced CSF absorption. There is communicating hydrocephalus in some cases with clinical features of raised ICP. Partially treated meningitis or sub-acute meningitis as well as chronic meningitis, all, present with progressive raised intracranial pressure due to the blockage of the sub-arachnoid spaces by the inflammatory exudates. [39-40]There are clinical syndromes (especially brain stem region) described in tuberculosis affecting the blood vessels and producing, vasculitis with focal cortico-subcotical ischemia and infarctions. In cases, where the middle and larger calibre sized arteries (ICA, MCA and ACAs) are involved then the presentations is that of acute ischemic stroke with focal neurological deficits. The tuberculosis produces arachnoiditis, tuberculomas, vasculitis and vascular occlusions. Each case is treated on its on merits. Even it may be a non-communicating obstructive hydrocephalus due to the blockage of foramen of Monro, aqueduct of Sylvius, foramina of Magendi and Luschka. The occurrence of the CSF obstruction at multiple sites including the spinal subarachnoid spaces is a rule rather than exception. Chronicity leads to organisation of the inflammatory exudates, formation of the fibrosis leading to a carpet of plaque over the dorsolateral aspect as well as at the basal parts of the brain. [42-47]

Brucellosis may manifest as meningitis but it has protean manifestations and the common presentation is that of granulomatous reaction in the CNS. Brucella organisms are small Gram negative coccobacilli that cause diseases in animals with B. abortus, B. melitensis, B. Suis and B. canis. Transmission of the infection occurs via direct exposure to the infected animals and indirectly by consuming the animal products such as the milk from the sheep, goat, camel and cattle, etc. About less than 5%of systemic brucellosis patients develop CNS disease. It is investigated on the similar lines as the tuberculosis. Treponema pallidum is a slender, tightly coiled spirochete that is usually acquired through the sexual contact and it may present as tertiary syphilis (meningo-encephalitis) if untreated effectively.

Differential diagnosis of bacterial meningitis will mainly include *other infective causes* (viral, tuberculosis, fungal, parasitic and rickettsial infections), vascular problems (intracranial subarachnoid hemorrhage, migraine), neoplastic lesions (carcinomatosis), medications (NSAIDs, allopurinol, azathioprine etc), systemic disorders (vasculitis, sarcoidosis), trauma, etc. Recurrent meningitis occurs in the patients with CSF fistulae, anatomical defects, persistence of primary foci, immunocompromised states, asplenia, etc and therefore special attention is needed in these cases. *Para-meningeal infections* (cranio-spinal epidural infections especially abscesses, osteo-myelitis & infected congenital dermal sinuses, mastoiditis and extensive long standing para-nasal sinusitis, pacchymeningitis, subdural empyemas and even brain abscesses) produce reactive changes in the sub-arachnoid CSF such as mild to moderate mononuclear and poly-morphonuclear pleocytosis (100-400 cells/mm^3) with normal glucose and mildly raised proteins but no bacteria on CSF analysis. Neuro-imaging studies such as CT head and the MRI scan will delineate these well. *Post-neurosurgical procedures* such as craniotomy for excision of the tumor or *post-neuro-radiological procedures* such as contrast myelography and cisternography, may produce CSF picture suggestive of meningitis with the findings of mild to moderate pleocytosis, mild protein rise, normal sugar and no bacteria present in the CSF analysis. These are managed with the symptomatic treatment. In the cases of meningitis following neurosurgical procedures and in the *partially treated bacterial meningitis*, the CSF picture may be same (mild to moderate pleocytosis , mild protein rise, normal sugar and no bacteria present in the CSF analysis) for some times and repeated re-cultures then may yield bacteria and if not then the alternative tests such as latex agglutination for bacterial antigens, CSF lactic acid measurement and measurement of CSF Ph may point to some evidence of infection. Radionuclide scanning may be required in some cases.

Investigations [11-43]

Three pronged investigations may be required:

1. Mandatory test to diagnose the bacterial meningitis per se remains the lumbar puncture and CSF analysis. It is imperative that the causative organism is isolated and identified on the urgent basis. Whenever, there is a suspicion of the raised ICP due to an intracranial lesion or an intracranial bleed then a CT scan of the head is initially performed prior to the lumbar puncture. The CSF analysis usually shows bacterial meningitis pattern: high polymorphonuclear pleocytosis (cell count more than 500 celle/mm^3), with low glucose levels (less than the 40% of the blood sugar levels) and highly raised protein levels(more than 100 mg/ dL) as well as bacterial organisms seen on microscopy or in the CSF cultures. The Gram stain is positive in majority (80-90 %) of meningitis cases due to NHS bacteria and in about 70% cases due to the Gram negative bacilli. If needed, bacterial antigens may be conclusively detected in the CSF studies especially on the latex agglutination for bacterial antigens. Lactic acid levels are higher (more than 35 mg/dl) in acute bacterial meningitis. Limulus lysate assay for endotoxins is positive in cases of meningitis due to Gram-negative bacilli. For the tubercular bacilli (Gram positive bacilli), ZN stain is positive more on spun CSF in tuberculous meningitis. In tubercular meningitis, the positive cultures are obtained in about 40-70 % cases. In post-neurosurgical infections, the CSF glucose level (less than the 40% of the blood sugar levels) is more important than the protein levels and cellular counts. Busting of a brain abscess in the ventricular system will result in serious fulminant meningitis with the CSF cell counts in the range of 10,000-20,000 cells / Cumm.

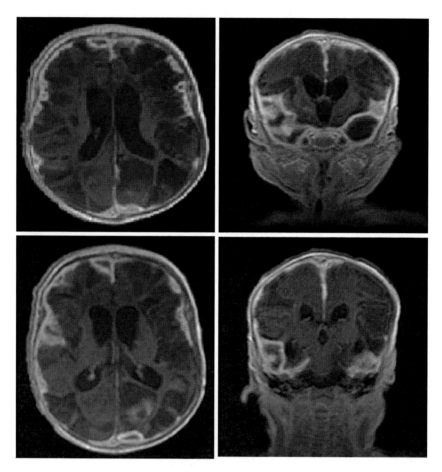

Figure 1. Newborn with proven B streptococcal meningitis. Contrast enhanced axial and coronal MRI shows bilateral, extensive nearly diffuse thick dural enhancement. Though, typically meningitis results in pia-arachnoid meningitis, rarely pachymeningeal enhancement can be seen, as in this case.

The CSF is sent periodically for routine analysis and bacterial cultures and antibiotic sensitivity of those organisms. Lumbar puncture is contraindicated in the presence of raised ICP and it should only be under taken once the ICP is well controlled. In partially treated meningitis where bacterial cultures are negative, the agglutination tests for the detection of bacterial antigens in the body fluid (blood, CSF, Urine , etc) are performed to detect the causative organisms, e.g., S pneumoniae, H influenzae-B, N meningitidis, E coli K1, etc. There is great potential in PCR technology in detecting the causative organism in the partially treated meningitis cases. In tuberculosis, definitive diagnosis is achieved following culture on Lowenstein Jensen medium, the Bactec radiometric system, mycobacterial growth indicator tube or luciferase reporter mycobacteriophage assays, PCR as well as serological tests. The cell wall of the Mycobacterium tuberculosis contains lipids mycolic acids, peptidoglycans and arabinomannans making it impervious to Gram stain where as the Ziehl-Neelsen stain reacts with the cell wall and makes a new bright red complex which is resistant to decolorization by the acids and alcohol and therefore the bacilli are seen distinctly against a blue back ground.

2. Tests to assess the general status of the patient-hematological, biochemical, coagulation screen, systemic infective screen including the blood cultures and assessment of intake and output. Culture may show bacteria involved and antibiotics can be instituted appropriately.

3. Neuro-imaging studies [Figures 1 to 6].

Meningitis is a clinical/laboratory diagnosis [CSF analysis by lumbar puncture]. Imaging is primarily to identify the complications and not to diagnose meningitis. Meningitis can occur in the presence of normal imaging and imaging findings are frequently non-specific. Contrast enhanced MRI is the investigation of choice for detection of meningitis/its complications. FLAIR and post-contrast T1W images are most useful and often provide complimentary information. Delayed contrast enhanced FLAIR images are useful for subtle diagnosis. Diffusion weighted images are invaluable in detecting complications of meningitis. CT is often helpful and viable alternative to detect complications. Abnormal Leptomeningeal/ pachymeningeal enhancement can be seen on post-contrast CT/MRI [Figure 1]. Main role of imaging in meningitis is to detect the complications- subdural hygroma/empyema [Figure 2], hydrocephalus [Figure 2/6], venous/arterial thrombosis and ischemia/infarction [Figure 3], cerebritis/abscess [Figure 4/5], ventriculitis/ependymitis [Figure 6].

Management [11-47]

The bacterial meningitis is one of the serious medical emergencies. Once it is suspected, it is rapidly investigated and its severity assessed and urgently treated in great speed. The clinical presentation of bacterial meningitis may be similar to the viral meningitis; but the CSF analysis differentiates these two. A greater caution is exercised as to not to miss the bacterial meningitis, where the delay in diagnosis may be life threatening and may be associated with high morbidity in the survivors.

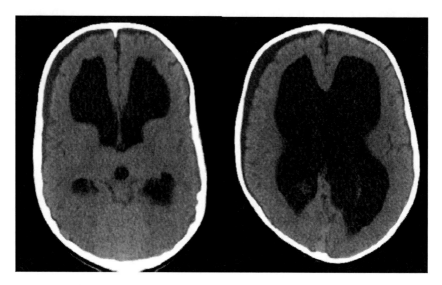

Figure 2. Axial Non-contrast CT scan of a patient with complicated meningitis. CT images show obstructive hydrocephalus and right fronto-parietal subdural collection. Subdural effusions associated with meningitis are sterile CSF collection and usually non-enhancing. In infants and young children, they can occur as a complication of meningitis without sinusitis/otomastoiditis.

The principles of management are as follows-

I. *Supportive symptomatic treatment of the bacterial meningitis:*
   1. Initial critical period (24 hours): a strict bed rest to the patient and the masterly vigilance of the physician with anticipation of the complications as well as their appropriate management, e.g.; such as endotoxic shock, DIC, ARDS, acute renal failure, status epilepticus, cerebral herniations, etc especially in patients with extremes of ages.
   2. An adequate re-hydration with electrolyte maintenance to replace intravascular volume and prevention of the shock state as well as limiting free water excess to avoid hyponatremia ,cerebral cellular

swelling and herniations. The serum sodium is kept slightly higher in the range of 145-150 meq /L.

3. An adequate control of the fever (antipyretics such as acetaminophen) and effective relief of concomitant headaches with acetaminophen, NSAIDs, Tramadol or even with opiate analgesia might be required.

4. An adequate airway management is mandatory. All necessary facilities to intubate and ventilate the patients should be readily available.

5. Effective management of the seizures with the help of phenytoin sodium, sodium valproate, barbiturates, diazepam, clonazepam, etc should be handy.

6. Cerebral edema is managed with mannitol, 3 % hypertonic saline infusion, dexamethasone, barbiturate coma etc to effectively control the raised ICP. Even in the absence of cerebral edema, in cases of bacterial meningitis under the cover of antibiotics, dexamethasone has been shown to be an excellent adjuvant therapy as it results in improvement in the clinical status & laboratory results as well as offers some protection to the cranial nerves from the meningitic inflammatory process.

7. Hematological, biochemical & coagulation parameters, arterial blood gas results, infection screening tests, intake/output chart maintenance and maintenance of ventilatory parameters are of utmost importance. Immunological status of the patient must be checked and if there is hypo-gamma-globulinemia then the needed immuno-globulins must be instituted.

8. Periodic CSF analysis and charting of their results on comparative basis along with the anti microbial antibiotic sensitivity.

9. Periodic neuro-imaging studies such as CT head and or MRI scan. A portable neuro-imaging CT/MRI scan is of immense help in critical care units.

10. Periodic charting of the patients clinical profile for the comparative purpose as to guide the treatment.

II. *Eradication of the causative organism with Anti-microbial therapy* : A large majority of the cases with uncomplicated bacterial meningitis recover completely with appropriate supportive therapy and prompt administration of an ideal antibiotic therapy whichever is indicated for a given bacterial organism. Ideality of the antibiotic depends on three important parameters: its high CSF penetration, effective bactericidal activity and well proven clinical efficacy.

A. *Antibiotic therapy in suspected cases of meningitis prior to the CSF analysis.* The empirical intravenous antibiotic therapy is, obviously, chosen from the predisposing factors in a given age group of patients prior to the results of the CSF analysis and cultures.

    1.   The Initial antimicrobial coverage is given for all the three common bacteria (NHS) causing meningitis in the patients' age group ranging from 4th month to 50 years. In acute bacterial meningitis of unknown origin in the immune competent healthy patients of these age groups, the antibiotic regime of choice is Vancomycin (60 mg/kg/day) with one of the cephalosporins (cefotaxime- 200-300 mg/kg/day or ceftriaxone- 100 mg/kg/day) in their high intravenous dosages. It is called double antibiotic regime. This combination also covers adequately for most penicillin resistant pneumococci and beta-lactamase resistant H influenzae type B. Only in cases of cephalosporin resistant pneumococci, rifampicin is usually added to increase the bactericidal activities in the CSF.

    2.   The vulnerable age groups (bordering the previous age group) as well as immunocompromised patients: these are early infancy (1-3 months) and old age (more than 50 years) group patients who need triple antibiotics. The best combination is made by just adding the ampicillin (200 mg/kg/day) to the aforementioned adult antibiotic regime of choice: Vancomycin with cephalosporins (cefotaxime- or ceftriaxone).

    3.   In neonates (age 0-4 weeks), ampicillin with cefotaxime or an aminoglycoside is used to cover common pathogens in that age group with effective results..

    4.   In the post operative neurosurgical infections, vancomycin plus Ceftazidime are commonly used with good results.

    5.   Immunocompromised patient due to impaired cellular immunity, a triple antibiotic combination, of ampicillin, Ceftazidime and vancomycin, is used.

    6.   In suspected cases of tuberculosis , antitubercular medications (Pyrizinamide, isoniazid, rifampicin, and

pyridoxine as a combination regime for 4 months and then only two selected drugs. Some times added ethambutol is added and rarely the streptomycin is given in the resistant cases) are effectively used maximum for a period of 18 months to 3 years.

B. *Antibiotic therapy after the CSF Gram staining results.* Following initial CSF analysis confirming the evidence of meningeal infection and when the Gram staining results are released but without identifying a specific bacterium, usually following general criteria are helpful in choosing the empirically effective combination of two antibiotics (double antibiotic policy) in the interim period:

1. *In the group of patients with cocci :* (a) Gram positive cocci are treated with vancomycin and a cephalosporin (cefotaxime or ceftriaxone); (b) Gram negative cocci are treated with Penicillin-G and if there is penicillin hypersensitivity or resistance, then ceftriaxone is used. In cases of Beta lactam (both, penicillins and cephalosporins) hypersensitivity or resistance , the antibiotics such as vancomycin , rifampicin (20 mg/kg/day for 4-5 days), carbapenem (imipenem and meropenem) and oxazolidinones (linezolid) are considered.

2. In the group of patients with bacilli, in general aminoglycoside is used effectively with one other broad spectrum antibiotic (double antibiotic policy): (a) Gram positive bacilli are treated with ampicillin and (b) Gram negative bacilli with cephalosporin (cefotaxime- or *ceftriaxone*; ceftazidime only if pseudomonas infection present).

C. *Antibiotic therapy following definitive identification of a specific bacterium on culture and sensitivity.* All antibiotics are given intravenously to achieve adequate blood and CSF levels and to have bacteriocidal effect at earliest.

1. S. pneumoniae is specifically treated with Penicillin-G, Cephalosporins((cefotaxime or ceftriaxone), Vancomycin and Rifampicin. Depending on the sensitivity, the antibiotic is selected for about 2 weeks of therapy.

2. H.influenzae has two types of strains: (i) beta lactamase positive H. influenzae are treated with cephalosporins (ceftriaxone or cefotaxime) for about one week, (ii) beta

lactamase negative H.influenzae is treated with ampicillin for about one week.

3. N. meningitidis is highly susceptible to Penicillin-G and ampicillin and these are given for about one week period.

4. L. monocytogenes responds well to a combination therapy using either penicillin-G or ampicillin with aminoglycoside for 2-3 weeks.

5. S. agalactiae is treated well with a combination therapy using either penicillin-G or ampicillin with aminoglycoside for 2-3 weeks.

6. Enterobacteriaceae is best managed with a combination therapy using one of the cephalosporins ((ceftriaxone or cefotaxime) and aminoglycoside for 3 weeks

7. P. aeruginosa is usually treated with a combination of ceftazidime and aminoglycoside for 3 weeks.

8. M. tuberculosis: In suspected cases of tuberculosis, antitubercular medications (Pyrizinamide, isoniazid, rifampicin, and pyridoxine as a combination regime for 4 months and then only two selected drugs. Some times added ethambutol is added and rarely the streptomycin is given in the resistant cases) are effectively used maximum for a period of 18 months to 3 years.

III. *Intensive Care Management* of the complicated bacterial meningitis is needed for the patient with recurrent seizures, altered state of consciousness, unstable vital parameters, neurological deficits, raised intracranial pressure, cerebral edema, intracranial hemorrhage or cerebral infarction, etc as in cases of viral meningitis which elaborated in that section.

IV. *Precautions to prevent the spread and recurrence* whilst receiving the treatment by using frequent hand washing, use of barriers (tissues) whilst coughing and sneezing, barrier nursing and universal methods of care by the health care professionals. Family members and friends should be evaluated for obvious reasons. For the prevention of the meningitis due to S. pneumoniae, H. influenzae, N. meningitidis and M. tuberculosis (BCG- Bacillus Calmette-Guerin vaccination) etc, the vaccinations are given. Therefore, the immunization, vaccination and chemoprophylaxis are important measures in prevention of the meningitis as well as its recurrence in the vulnerable groups. The vaccines are used against H. influenzae B (three doses in the first 6 months and fourth at one or one and half year of age), N. meningitidis (antibiotics to close contacts and vaccines to control out breaks as well as vaccines to travelers about one week prior to the areas where the meningococcal disease is prevalent such as in African countries), S. pneumoniae (for persons prone to recurrent S pneumoniae infection and elderly people) and Mycobacterium tuberculosis. Meningitis cases are reported to the central registry in local health authority as well as to the state health authority.

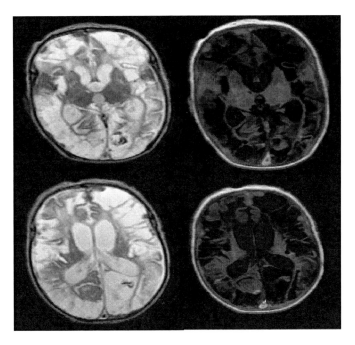

Figure 3. Newborn with complicated B streptococcal meningitis. MRI at the age of six months- T1/T2W axial images show bilateral extensive encephalomalacia, as a sequel of bilateral cerebral infarction, complication of meningitis.

Prognosis: Morbidities and Mortality

Prognosis including mortality and morbidities in cases of bacterial meningitis depends on basic fundamental factors such as age and immunity of the patient, type and virulence of the pathogen, dose of the inoculums and clinical severity. No amount of intensive care treatment, even in time, can guarantee a successful outcome in a given case. Acute bacterial meningitis is akin to a clinical state where suddenly the cerebrospinal axis is set on (bacterial) fire. Management is akin to the fire-fighters' controlling exercise and salvaging what we can with best efforts and then the patient, family and society face the challenges there onwards for whatever is left out of the episode.

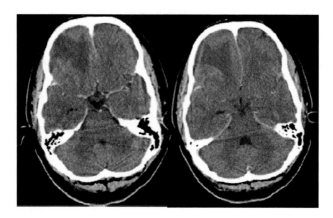

Figure 4. A young woman with meningitis complicated by convulsions. Axial post-contrast CT scan shows right frontal ill-defined subcortical hypodense lesion mass effect and shows mild irregular patchy peripheral enhancement. This could represent an infraction/cerebritis as a complication of meningitis. Clinical correlation and follow up imaging will be able to help to differentiate infarction vs. cerebritis.

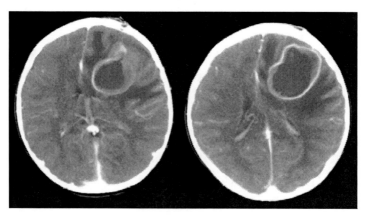

Figure 5. Axial post-contrast CT scan of a child with meningitis shows a left frontal lobe large sharply marginated, ringed lesion with surrounding perilesional vasogenic edema- keeping with cerebral abscess. Cerebritis and cerebral abscesses are complications of meningitis and imaging plays a very important role in diagnosis/management.

Following facts must be born in mind---

1. Fortunately following meningitis with early effective management, many patients recover without any clinical residual squeal / disability. The overall mortality in bacterial meningitis is about 10-20% and the morbidity 15-25 %.

2. In general predictions, the extremes of ages, clinically prolonged seizures (more than 3 days), altered state of consciousness/coma, focal neurological deficits, leucopenia, immune compromised state, endotoxic shock & disseminated intravascular coagulopathy (4-6%cases), ventriculitis with hydrocephalus, extensive cerebral edema-hemorrhage-raised intracranial pressure and cerebral infarction are the factors predicting overall poor outcome in bacterial meningitis. Apart from these factors in tubercular meningitis, the poor prognosis is also related to the development of low GCS, focal neurological deficits, SIADH, opto-chiasmatic arachnoiditis and opto-chiasmal tuberculoma, and the advanced clinical stage of the disease procession at the time of the diagnosis.

3. Among the various age groups, neonates and infants under the age of one year have highest mortality (10-20%) and morbidity rates (20-30 %) with long term disabilities in the survivors. The same is nearly true for the elderly people. In adults, the mortality is about 10% and morbidity 12-15%.

4. Currently among the organisms responsible for bacterial meningitis, Streptococcus pneumoniae is responsible for one of the highest combined mortality and morbidity rates (30-40%); followed by Listeria monocytogenes (25-30 %), Neisseria meningitidis (15-20 %), Hemophilus influenzae (5-10 %), etc. Tuberculous meningitis, despite appropriate anti-tuberculous therapy, is associated with appreciable mortality and significant morbidity in the surviving cases.

5. The short and long term complications, sequalae and residual effects with dys-functionalities and disabilities take the shapes of many type of clinical presentations related to the changes, alterations and loss of functions in the higher mental faculties, speech, crania nerves , motor sensory functions in the limbs and sphincter disturbances. These ranges from mental and physical retardation, behavioral problems, aphasia/dysphasias, seizures disorders, focal paralysis in cranio-spinal regions, cranial nerve dysfunction (hearing loss, cortical blindness, abducent palsy, multiple cranial nerve palsy, etc),ataxia, muscular

spasticity, and intracranial sequalae such as subdural effusions, hydrocephalus & cerebral atrophy, etc. These conditions are managed on their own individual merits.

3. Fungal Meningitis [48]

Fungal infections of the central nervous system (CNS) are rare clinical entities presenting with protean clinical manifestations, difficult diagnostic dilemmas and special therapeutic challenges. [1, 2] Mostly, the fungi have low pathogenicity and therefore rarely infect normal subjects. In recent times, the incidence of opportunistic CNS mycosis has greatly increased especially in immuno-compromised hosts and in patients taking broad-spectrum antibiotics. The CNS fungal infections present with varied clinical syndromes; however, basal meningitis and or hydrocephalus (candidiasis, cryptococcosis, coccidioidomycosis) being the commonest among them. [49-51]

Epidemiology and Classification [51]

Fungal infections are not notifiable diseases and precise information on their prevalence through out the world is not available. Although, in general, fungi are cited to be ubiquitous; however, some forms have a more restricted geographical distribution than others. More than 100 thousand fungal species are recognized by now and only a couple of hundreds are found to be pathogenic to humans. Fortunately, only about 10-15% of pathological fungi usually produce systemic/CNS mycosis. True pathogenic fungi (having a restricted geographic distribution, mostly in USA) are Blastomycetes, Coccidioides, Paracoccidioides, Histoplasma, Sporothrix etc. They produce clinical lesions in normal individuals and then provide long term immunity to the patients recovered from the active infections. Whereas the opportunistic fungi (having ubiquitous distribution) are Aspergillus fumigatus, Candida albicans, Cryptococcus neoformans, Rhizopus arrhizus etc and these provide no long term immunity to the patients and hence relapses are noted. Histoplasma capsulatum is a soil contaminant with bird and bat droppings in endemic areas (Eastern Canada, eastern-central USA, Central &South America, Africa and South-East Asia). Blastomyces dermatididis is indigenous to Mississippi, Ohio, St Lawrence River valleys etc.

Etio-pathogenesis

Fungi are broadly classified in three major groups as follows: 1. Pseudo-mycetes /yeast (smaller and larger groups): Blastomycetes, Candida, Coccidioides, Cryptococcus, Histoplasma, Paracoccidioides, and

Sporotrichum; 2. Septate mycetes: Aspergillus, Cephalosporium, Cladosporium, Diplorhinotrichum, Homodendrum Paecilomyces, Penicillium; 3. Non-septate mycetes: Absidia, Basidiobolus, Cunninghamella, Mucor, & Rhizopus.

The important predisposing risk factors are as follows: severe systemic disorders with malnutrition, immune-suppression and organ transplants, HIV-AIDS infection, systemic malignancy, Hodgkins disease, collagen vascular diseases, uncontrolled diabetes mellitus, alcohol or intravenous drug abuse, long term antibiotic therapy or corticosteroid uses and prolonged parenteral nutrition. In critically ill patients from infancy to old age needing invasive interventions in the intensive care units, candidiasis is emerging as a frequently diagnosed nosocomial infection due to hematogenous dissemination with high morbidities and mortality. Aspergillosis is also a frequent opportunistic infection (look for chronic paranasal sinusitis) in such cases with impaired immunity.

Usually, the inhaled aerosolized fungi initiate a primary mycotic infection in the lungs and or paranasal sinuses which is usually self-limiting but may spread to other organs. Frequently, *hematogenous dissemination* (from lungs, intestine or prosthetic heart valves) results frequently in the systemic mycosis and less frequently in the CNS.

Direct contiguous spread to the CNS occurs from the paranasal sinuses, orbits, petro-mastoid region and retro-pharyngeal area in some patients. *Direct implantation* may result during the period of craniospinal trauma and nosocomial infection due to intensive care procedures and intracranial operations.

Fungi profoundly grow in the environment with abundance of organic matter and water. The enzymes produced by the fungal cell wall act on the organic matter and break down their protein, carbohydrates and other macromolecules into micro-molecules which are then easily used by the fungi to maintain their life processes.

The impermeable blood brain barrier (BBB) and effective meningeal barriers provide effective resistance to fungal infections. For immune surveillance, mainly activated T-lymphocytes are usually permitted across the BBB in normal individual. However in immune-compromised states these anatomical and functional barriers are easily overcome by common opportunistic and or pathogenic fungi to produce clinical manifestations.

Fungal infections of the CNS also evoke humoral and cellular responses to enable the host to eliminate the pathogen. Activation of the resident brain cells by fungi combined with relative expression of immune-enhancing and immune-suppressing cytokines and chemokines may play a determinant role. Activated resident brain cells such as microglia, astrocytes and endothelial cells express major histocompatibility complex (MHC) Class I and Class II molecules and therefore act as antigen presenting cells. In addition, they express complement receptors and produce cytokines, chemokines and molecules with antifungal activity such as nitric oxide (NO).They are also capable of phagocytosis.

Microglia acting as antigen presenting cells stimulates T-cell proliferation and cytokine secretion which in turn stimulate these microglial cells to ingest and more effectively kill invading fungi. The compliment (C) system is a key component of innate immune system, playing a central role in host defense against pathogens. It is also a powerful drive to initiate inflammation and if unregulated can result in pathological changes leading to severe tissue damage. It is generally accepted that the C system is essential to mediate cytolysis of fungi. Furthermore, it is well known that C-receptors expressed by activated microglial cells are important to mediate phagocytosis. Fungi produce diseases due to their allergeniety, toxigenicity, pathogenicity, neurotoxicity and or virulence.

Small pseudomycetes (yeasts) are usually causing leptomeningitis. Because of their small size (cryptococcosis, blastomycosis, histoplasmosis, coccidioidomycosis etc) these fungi gain access to the cerebral microcirculation. From there, they seed n' infect the CSF and its containing leptomeninges. Fungi may reach the brain parenchyma along the Virchow Robin spaces around the penetrating and perforating small cortical/cerebral vessels arising from the major vessels in the sub-arachnoid spaces. Therefore, these fungi may result in meningitis and or meningoencephalitis. Larger pseudomycetes (candidiasis) are capable of producing cerebral abscesses and granulomas. Septate (aspergillosis)and nonseptate(zygomycosis) mycetes are very large in size and normally grow with large branched hyphae. Usually they infect paranasal sinuses, orbits, oral cavity etc for a considerable period of time before invading contiguous cranial bones, meningeal tissues, basal cerebral venous sinuses etc. These fungi then invade intermediate and large sized intracranial arteries, and cause arterial thrombosis and occlusions which in turn result in extensive cerebral infarctions. These patients clinically present with cerebral strokes. The evolving hemorrhagic cerebral infarct is then converted to septic infarcts with associated cerebritis and abscesses whereas a good host defense result in granuloma formation.

Clinical Presentations , Diagnoses and Differential Diagnoses

Chronic fungal meningitis is far common, whereas subacute meningitis relatively less common, and the acute fungal meningitis distinctively rare except in ICU patients or prolonged ventilatory cases with severely immuno-compromised states. Most of the pseudo-mycetes (yeasts) are capable of producing meningitis or meningo-encephalitis. Fungal meningitis ranges from the relatively common cryptococcal meningitis to the rare meningitis due to large pseudomycetes (diamorphic) or filamentous (septate and non-septate) fungi. Therefore, the fungal meningitis more frequently occurs with Cryptococcus, Coccidioides, Blastomyces, Paracoccidioides, Sporotrichum, Histoplasma and Candida as compared to Filamentous fungi such as Aspergillus, Phaeohyphomycosis and Zygomycetes. In critically ill patients from infancy to old age needing invasive interventions in the intensive care units, candidiasis is emerging as a frequently diagnosed nosocomial infection due to hematogenous dissemination with high morbidities and mortality. Aspergillosis is also a frequent opportunistic infection (look for chronic paranasal sinusitis) in such cases with impaired immunity.

A good clinical history to uncover predisposing factors is of paramount importance. Fungemia, hematogenous dissemination of fungal infections, causes constitutional symptoms of fever, headache, malaise, anorexia, night sweats, lethargy, & musculoskeletal pains.

Clinical features of fungal meningitis and meningo-encephalitis usually are headaches, nausea, vomiting, visual impairment, and papilledema and later neck stiffness with fever, personality changes, and then the seizures, deterioration in sensorium, cranial nerve palsies (deafness, ocular palsies, middle and lower cranial palsies) and hydrocephalus. In many patients, there are no focal or generalized physical signs. The CSF analysis

Cryptococcus [48-51] is ubiquitous in distribution, mainly around the areas of avian (pigeons droppings) habitates contaminating the soil and is involved in opportunistic infections more commonly in males with immunocompromised states. The inhalation of the air borne Cryptococcus neoformans results in pulmonary infection which may or may not cause significant symptoms. It has a protective capsule around the cell wall. Cryptococcal infection (European Blastomycosis) of the CNS commonly presents with insidious onset and then manifest with typical clinical symptoms of meningitis (subacute or chronic) or meningo-encephalitis.

Headaches, vomiting, papilledema, seizures, disturbances of higher mental faculties and cranial nerve deficits (visual impairment, double vision, facial weakness, hearing loss) are common complaints. Acute fatal meningitis is rare in cryptococcosis; but the periods of remissions and relapses are well known. Cryoptcoccosis is one of the most common CNS fungal infections in immuno-compromised patients. Nearly one tenth of the patients with HIV develop cryptococcosis and in significant number of patients, cryptococcosis manifest as an initial presentation of HIV infection. Intraparenchymal cysts occur commonly in basal ganglia in cryptococcal infection as compared to other mycosis. Cryptococcal meningitis may be complicated by the appearance of cerebral abscesses, cryptococcoma, Intraparenchymal basal ganglia cysts filled with slimy gelatinous material.

The CSF analysis shows typical picture of chronic meningitis and if HIV-AIDS is coexisting than the pleocytosis may not be significant. The best method is the India ink preparation of the post centrifuged CSF sediments which shows double-refracting spherules. The latex cryptococcal agglutination test is positive for the capsular antigen in about 95%patients.The Cryptococcus is well stained with PAS and Gomori methanamine silver stains.

Coccidioides immitis [50-51] is probably the most virulent of the fungi causing human fungal infections. Coccidioides immitis is a dimorphic fungus, a soil contaminant in the southwestern USA (California and Arizona), Mexico and Central and South America. Commonly initial infection is in the respiratory system and then to the skin and bones. Uncommonly the disease spread via hematogenous dissemination from the pulmonary lesions and in about 30% of these cases, CNS involvement occurs, mostly, in the form of chronic or subacute meningitis.

Meningeal inflammation due to coccidioidomycosis results in accumulation of exudates, opacification of lepto-meninges and obliteration of sulci with caseous granulomatous nodules at the base of the brain and in the cervical region. Extensive fibrosis causes obstructive hydrocephalus and invasion of cranial nerves and basal blood vessels leads to cranial neuro-vascular syndromes and rarely multiple cerebral aneurysms. These patients, therefore, present in initial stages with headaches, vomiting, neck stiffness, and features of raised ICP if there is an associated hydrocephalus and in later stages with neurovascular syndromes and hydrocephalus. The diagnosis may be difficult on the CSF studies as the results may show only the typical features of a chronic meningeal inflammation. The CSF microscopy and culture may be positive in some patients only. If positive, then the fungi will be well demonstrated on all the routine staining preparations for the fungi: H &E stain, PAS, and Gomori methanimine silver stains on the biopsy materials with its pathognomonic features of encapsulated spherules with endospores. However, immunological tests initially (up to 3 weeks) for IgM antibodies (latex particle agglutination, immuno-diffusion methods) and later on (up to 8 months) the serological tests for compliment-fixing antibodies in the blood and the CSF. Neuro-imaging studies (the CT scan and MRI scans) demonstrate frank basal granulomatous meningitis.

Candidiasis, [52-54] in the autopsy studies, is the most common cerebral mycosis whether community acquired or nosocomial infection. Candida albicans is a normal oral and vaginal flora but an opportunist pathogen commonly causing esophagitis and vaginitis. Mucosal injury predisposes to local candidiasis and then invades sub-mucosal blood vessels. Fungemia disseminates hematogenously to the CNS and systemic consequences in immuno-compromised or in high risk patients or following prolonged antibiotic treatment. The presenting symptoms of candidial esophagitis are substernal odynophagia, gastro-esophageal reflex, nausea, etc. The diagnosis of candidial esophagitis is performed with endoscopy, biopsy and fungal culture. Hematogenous spread results in CNS candidiasis, where the commonest presentation is candidial meningitis, less common being candidial cerebral abscess, uncommonly granulomas and rarely chronic granulomatous meningitis, ventriculitis and mycotic aneurysms. Direct invasion, from the skull base infections and during intensive care procedures or neurosurgical operations, is also possible. The latter may be caused via colonization of the ventricular drains, shunt tubing and central venous lines. The clinical presentation is typical: fever, headaches, vomiting, neck stiffness, and features of raised ICP if there is an associated hydrocephalus. The CSF Study is essential to confirm candidial meningitis. The fungal stains show a Gram positive yeasts in the CSF which are more clearly visualized with PAS and Methanamine silver stains.

.Blastomyces dermatididis [50,51] is a soil contaminant and its portal of entry may be cutaneous inoculation or respiratory system and then hematogenous dissemination leads to CNS infection in only a small percentage of patients (6 %) with systemic infections.

Usually chronic but infrequently sub-acute, basal fungal meningitis causes obliteration of intracranial sub-arachnoid spaces and results in the clinical presentation of the features of increased intracranial pressure (headaches, vomiting, neck stiffness and visual impairment) with or without hydrocephalus. Brain lesions such as cerebritis, abscesses, granulomas etc or extradural abscess or osteomyelitis are rare and are associated usually with meningitis. The diagnosis is made by the CSF analysis and microscopic examination of a wet preparation of the exudates in 10%KOH clearly showing the yeast like fungi.

All the other major fungi (i.e., histoplasmosis, Phaeohyphomycosis, and aspergillosis) can also produce life threatening meningitis and therefore high index of suspicion, prompt diagnosis and vigorous therapies are required to reduce morbidities and mortality.

Histoplasma capsulatum [55-59] is also a soil contaminant. Inhalation of its spores results in upper respiratory infection-influenza type, fever, nasal discharge, cough and constitutional symptoms. Frequently, residual calcified lung lesions are noted in these cases. It gives immunity with a positive skin test. Active lung lesion (Ghon complex on the chest x-rays) may cause hematogenous dissemination to other organ systems. Only in less than one fifth of cases of systemic infection develop CNS histoplasmosis in the form of meningitis and solitary or multiple cerebral granulomas. In the Histoplasma meningitis, the process of meningeal inflammation excites fibroblastic proliferation with obliteration of the sub-arachnoid spaces (hydrocephalus), vasculopathy (ischemia and infarctions) with varied presentations. The CSF picture is that of a chronic meningitis. The staining of the CSF sediments with Wright or Gemsa stain shows the organisms clearly. Compliment fixing antibody tests are positive in 4/5 patients and the CSF histoplasma polysaccharide antigen is positive in about 90% of patients.

Aspergillus and zygomycetes [57-61] colonize paranasal sinuses as well as the upper respiratory tree; and then the local tissue and vascular invasion proceeds to hematogenous dissemination from these sites or there may be a direct extension from the para-nasal sinuses occurs [Figure 7]. These infections spread by direct extension across the bones, nerves, blood vessels and the cartilage. These infections usually take the form of cerebral granulomas, or abscesses, thrombophlebitis, arteritis or *rarely meningitis.* [62] Invasion of the cerebral vessels results in cerebral infarction and tissue necrosis. Cranio-sino-orbital syndrome progressing to cavernous sinus syndrome and orbital apex syndrome may initially present with nasal stuffiness and rhinorrhea or nasal blockage with periorbital pains. Epistaxis is very common due to the vascular invasion. Once the sinuses are full, then the infection spreads to the orbit, cavernous sinuses and the meninges. The progressive symptoms are recurrent headaches, proposes, impaired ocular movements, progressive visual loss, and sensory impairment in ophthalmic (frequently) and maxillary (infrequently) divisions of the trigeminal nerve, chemo sis then further progressing to ophthalmologic, blindness and periorbital-facial swelling. Headaches, confusion, irritability, seizures, speech disturbances, focal signs, ipsilateral facial palsy, etc herald either direct cerebral involvement or invasion of major vascular structures at the skull base-internal carotids and vertebro-basilar systems and then overall clinical picture leads to a poor prognosis. These are basically diagnosed by tissue biopsies and septated and non-septated hyphae are best demonstrated on Periodic Acid Schiff and Gomori methanamine silver stains. The methods of radioimmunoassay for circulating antigens and the PCR for antigens in the CSF are helpful in diagnosis. A serum immunodiffusion test for antibodies also can be done. Neuro-imaging studies (CT/MRI with angiography) show sinusitis, meningitis, subdural empyema, hydrocephalus, ischemia-infarction, vascular occlusions, filling defects and cerebral aneurysms. Majority of these patients usually progress to coma and death within a few days or weeks. Therefore early diagnosis and intensive treatment are necessary to make the management effective in some patients at least.

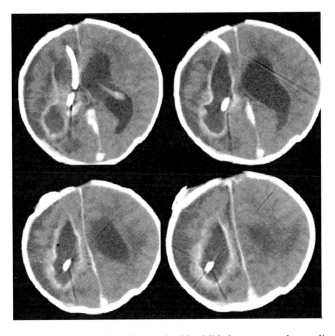

Figure 6. A child with meningitis. CT scan in this child shows several complications of meningitis. Contrast enhanced axial CT of head shows shunted obstructive hydrocephalus. There is thick ventricular rim enhancement keeping with changes of ventriculitis/ependymitis. There is presence of right cerebral hemisphere infarction with volume loss of gliotic changes- sequel of old infarction as a sequel to meningitis. Patients with ventricular shunt catheters may also develop ventriculitis from an ascending infection in the shunt tubing.

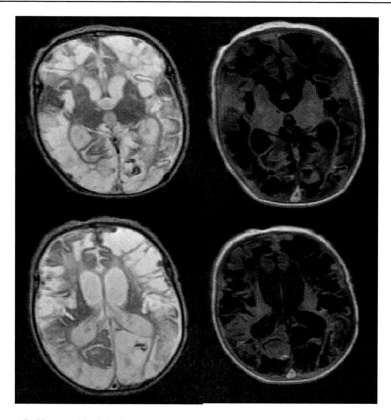

Figure 7. 50 year old Diabetic woman with left eye proptosis. Contrast enhanced FAT SAT T1W axial images of orbits and skull base shows- invasive rhinocerebral mucormycosis- suggested by diffusely inflamed ethmoid and sphenoid sinuses with inflammation of left orbit and periorbital soft tissue. Intracranial extension of the fungal infection- resulting in mixed pachymeningeal and Leptomeningeal enhancement- suggested by extraaxial enhancement adjacent to the left cavernous sinus and left anterior temporal lobes. Left cavernous sinus thrombosis is also noted. Left temporal lobe shows a small subcortical rim enhancing lesion- suggestive of brain abscess as a complication of adjacent fungal meningitis.

Spinal intramural involvement usually occurs as a part of generalized cerebro-spinal fungal lepto-meningitis but other intramural lesions are extremely rare such as localized spinal meningitis, spinal arachnoiditis{(aspergillosis , cryptococcosis) presenting as radiculopathy and or myelo-radiculopathy} and fungal myelitis. The management primarily depends on the antifungal drug therapy in these patients and in only some cases of granulomas /abscesses, where indicated, neurosurgical decompression is needed. [61-68]

Differential diagnosis of fungal meningitis will mainly include to differentiate it from other infective causes (viral ,bacterial including tuberculosis, parasitic and rickettsial infections), post vaccinal causes (especially in cases of measles and rubella vaccines), vascular causes(intracranial subarachnoid hemorrhage, migraine), neoplastic causes (carcinomatosis),drugs(NSAIDs, allopurinol, azathioprine etc), systemic disorders (vasculitis, sarcoidosis), trauma, etc. *Identifying the etiological agent as fungal and not bacterial is vital since antibacterial therapy is not effective against fungi* and CNS mycoses leads to high morbidity and mortality.

Management [69-70]

In general, symptomatic CNS fungal infection carries higher risks of morbidities and mortality as compared to viral, bacterial, or parasitic CNS disorders. An early recognition and an appropriate medical and surgical management strategies are therefore of paramount importance in improving the overall prognosis in CNS mycosis. Many advances have been made in the diagnostic armamentarium of the fungal infections. Medical advancements paralleled increase in fungal infections as a result of medical therapy of various diseases and have produced many more cases of immunocompromised status which are prone to opportunistic systemic mycosis.

The principles of the management of the fungal Infections of the CNS are as follows- [50,51,71,72]

1. Identifying and then controlling the predisposing risk factors and co-existing enhancing medical conditions wherever possible, i.e.,
2. Establishing that the fungal infection exists and then the type of the infection is identified for an appropriate antifungal drug therapy.
3. Early empirical broad spectrum antifungal drug therapy started even if fungal infection of the CNS is strongly suspected and take further from there.
4. Radical surgical procedures are under taken to excise the fungal mass in the orbit and paranasal sinuses, and active neurosurgical interventions are performed for intracranial infective lesions or hydrocephalus. Excision of necrotic and infected tissues as well as the drainage of paranasal sinuses is needed in these patients.
5. Aggressive antifungal drug therapy including irrigation of aerated paranasal sinuses with antifungal agents is needed for a prolonged period (more than 3 months).

6.   Periodic clinical assessments, laboratory tests and neuro-imaging studies are needed for the monitoring of the progress and management.

Still Amphotericin-B remained as one of the most useful broad spectrum anti fungal medication but with many toxic side effects and limitations. Fortunately, during the last two decades, many useful antifungal drugs were introduced. Initially, the lipid based formulations of the Amphotericin B, then the new triazoles and most recently, echinocandins. These medications are used, more and more effectively in combinations. Initial experiences are encouraging in favor of their useful roles in the management of invasive fungal infections. But still, many questions are unanswered and controversies are persisting in relation to their selection and use.

The antifungal therapy for candidal meningitis is still evolving. Various medications are used to deal with systemic and CNS candidiasis, singly or in combination: amphotericin-B 0.3-0.5 mg/kg/day; caspofungin 50 mg/day, micafungin 100 mg/day, voriconazole, 200- 400 mg daily, fluconazole 400-800 mg daily, and flucytosin 150 mg/kg/day in four divided doses (especially in CNS candidiasis).Therapy is continued for about 2 weeks following resolution of symptoms and a negative blood and or CSF culture. Oral fluconazole therapy is better once the patient is clinically stabilized. Appropriate antifungal medication with reversal of the underlying predisposing factor even with the performance of bone marrow or liver transplants, where indicated, will prevent further relapses. Caspofungin is licensed for the empirical treatment of systemic fungal infections (Candida, Aspergillus, etc) with neutropenia.

In CNS blastomycosis, amphotericin-B (0.3-0.6 mg/kg/day for a total dose of 1.5-2.5 gm) is the first choice. If there is failure then, 2-hydroxystilbamidine isethionate is effectively used in 2/3rd of patients.

In acute cryptococcal meningitis, amphotericin-B (0.7-1.0 mg/kg/day) for about 2-3 weeks and then fluconazole (400mg/day) for 2 months achieve good results. Lipid formulations of the amphotericin-B are effective in patients where amphotericin-B is not well tolerated. Addition of Flucytosin(100 mg/kg/day in four divided doses per day) to the primary therapy is used to prevent early relapses

Fluconazole (200mg/day as maintenance therapy of choice for at least 3 months following successful primary therapy) is often used in prevention of the late relapses of cryptococcal meningitis especially in AIDS patients after completion of the primary therapy.

Coccidioidal meningitis is treated with oral fluconazole in high doses (400-800mg/day). In refractory cases, either intrathecal administration of amphotericin-B (1.0-1.5 mg/day) along with intravenous amphotericin-B (0.6 mg/kg/day) or alternatively triazoles (voriconazole / posaconazole) are used. Once the patient is stable then the fluconazole is given for a prolonged period (at least 6 months or more) to prevent the relapse.

Histoplasma meningitis is best treated with amphotericin-B (1.0 – 1.2 mg/kg four times a day) for a period of 3 months to start with and then it is better to evaluate the antibody and antigen titers with the progress of the clinical response. Ventriculo-peritoneal shunts may be needed for the hydrocephalus with the potential risks of fungal peritonitis. Intraparenchymal brain lesions may need excision.

Either in the confirmed cases or in cases where the possibility of CNS aspergillosis is considered high then the urgent administration of high doses of amphotericin-B, voriconazole or caspofungin may be life saving. Lipid preparations of the amphotericin-B are preferred because of their better tolerance and less side effects; and these can be used in the higher doses with better effectiveness. In patients with systemic medical disorders, comparatively voriconazole (6 mg /kg, twice on the first day and then about 6-8 mg/kg/day for the maintenance) might be a better option because of far better tolerability(both, oral and intravenous preparations are available), least side effects and improved survival than amphotericin-B. If there is allergic reaction to both aforementioned drugs then Caspofungin acetate (1 mg/ kg loading dose and then about 50 mg /day intravenously) is used. However, mortality remains high.

In patients with cerebral mucormycosis, a prolonged course of amphotericin-B (1-1.5 mg/kg/day) or one of the lipid preparation of the amphotericin-B given. In some cases of allergy, posaconazole may be the next choice.

It is difficult to eradicate fungal infection and therefore, lifelong watch and may be prophylactic therapy needed. Rapid control of the primary and coexistent medical conditions including diabetes, and extensive removal of the necrotic material are necessary in the salvage therapy. The antifungal treatment is given until the compliment fixation tests become negative for 3 months. There is high risk of fungal infections in immunocompromised patients Prophylactic antifungal drug therapy using oral azoles (fluconazole, itraconazole, ketoconazole) is given in such cases. Fluconazole is the drug of choice for long term use. If the fungal infection is confirmed in a given case, then the Amphotericin is used initially on the empirical basis. Once the type of the opportunistic fungal infection is established, than the more specific antifungal drugs for that particular fungal infection are given such as in Candidiasis (Triazoles, Echinocandins), Cryptococcosis (Amphotericin and Flucytosine in synergistic combination), Aspergillosis (Amphotericin, Voriconazole, Posaconazole, and Caspofungin), Mucormycosis (Amphotericin), etc.

The main end points for intravenous primary antifungal therapy and then switching it over to secondary prophylactic therapy are a favourable clinical response (normo-thermia with no headaches, nausea and vomiting; and significant relief in neck stiffness and photophobia as well as improved mini mental scores), normal intracranial pressure (diamox, periodic lumbar punctures or CSF shunting), improving CSF picture (decreasing pleocytosis and protein concentrations in the CSF ,and normo-glycorrachia and no fungal organism on fungal stainings), negative compliment fixation tests, improving CSF fungal antigen titers (below 1:8) and sterile CSF cultures as well as resolution of the intracranial infections on neuroimaging studies..

The factors predicting the poor prognosis are extremes of ages, organ failures, acuity of clinical presentation, type and virulence of the fungal organism, complicated forms of meningitis, cerebral-vascular involvement, infarction, raised ICP, increased antigen titers in the blood and CSF, extensive extra-cranial mycosis, and co-existing medical disorders such as immune-compromising states.

Among the antifungal medications, the lipid formulations of the amphotericin-B are primarily indicated for life threatening invasive fungal infections such as systemic candidiasis, cryptococcosis and the endemic mycoses (blastomycosis, histoplasmosis, coccidioidomycosis and paracoccidioidomycosis). In these infections, alternatively, Amphotericin-B and triazoles antifungal such as Voriconazole, Fluconazole, and Posaconazole, are advised either singly or in combinations.

Flucytosine (5-fluorocytosine) is the only commonly used drug (usually in combination with Amphotericin-B) among the pyrimidine class of antifungal drugs especially in infections such as invasive candidiasis, cryptococcosis, aspergillosis etc with significant bone marrow toxicity, hepatotoxicity and drug resistance.

Among the azoles group of antifungal medications, triazoles (fluconazole, voriconazole, posaconazole) are used for invasive life threatening fungal infections because of their ease of administration(oral preparations), high bioavailability, water solubility, low protein binding and a good body fluid distribution, relatively low toxicity and long half life. A good CSF penetration is usually achieved. Triazoles have a relatively broad spectrum of activity against common fungal pathogens e.g., Aspergillus, Blastomyces, Candida, Cryptococcus, Coccidioides, Paracoccidioides, Histoplasma etc. However, their limitations lie in the interactions with co-administered drugs, development of the resistance of fungal organisms (Candida) especially with fluconazole and hepato-toxicity.

4. Parasitic Meningitis [73-74]

Parasitic infections are generally causing focal (amoebic meningo-encephalitis, cysticercosis), multi-focal (toxoplasmosis), or generalized meningo-encephalitis (falciparum malaria, trypnosomiasis) and these may respond to timely interventions and long term chemotherapy with overall good prognosis. But, unfortunately, the timely interventions do not happen in majority of the patient in the underdeveloped countries and therefore the morbidity and mortality associated with them are still very high.

Epidemiology and Etiopathogenesis [73,75-78]

In comparison to the viral, bacterial and fungal infections, the parasitic infections of the CNS are relatively rare especially in the developed countries. Parasitic infections/infestations are far more common in the economically underdeveloped and developing countries especially in the warm climatic regions in the world. Low socio-economic conditions, poor standard of hygiene, lack of medical facilities, lack of education and awareness of preventive measures are main factors responsible. These infections are mainly transmitted and spread via vectors, excretions, contamination of food and direct contact. Higher environmental temperature helps in completion of the life cycle of the infectious agents in their vectors as well as maintenance of the population of the vectors.

These parasites may produce focal or generalized systemic infections and the involvement of the CNS is not specific but co-incidental. In the tropical and subtropical regions, the morbidity and mortality due to these infections (amoebic meningo-encephalitis, cerebral malaria, cerebral schistosomiasis and trypnosomiasis) are substantial. Parasites are mainly of two categories such as protozoa and helminthes.

Among the protozoans, various forms of amoeba, malaria, and trypnosoma are more frequently involved. Whereas in helminthes, Taenia solium, Coenurus cerebralis, Echinococcus granulosus, Diphyllobothrium latum, Schistosoma species, Paragonimus westermani, Heterophydiasis,

Toxocariasis, Cerebral angiostrongyliasis (eosinophilic meningitis), strongyloidiasis, Gnathostomiasis, Trichinosis, etc.

Interestingly, once the parasitic infections are established in the human body, some of these (angiostrongyliasis, Gnathostomiasis) may cause recurrent , intermittent or relapsing type of symptomatology with diagnostic and therapeutic challenges. In USA about 6-8 cases of amoebic meningo-encephalitis are noted annually and only about 200-300 cases are recorded so far in the medical literature. [78-80] Malaria is widespread in tropical and subtropical areas of Africa, South America and Asia. About 200-300 million cases occur annually with an estimated mortality of at least one percent of cases due to cerebral malaria. Trypnosomiasis affect about 10 million people in South and Central America alone. The disease is more pronounced in African countries. Trichinosis is widespread in USA, South America, and African countries such as Kenya, Tanzania and Far East. Cysticercosis is ubiquitous in distribution especially in the pork eating communities especially in South and Central America, South East Asia and Eastern Europe.. Hydatid disease is common in the Middle East, Southeast Africa and Asia, South America, etc. Schistosomiasis occurs in many countries in the tropical Africa, South America and the Far East and affects over 200 million people. Angiostrongylus cantonensis is present in Mudagascar, Far East countries, Japan, Australia, Tahiti, etc. Gnathostomiasis is mainly occur in South East and Far East Asia particularly in Thailand and Japan, although sporadic cases are reported from many parts of the world including Middle East, Africa, America, Europe, etc. [78-82]*Among the protozoans,* amoebae naegleria fowleri and acanthamoebata are present ubiquitously in the soil and in the warm (at least 20 ^{0} C), stagnant, fresh water in the swimming pools or natural resources and mostly affect the swimmers. These are thermophilic, free living natural fresh water organisms in the tropical and subtropical regions and are highly sensitive to chlorine even in concentrations less than 0.5 ppm. These organisms first enter the nose and then through the olfactory nerves reach intracranial cavity and cause necrosis of the brain tissues very rapidly. However, acanthamoebata infections usually occur in patients with lymphoma, immuno-suppression, diabetes mellitus, malnutrition, etc. The pathological process in the amoebae naegleria fowleri is far more rapid and extensive than in cases of acanthamoebata. Pathologically, wide spread necrosis involving the olfactory lobes, front temporal lobes, petechial hemorrhages amoeba in the peri-vascular spaces and purulent meningeal inflammation with exudates are noted and in case of acanthamoebata, in addition, necrotising granulomatous meningeal reaction also present. The CSF examination is positive for the pleocytosis and the amoeba organisms are well seen in these cases and in, acanthamoebata infections, spiny amoeba is very well recognized. [73-80]

Malaria [83] is caused by four species of the genus plasmodium: P.falciparum, P.vivex, [84,85] P.ovale and P.malariae. Among these, P.falciparum (need at least 18^0 C temperature to complete its sexual cycle in mosquitoes) is mainly responsible for cerebral malaria and serious morbidities and mortality. It is usually transmitted by the infected female anopheline mosquito bite; however, rarely via blood transfusion, or the syringes used by the drug addicts, etc. Hematogenous spread leads to systemic problems and involvement of the CNS is although rare but once it happens then the prognosis is guarded. In cerebral malaria, the cerebral microcirculation is grossly affected. Both capillary sequestration and non-sequestration related cerebral complications may occur in cerebral malaria. The central capillary vessels are occluded with the swollen parasitized red blood cells and then there are peri-capillary ring hemorrhages along with peri-capillary infarction in the form of numerous petechial hemorrhages. Recurrent seizures exacerbate these changes. The surrounding brain parenchyma responds to these pathological changes with reactive gliosis and development of profound cerebral edema and these changes in turn result in highly raised ICP and further lead to grave consequences. The CSF may show mild lymphocytic pleocytosis with mildly increased CSF proteins. Detailed hematological investigations, including thick blood film analysis ,will yield the diagnosis. [83-87]

Various forms of Trypnosomiasis are common in Africa { hem flagellate protozoans: (a)Trypanosoma brucei gambience –transmitted by tsetse flies at the river side; and (b) Trypanosoma brucei rhodesiense- transmitted by the vectors-savannah dwelling tsetses such as G. morsitans } and America (Trypnosoma cruzi-transmitted by the bites of the large reduviid bugs, blood transfusion and congenitally). In African trypanosomiasis, primarily at the site of the bite, there is a subcutaneous tender itchy, inflammatory lesion called bite chancre which gradually enlarge due to multiplication of the trypnosomes in 2 weeks and then gradually disappears also in further 2 weeks. During this later period, there are febrile episodes with headaches, erythematous rashes, lymph-adenopathy (marked in the cervical regions), joint pains, anemia, weight loss etc. Then there may be a period of remission for a variable period of time but eventually in almost all cases, there is CNS involvement. Pathologically, the CNS trypanosomiasis presents with typical features of meningo-encephalitis. These changes are mediated by inflammatory processes, immunology, and allergy, and vascular invasions. Immunological inflammatory processes lead to central vasculitis, perivascular infiltration of mononuclear cells, lymphocytes, plasma cells (progressive arthus reactions). The process of endarteritis, further, results in neurolglial proliferation with cerebral edema, granulomatous lesions as well as thrombotic occlusions with multiple hemorrhages and consequent multiple areas of infarctions. The characteristic findings are Morular cells of Mott which are, in fact, large plasma cells containing eosinophilic inclusions of IgG. There may be changes in the surface antigens and polyclonal stimulation of B cells. The large amount of IgM antibodies result in hyper-gammaglobulinaemia. Obviously the RBCs are destroyed and there is enlargement of lymph glands, spleen and liver. [83-88]

American trypanosomiasis (Chagas 'disease) is a zoonotic disease infecting wild and domestic animals (cats, dogs, chickens, etc) which are acting as the reservoir of human infection. Usually, if once infected, the subject is infected forever. There is primary inflammatory lesion at the site of bite of the large reduviid bugs. Later, the parasites multiply over there and are discharged in the blood stream as trypomastigotes in the significant number of patients. These have affinity towards parasympathetic nerves in the smooth muscles of the GIT and urinary systems, cardiac muscles (carditis), reticuloendothelial cells (facial hyperpigmented area, rashes, scaly nodule, lymphadopathy, hepato-splenomegaly) and neuroglial cell in the CNS(meningoencephalitis). Patients develop problems in these systems such as "mega" syndromes in the GIT and urinary system as well as myocarditis.

Among the helminthes, acute encephalitis or meningoencephalitis is rare but it may be caused by Trichinella spiralis, angiostrongylis cantonensis, strongyloides stercolis, Toxocara canis ,Gnathostomiasis and chronic encephalitis may result due to Schistosomiasis japonicum or mansoni, Paragonimus, cysticercosis and Heterophyces. [89]

Trichinosis is caused by Trichinella spiralis present in the undercooked *pork* or wild animal (bear, pig) meat. The larvae are liberated in the stomach and then these penetrate through the wall of the intestine to become adult worms which discharge larvae in the blood stream. Hematogenous spread leads to systemic illness. Symptomatology is due to inflammatory reaction to these larvae and the cysts they produce. Interestingly, larvae of the Trichinella spiralis do not produce cysts in the brain and mainly give rise to vasculitis. Ischemic occlusions and hemorrhagic effects lead to micro-infarcts and petechial hemorrhages. The clinical picture is that of meningo-encephalitis.

Angiostrongylus cantonensis and Gnathostoma spinigerum cause eosinophilic meningitis. [78-82] *Angiostrongylus cantonensis* is a parasite of *rodents* which excrete it in their faeces and contaminate the water. The adult worm lives in the pulmonary arteries of the rodents where they lay their eggs comfortably. Once the eggs are hatched to liberate larvae in the lungs and then the larvae penetrate the alveoli and migrate to pharynx and swallowed. The larvae are then reach to the intestine and passed in the stool. These second and third stage larvae then infect snails. Snail is inter mediate host and eating the snails or the other animals consuming snails would transmit the infection to the humans. Once the contaminated food is ingested, the larvae are liberated in the intestine and then these penetrate the intestinal wall and later migrate to other organs including the brain. The incubation period is about one week to four weeks. These larvae migrate through the tissues and there is strong eosinophilic reaction to these larvae along their tracks and tunnels in the brain with the formation of the cavities in some places, as well as, granulomatous reactions at other parts. [89]

*Gnathostomiasis [78-82,89]*may present rarely with myelo-encephalitis or meningoencephalitis when its larvae travel through the brain and spinal cord tissues and the CSF may show eosinophilic pleocytosis. It is caused by Gnathostoma spinigerum which is a nematode parasite of domestic animals such as dogs and cats. They pass parasitic eggs in their feces and second stage larvae so hatched in the fresh water are ingested by the cyclopses who are in turn eaten by the paratenic animals such as fishes, frogs, eels, snakes, etc. The larvae further develop in their muscles as their third stage. After ingesting raw or poorly cooked infested muscles of these animals, the humans get infected with these larvae which fortunately do not mature in to adult forms but unfortunately behave like aggressive wanderers through the tissues. The damage is basically done along the uncontrolled migratory path of these larvae in the form of tissue inflammation, necrosis, hemorrhage, and granulomatous reactions due to local inflammatory reaction, direct mechanical injuries, allergic reactions, etc.

Paragonimiasis is caused by the lung fluke. Infected human and animal excreta release the eggs in the water and the larvae (miracidia) from these eggs and animal infect snails and in the *snails* these larvae develop into metacercariae which are then released in the water. These metacercariae then infect crustaceans. The infection is then contracted by ingestion of the infected crabs and crayfish. These metacercariae penetrate the intestinal walls and travel through the tissues to reach the lungs where they form small cysts. Some larvae enter the blood stream and reach brain and hence in endemic areas cerebral paragonimiasis is a common neurological manifestation.

Cysticercosis [90-93] caused by the Taenia solium (an adult pork tapeworm) is the commonest helminthic parasite infecting the CNS. *Man-Pig cycle* is typical of this infestation. In the man's intestine, eggs of the Taenia solium are hatched and the larvae migrate through the intestinal walls to enter the blood stream and the hematogenous transmission occur to various organ systems., mostly to the skeletal muscles and subcutaneous tissues but rarely to CNS, eyes and heart. These larvae form cysts in the organs (called cysticercosis) wherever they lodge in about 3 month period and thereafter, these cysts remain active for about 4-5 years and then these die and calcify over a time period of 1-2 years. Neuro-cysticercosis may develop in to following pathological entities: meningeal-recemose variety resulting in meningoencephalitis or granulomatous meningitis; parenchymal solitary or multiple cysticercus cysts or granulomas; ventricular cysticercosis with communicating or non-communicating hydrocephalus as well as allergic-immune responses presenting with arteritis.

Echinococcosis (hydatid disease) is caused by the infection with the larvae of *the dog's tapeworm* called echinococcus granulosus. Handling of the dogs, eating contaminated food with the echinococcus eggs, etc transmits the disease to humans. In human intestine the embryos are liberated from the eggs and these penetrate the intestinal wall to enter the blood stream and get lodged in the portal venous system. Then, the larvae form hydatid cysts in the liver. The larvae which are filtered out of the liver and get in the general vascular system reach various organ systems and only 1% of hydatid cysts are found in the CNS. Hydatid disease is usually causing cystic mass lesions in the brain and the spinal canal and therefore present with the compressive symptoms rather then meningo-encephalitis.

Schistosomiasis is usually caused by the Schistosoma japonicum, Schistosoma mansoni and Schistosoma haematobium. Among these, cerebral schistosomiasis is usually caused by S. japonicum and the spinal schistosomiasis by S. mansoni. These parasites infest the human bowel and the ova penetrate the bowel wall and reach blood vessels and then hematogenously transmitted to the brain and the spinal cord.

There ova are lodged in the small vessels and then produce host reaction there to form granulomatous lesions rather than meningo-encephalitis. Praziquantal is effective in 40-60 mg /kg for 2 doses. Niridazole (25 mg/kg tid for one week) may be more beneficial for its additional anti-inflammatory actions in the patients with neurological manifestations. *Coenuriasis* due to Coennurus cerebralis mainly produces a single cyst of a variable size in the posterior fossa and has no specific chemotherapy but surgery may be helpful. *Heterophydiasis and toxocariasis* rarely produce cerebral granulomas causing epilepsy in humans as compared to extremely rarely the features of meningo-encephalitis. *Diphyllobothrium latum* (largest tapeworm) usually consume Vit-B12 in the man's intestine and produce deficiency syndromes of megaloblastic anaemia and sub-acute combined degeneration of the spinal cord rather than any form of meningo-encephalitis. In *massive strongyloidiasis*, larval invasion of the blood stream and hematogenous spread leading to serious or fatal meningo-encephalitis may result especially in cases who are receiving cortico-steroid therapy or immuno-suppressants.

Clinical Presentations and their Management [73-93]

Protozoans infect the CNS more commonly as compared to the helminthes. Protozoans usually cause diffuse or wide spread CNS involvement where as the CNS helminthic infections are either focal or multifocal in nature and mostly in the form of parasitic cerebral cysts or granulomata. Occurrence of a pure parasitic meningitis or meningoencephalitis is extremely rare. It is mostly in the form of eosinophilic meningeal reaction with some clinical features of meningeal irritation. Among many aforementioned parasites, clinically only a few of them are more commonly causing the meningitis or meningoencephalitis, e.g., Amoebae naegleria fowleri, Acanthamoebata, Malaria, Trypnosomiasis, Trichinella spiralis, Angiostrongylus cantonensis, Paragonimiasis, cysticercosis, etc. These organisms are therefore discussed here.

Primary amebic meningo-encephalitis (PAM) is a water recreational disease and it occurs in young swimmers when the infected water (commonly with Ameba Naegleria fowleri) is insufflated in the nose. Initially, these organisms get attached to the mucosa and then to the olfactory endings over the mucosa.

These organisms have ability to multiply and migrate via neural pathways mainly by destroying the nerve endings and reach olfactory bulbs via necrosis of these through the cribriform plate. The consumption of the main mitral cell over there, leads to the initial stage of altered sense of smell (parosmia), and followed later by anosmia and ageusia. As the destruction spread from the olfactory bulb to the anterior perforated substances and fronto-temporal lobes, the clinical features become apparent such as headaches, nausea-vomits, neck stiffness, cerebral irritation phenomenon and altered state of consciousness. Patient passes into the repetitive seizures, status epilepticus, anoxia and irreversible coma. The brain stem damage leads to respiratory failure and mortality with in two weeks of infection. The neuro-imaging studies show nonspecific meningo-encephalitic changes initially in the medial fronto-temporal regions and then in the later stages, in many parts of the brain. The

CSF studies including the microbial cultures (Nelson's medium)are the main basis of the early diagnosis of PAM. Amoeba are better seen in centrifuged CSF deposit stained with Giemsa stain or Gomaris' trichrome stain after adding few drops of polyvinyl alcohol. Early medical therapy (including Amphotericin-B, rifampicin, azithromycin, azoles,etc) for the PAM is the only chance (3-4%) of survival in this highly aggressive and mostly lethal condition with terminal hemorrhagic cerebral necrosis. Unfortunately, being a rare cause of meningo-encephalitis it does not raises awareness and is less likely to generate high index of suspicion until unless the positive public health awareness measures are undertaken in this regard by the appropriate governmental institutions considering the fact that the diagnosis is usually reached in majority of cases only after the postmortem studies.

Cerebral malaria is usually caused by intracellular protozoa called falciparum malaria. Incubation period, after the anopheles mosquito bite and transmission of the parasite, is about 1- 2 weeks. Initially, high grade remittent fever for about 1 week occurs with malaise, headaches, body pains, chills and rigors as well as frequent vomiting. Laboratory investigations including the CSF studies may be done to rule out bacterial meningitis. Then, it is followed by classic tertian form of febrile episodes each lasting for 12-24 hours every alternate day: cold stage followed by hot stage and then the sweat stage (ague attacks) resulting in severe exhaustion. The liver and spleen may become palpable. Three types of the outcome are possible in such cases: (A).gradual recovery due to an acquired immunity; (B) Further worsening to become complicated malaria such as the occurrence of the cerebral malaria; and (C) mortality in about 35-40% of the untreated patients due to one or more of the following causes: acute renal failure, black water fever, algid malaria, pulmonary failure, hepatic failure, shock and hemolytic anaemia etc. In cases of cerebral malaria, severe unremitting headaches with agitation and behavioral changes followed by confusional stages and recurrent seizures and then it may lead to stupor and coma. Raised ICP with features of intrinsic brain stem disturbances and cerebral herniations (decerebrate posture and cardio-respiratory changes) are features of grave consequences.. There may be one or more co-existing systemic complications as described earlier. Thick blood (collected during the febrile episode) films stained with the routine Field's stain or Giemsa stains will yield the diagnosis. Cerebral malaria is often fatal unless timely intensive management is undertaken.

American trypnosomiasis is caused by Trypanosoma cruzi. In these cases, the clinical features of the meningo-encephalitis develop very early in some patients. Trypanosomes infect meningeal cells and glial cells to cause meningeal inflammation and glial nodules. Acute meningo-encephalitis initially presents with fever, headaches, nausea, vomit, neck stiffness, confusional state, agitation and recurrent seizures. These lead to disorganized mental functions and then deterioration in the level of consciousness followed by coma and high mortality. In surviving patients of meningo-encephalitis, involvement of the brain leads to dementia, pyramidal system and the spinal cord to spastic paralysis and Chronic involvement of the nerves to peripheral neuropathy. Blood films prepared during the periods of high fever may show trypanosomes. Blood cultures on NNN medium as well as the Xeno-diagnosis are more sensitive tests for the diagnosis of trypanosomes. Sero-diagnostics such as indirect fluorescent antibody, CFT and indirect hemagglutination are also helpful in chronic stages. There is no universally effective Chemotherapy available in Trypnosomiasis. In acute cases, Nifurtimox (a nitrofurazone derivative, 8-10mg/kg/day for 3 months with side effects such as skin rashes dementia and peripheral neuropathy), benzonidazole (a nitroimidazole, 6-8 mg/ kg/ day for one month with similar side effects as to nifurtimox plus hematological problems).

The overall prognosis is poor.

African trypanosomiasis is caused by T. brucei gambiense and T. brucei rhodesiense as mentioned above. Initially, patients develop lethargy, lassitude, apathy, depression for months and then develop somnolence and dementia. Some patients develop generalized seizures, extra-pyramidal features (tremors, choreiform movements, rigidity) as well as speech and cerebellar disturbances. This may progress to stupor, incontinence and coma. This condition is invariably fatal in untreated cases. The diagnosis may be established by seeing trypanosomes in the blood or tissue fluids including CSF. Melarsoprol (mel B), Dimercaprol and dexamethasone, Suramin are the medications used in the pharmacological management.

Eosinophils are not usually present in the CSF. However, these are well very demonstrable in tissue fluid preparations with Giemsa or write's staining. Commonly, the CNS helminthiasis (angiostrogyliasis, gnathostomiasis, toxocariasis, baylisascariasis, cysticercocsis, etc) can cause eosinophilic meningitis (10 eosinophils /microlitre of the CSF or eosinophils more than 10% of the CSF cell counts). Currently, the management of the CNS helminthiasis is faced with diagnostic challenges and controversial therapeutic recommendations.

Angiostrogyliasis is a neurotropic helminthic infection and one of the most common causes of eosinophilic meningitis. It is basically a self limiting disease. It is mainly due to the larvae of the A. cantonensis which migrate through the human meninges and the brain substances. These larvae can not develop further and whilst migrating through the meninges excite eosinophilic meningitis and through the brain substances excite granulomatous reactions. These reactions are there even to the dying or dead larvae. The patients develop low grade fever, nausea, vomiting, severe bi-temporal and fronto-occipital headaches lasting for weeks as well as neck stiffness in the severe cases. Interestingly, fairly commonly, the noteworthy migrating painful paresthesia or dysaesthesia occurs. Uncommonly, the cranial nerve palsies (facial, abducent and auditory nerves) result due to migrating larvae and rarely the loss of vision, and mortality(less than 1%).The parasites produce clinico-pathological changes due to inflammatory reaction, allergic reaction, foreign body reaction, etc. Peripheral eosinophilia and CSF eosinophilia along with the h/o exposure sea food and neurological manifestations raise the possibility of CNS parasitic infection. The neuro-imaging studies may be normal and the CSF studies via lumbar puncture show higher CSF pressure, cloudy CSF, increased proteins but normal glucose levels and pleocytosis with eosinophilia. The management is basically consisting of the treatment of the presenting symptoms, anti-helminthic medications (a course of albendazole or mebendazole for 2 weeks), steroid therapy (a course of prednisolone for 2 weeks) and relief of the raised CSF pressure (periodic lumbar punctures).These measure help in shortening the duration of the symptomatology and lessening the inflammatory effects with better symptomatic outcome in these patients.

Gnathostomiasis is caused by Gnathostoma spinigerum which is a nematode parasite of dogs and cats as mentioned earlier. There are three types of clinical presentations occur singly or in various combinations: dermatological, systemic and CNS manifestations. Generally, patients have intermittent fever, colicky pains, subcutaneous swellings and eosinophilia. The cutaneous features include local pains, pruritis, skin rashes, panniculitis, migratory subcutaneous swellings, furunculosis, etc. Among the systemic problems, various organ systems may be involved due to these migratory larvae and result in their functional derangements, e.g., blindness due to the invasion of the eyeball. Due to its aggressive behavior, the CNS manifestations are more severe. Initially, the peripheral nerves are affected by the migratory larvae and present with radicular pains and paresthesia in spinal or cranial nerve territories. Involvement of the meninges leads to the features of meningeal inflammation such as fever, headaches, and neck stiffness. Later, direct involvement of the larvae in the spinal cord and brain tissue leads to encephalo-myelitis, meningo-myelitis, and meningo-encephalitis with features of focal neurological deficits, paralysis, and disturbances of higher mental functions. Injury to the cerebral vessels may lead to severe intracranial hemorrhages. These pathological changes lead to recurrent seizures and coma with poor prognosis in some patients. The CSF picture is almost similar to as in cases of angiostrogyliasis. However the neuro-imaging studies may show focal inflammatory lesions in the spinal cord and brain as well as the areas of hemorrhages. The management revolves around the supportive care, anti-helminthics [albendazole or ivermectin (for dermatological manifestations) mainly for cutaneous and general systemic gnathostomiasis for a period of three weeks; however, for the CNS manifestations such regime is undertaken on case to case basis with strict monitoring of the clinical profile and laboratory studies due to the exacerbation of the clinical manifestations owing to severe inflammatory reaction to dying larvae], steroids and management of increased ICP with guarded prognosis.

Trichinosis is caused by Trichinella spiralis as discussed above. During the initial period (one week) of formation of the adult worms from the ingested larvae in uncooked meat, the patient present with abdominal symptoms of pains, nausea-vomiting, diarrhea and fever. Once the larvae are liberated from the adult worms in the blood stream, it leads to systemic illness. Symptomatology is due to inflammatory reaction to these larvae in various organ systems and the formation of cysts there. The symptoms of muscle involvement, orbital inflammatory changes, pneumonitis, carditis and encephalitis are present in various combinations.. Interestingly, larvae of the Trichinella spiralis do not produce cysts in the brain and mainly give rise to vasculitis. Severe headaches, meningitis, encephalitis with convulsions and coma. Ischemic occlusions and hemorrhagic effects lead to micro-infarcts and petechial hemorrhages. The clinical picture is that of severe meningo-encephalitis with high morbidity and mortality in such subset of patients. The diagnosis may be achieves with muscle biopsy and antibody detection by ELISA and bentonite flocculation method. The main management comprises of the treatment of the symptoms, antihelminthics (mebendazole 200 mg /day for 4-5 days or thiabendazole 2-3 gm/day for 5 days), prednisolone to moderate allergic reactions. Relatively, it has a better prognosis as compared to other parasitic disorders.

Cysticercosis, caused by the Taenia solium, is the commonest helminthic parasite infecting the CNS. The formation of the cysts in various tissues by the larvae of the Taenia solium is known as cysticercosis. These may be subcutaneous cysts, cardiac muscle cysts, CNS cysts, etc. No body part is immune to cysticercosis and wherever it occurs it causes loss or disturbed functions. Neuro-cysticercosis is a serious condition posing special management challenge due to diversity in clinical presentations. Following clinical forms are common:(a) raised intracranial pressure without hydrocephalus presenting with recurrent headaches, vomiting and papilledema due to diffuse parenchymal cysticercosis with small ventricles;(b) hydrocephalus-non communicating hydrocephalus due to intraventricular cysticercosis or communicating hydrocephalus due to recemose meningeal cysts;(c) recurrent seizures due to focal or multifocal granulomas or cysts;(d) meningo-encephalitis due to allergic-immunological responses , and (e) intra-parenchymal solitary or multiple large cysts. Dying or dead cysts excite more pronounced inflammatory reactions and the adult cysts are usually surrounded by the neuroglial reactive cells. Dead cysts may be completely calcified.

On clinical grounds, these patients present with features of seizures (80 %cases), focal neurological deficits (20-30%cases)and raised ICP(in 10-20 % cases; headaches, vomiting, visual obscurations, papilledema, and slowness of mental faculties).Patients may present with strokes due to the arteritis caused by the recemose variety of cysticercosis which also causes hydrocephalus. The spinal cysts with clinical features of radiculopathy, and severe spinal cord compression are not unusual. There is non-specific peripheral as well as CSF eosinophilia. Plain X-rays of the muscular tissues in the limbs or body show multiple about one centimeter long, calcified, oval, oat-shaped cysts. The CT head and MRI scan of the Brain show characteristics of the cystic or granulomatous lesions as well as hydrocephalus.. Immunological tests with variable success are utilized such as indirect hemagglutination, complement fixation, agar gel precipitation, immuno-electrophoresis, counter electrophoresis, indirect immuno-fluorescence, ELISA and PCR. These are strong cross reactions between sera of patients with cysticercosis and antigen of taenia saginata, taenia crassiceps and echinococcus granulosus, etc. Neuroimaging studies with MR spectroscopy further help in arriving at the diagnosis. Management basically comprises of antihelminthics (a course of Praziquantal or a course of mebendazole, 400-600 mg/day for 4-6 weeks), anticonvulsants, antiedema measures (prednisolone) where indicated and surgical treatment in form of CSF diversion procedures and microsurgical excision of the intracranial or intraspinal cysts with overall good prognosis. Especially, Praziquantal kills cysticercus in the CNS and improves the parenchymal changes but with intense allergic-immunological reactions in the surrounding tissues due to dying parasite and hence concurrently the steroid therapy (prednisolone 40 mg daily for the period of therapy) is given as an inpatient in the hospital. The overall mortality is about 8-10% cases.

Strongyloidiasis is caused by Strongyloides stercoralis infection in the small intestines. It is ubiquitous in distribution and about 800 million people is estimated to be infected in the world over, being endemic in South East USA and tropical parts of the world. Usually, the infective focus in the small intestine is asymptomatic; however, once the infection becomes heavy then intestinal symptoms of abdominal pains, diarrhea, and malabsorption syndromes develop and if unchecked then features such as Crohn disease and even necrotizing bowel disease may present as dire emergency. The patients may present with cutaneous manifestations once the infection become heavy and the larvae migrate under the skin. The laboratory diagnosis is usually made by observing motile rhabditiform larvae in the stool preparations. These larvae commonly penetrate skin and present with cutaneous manifestations such as dermatitis, urticarial rashes or subcutaneous swellings. Pulmonary involvement leads to non-bacterial pneumonia, chest pains, dyspnea, hemoptysis, wheezing and eosinophilia with a sputum sample positive for S. stercoralis. Immuno-suppressants and long term corticosteroid therapy are two most important vulnerability increasing factors leading to a massive disseminated strongyloidiasis or hyperinfection syndrome. The larval invasion of the blood stream leads to peritonitis, severe pneumonitis and meningoencephalitis. Rapidly developing raised intracranial pressure with headaches, vomiting, and neck rigidity, progresses to the deterioration in level of consciousness, coma and fatality. The worse scenario is the frequent association of the gram negative sepsis with this heavy infection syndrome with very high mortality. The treatment of choice is supportive intensive care management with medical therapy including the drugs such as antibacterial antibiotics as well as thiabendazole, 25 mg/kg every 12 hours for 2 days. Therefore the patients living in tropical areas should be carefully evaluated and forewarned before giving steroids or immuno-suppressants.

Toxocariasis is a self limiting disease caused by the larvae of the Toxocara canis, dog's roundworm. It is a form of visceral larva migrans (VLM). Dogs may be heavily infected in their intestines and they pass ova in their faeces. Humans' contract these ova through the contaminated food items. Once ingested, the eggs hatch larvae in the intestine. These larvae penetrate the intestinal walls and enter the blood stream to cause dissemination of larvae. These larvae again penetrate the capillary walls from within causing microhemorrhages and come out to enter various tissues. They produce damage along their course of migration for one to two years before dying. At some stage of migration, these are contained by a granulomatous reaction comprising of eosinophils, lymphocytes, plasma cells, microglial cells and astrocytes. In the craniospinal region, meningo-encephalitic symptoms predominate in the form of headaches, vomiting, seizures, focal neurological deficits (aphasia, ataxia, hemiparesis) as well as features of Guillain Barré syndrome).Stool examination for eggs and larvae, peripheral eosinophilia, hemagglutination and intradermal tests are non-specific and the best is ELISA. Medical management includes symptomatic treatment (including anticonvulsants), DEC(a full course of diethylcarbamazine, 1 mg/kg on first day, 2 mg/kg on second day, 3mg/kg on third and fourth days and then 3 mg /kg TID for 3 weeks) along with Thiabendazole, 25 mg/kg BID for 5 days and steroids where indicated. The overall prognosis is good and the mortality is extremely rare.

5. Chemical Meningitis [94]

Meningitis due to the pathological effects of the chemical substances on the meninges is called chemical meningitis and it is in fact one of the uncommon or rare form of meningeal inflammatory disorder. Initially, Lepto-meningeal (pia-arachnoid compartment) inflammation per se without obliteration of the CSF spaces or cisterns but with reactive changes in the CSF is referred as lepto- meningitis or simply as meningitis. By enlarge, then the late stage of this condition, based on the neuro-imaging studies showing obvious obliteration of the sub-arachnoid spaces and histo-pathology confirming the leptomeningeal scarring due to the inflammatory processes, is termed as adhesive meningitis, obliterative lepto- meningitis, plastic arachnoiditis or chemical arachnoiditis. [95, 96]

Epidemiology and Etiopathogenesis [97,98]

Chemical meningitis is reported from all over the Globe although mainly as anecdotal cases or reports of small series with few patients. There is no specific evidence to postulate any bar to age, sex, race, ethnicity and geographical locations. It appears to be either an uncommon or a rare event. There are many types of the chemical substances used by the patients during the course of their illness which can cause chemical meningitis such as analgesics (NSAIDs), antibiotics, blood products, other medications (baclofen, methotrexate, cytarabine), immuno-globulins, vaccines, intra-ventricular and intra-thecal medications (baclofen, methotrexate{IT-MXT),cytarabine, steroids-methylprednisolone, hydrocortisone, vincristine) radiological contrast mediums(both, oil based and water soluble for examples myodil, metrizamide, iohexol, iopamidol, gadolinium), anesthetic medications, diluents, preservatives, contaminants(during spinal anesthesia), etc. All these medications are capable of inducing various grades of chemical meningitis in different time spans along with their protein manifestations. Among the NSAIDs, ibuprofen results in maximum number of cases with chemical meningitis. [99]

Among the pre-existing medical illnesses, some patients with lupus erythematosus and occasional patient with rheumatoid arthritis are particularly vulnerable for chemical meningitis on ingestion of ibuprofen. Following intracranial mass lesions result in the chemical meningitis due to the spillage of their contents in the leptomeningeal spaces: cystic craniopharyngiomas, epidermoid and dermoid cysts, pineal cysts, colloid cysts of the third ventricle, etc. [100]The rupture of these cystic lesions discharges proteinaceous material in the leptomeningeal spaces and excites strong inflammatory responses to start with and then the severe reactive CSF changes with further consequences.

The possible pathological mechanisms may be as follows: (a) direct meningeal irritation / inflammatory response against the medications or chemicals, [101] (b) immunological response to the medications, [102, 103] (c) allergic responses to the preservatives, and (d) chronic infections where the organisms or their components are not identified. Idiosyncratic immunologic meningitis may result especially from NSAIDs and intravenous immuno-globulins. [99-104]

Clinical Presentations, Management and Prognosis

The patients with chemical meningitis present with the similar symptoms as the patients with bacterial meningitis but in slightly milder form. After the ingestion or application of the medications, the patient usually develops meningeal inflammatory symptoms such as headaches, fever, nausea, neck stiffness and photophobia. However, the headaches are like generalized cephalic discomfort and the vomiting is uncommon but nausea is commonly present. The fever is not very high. The neck stiffness is marginal. There are usually no focal neurological deficits or any signs or symptoms of raised ICP. However in severe cases, there may be altered higher mental functions including the confusional state and cloudy level of consciousness and recurrent seizures with their consequences.

The neuro-imaging studies [100] are normal in the initial stages of the chemical meningitis; however, in the late stages when the arachnoiditis sets in then the clinico-pathological picture will change along with the typical features of arachnoiditis on the CT scans and the MRI scans of the neuraxis or of the region of interest. The CSF studies in these cases show consistently negative culture studies; however, white cell counts are slightly higher, as is the protein estimations but the CSF glucose may be slightly low. [101]

Chemical meningitis [102,103]due to the drug ingestion usually subsides after the withdrawal of the medications in few hours to few days without significant sequalae in the majority of the patients. However, if it is due to the intrathecal injection of the medications then its severity will depend upon the concentration of the medication, lipid solubility, drug particle size, duration of the contact with the lepto-meninges, etc. These patients are usually recovered without antibiotic therapy. The management of the significant cystic intracranial mass lesions is the microsurgical excision of these lesions so as to prevent spillage in the sub-arachnoid spaces. Every case of the chemical meningitis is treated on its on merit with the treatment strategy most suitable for the type of chemical meningitis the patient is having. The principles of management of chemical meningitis remain as follows: symptomatic supportive therapy including periodic CSF assessments, analgesics, antipyretics, fluid and electrolyte supplements, anticonvulsants where indicated, control of raised ICP (carbonic anhydrase inhibitor, mannitol, etc), checking super infections, and effectively dealing with the causative factors. The overall prognosis in cases of chemical meningitis is good to excellent if the condition is recognised early and effectively treated in time.

6. Carcinomatous Meningitis [104]

Among the various etiological factors, carcinomatous lesions are rare cause of the meningitis affecting the entire neuraxis. However, nowadays in the oncology setups around the world, carcinomatous meningitis is more frequently (4-6% of all cancer patients) recognised and managed more effectively then ever before to provide mainly the palliative therapy in majority of such patients. Usually, carcinomatous meningitis is due to the metastatic deposits from the extracranial sites but rarely intracranial lesions may spread to result in the malignant meningeal inflammation. [105, 106]

Epidemiology and Etio-pathogenesis [107]

Carcinomas and sarcomas may lead to CNS metastasis but the former is far more common as compared to the latter. Carcinomatous meningitis [108,109]is basically leptomeningeal metastasis by a variety of primary (rare) and secondary (common) intracranial lesions such as carcinomas and hematological malignancies. More commonly the disseminated systemic extracranial malignancies (about two third cases) reach meninges via hematogenous spread and less commonly, the cells from the primary brain tumors in the ventricles(choroids plexus carcinomas), near the ventricular surface (ependymomas, lymphomas) or meningeal surface (astrocytomas, medulloblastomas)invade subarachnoid spaces to cause malignant meningitis and rarely the perineural and perivascular migration of the systemic malignancies occur. Two types of leptomeningeal spread from the solid tumors are recognized: (1) nodular infiltration of the meninges with long time survival and better prognosis and (2) free floating-thin carpeting carcinomatous cells over the surface of the lepto-meninges with infiltrations of the Virchow- Robin spaces (vascular and neural invasions) and thereby relatively unfavorable prognosis.

Mostly, these are solid adenocarcinomas from the breast, lungs and stomach which are resulting in carcinomatous meningitis in approximately one in 15 to 20 patients. Malenomatous meningitis is also frequent as it develops in one in five patients of extracranial malenomas. Hematological malignancies are the commonest to cause neoplastic meningitis in about one in five to ten patients of leukemia and lymphomas. Among the hematological neoplasms, the incidence of lymphomas and lymphoblastic leukemia are common. Among the primary brain tumors(1-2%), choroid plexus carcinomas, malignant ependymomas and pituitary adeno-carcinoma are more frequently implicated. Meningeal carpeting (layering /infiltration) is usually is about one-three cells thick. Widespread few cell thick layered meningeal infiltrations may result in blockage of the sub-arachnoid spaces, hydrocephalus, vasculitis and cranial neuritis. There is meningeal inflammatory reaction to the neoplastic cells.

Macroscopically, there may be nodules on the meningeal surfaces especially in the CSF cisterns such as lumbar cistern, CP angle cistern, and basal cisterns. Once the tumor seeding establish themselves in the meningeal layers, these establish their blood supply as well and breaks blood brain barrier and blood CSF barrier and their by spread more rapidly. These malignant cells usually extend in the perivascular spaces and then the pial invasion lead to intra-parenchymal spread. There is beading appearances of the vessels and consequently decreased regional blood flow with ischemia. This results in vascular occlusion, thrombosis and infarctions along with the multifocal spread in the brain as well as cranial neuritis monoplex or multiplex.

Clinical Symptomatology [110,111]

Usually the clinical picture is that of insidious in onset with chronic course but in a significant number of cases acute presentations results due to focal radiculopathy, neurological deficits, stroke and neuropathy. In the majority of cases of cranial malignant meningitis (two in five cases of neoplastic meningitis), the patients present initially with progressive generalized headaches, nausea and then recurrent vomiting, cervico-occipital or fronto-orbital headaches, seizures, focal neurological deficits and cranial nerve palsies(ocular nerve palsies especially the abducent palsy, trigeminal sensory-motor disturbances, hearing impairment and visual loss). These are followed by general constitutional symptoms or malaise, lassitude, generalized myalgia, confusion, memory disturbances, etc. The patient may present with frank features of raised intracranial pressure needing immediate relief. The spinal carcinomatous meningitis (three out of every five patients with neoplastic meningitis) usually presents with the features of radiculopathy (cervicalgia with brachialgia and lumbago with sciatica), cauda equina syndrome (sensory motor weakness in the lower limbs with sphincter disturbances) and frank acute or subacute myelopathy. The involvement of more than one cerebro-spinal region points towards the possibility of neoplastic meningitis in a known case of disseminated systemic malignancy.

Diagnosis and Differential Diagnosis [104-112]

The primary choice among the diagnostic investigations is the lumbar puncture with CSF analysis. However, if there are features of raised ICP, then the CT scan of the head (plain and contrast studies) is the investigation of first choice to rule out a significant intracranial space occupying lesion or hydrocephalus and then followed by the CSF studies via cisternal or lumbar puncture. In about half of cases, the CSF pressure is elevated with raised proteins and slightly low sugar levels. On the cytological studies, the malignant cells are larger in size with larger-denser nuclei as compared to the normal lymphocytes. The malignant cells and reactive leucocytes-lymphocytes are, at time, difficult to be differentiated with the morphological histo-pathological studies and therefore these are well differentiated with electron microscopic studies and special immuno-histo-chemistry using monoclonal antibodies. These monoclonal antibodies are basically markers for leucocytes, epithelial cells, neuroblasts and neuro-ectodermal tissues. These studies can very well differentiate and categorize these lesions such as carcinomas, lymphomas and neuro-ectodermal tumors.

Obviously the CNS staging of the carcinomatous/ neoplastic meningitis will need a detailed workup of the whole neuraxis and the entire leptomeningeal encompassing sub-arachnoid spaces.

Neuro-imaging studies such as the CT and MRI scanning (both, plain and contrast enhanced) are of prime importance in precisely defining the malignant lesions along with their spread across the tissues [Figure 8]. Apart from the morphological characteristics, these show meningeal enhancement and carpeting of the lesion in the sub-arachnoid spaces, obliteration of the superficial sulci and basal cisterns with intense contrast enhancements, intra-parenchymal neoplastic lesions and ischemic cortico-subcortical changes, hydrocephalus and trans-ependymal edema. Spinal imaging may show deposits, nodules, beading and thickening of the spinal roots, infiltration and obliteration of the sub-arachnoid spaces and compressive and infiltrative myelopathic changes. Solitary or multiple cranio-spinal metastases may be apparent in cases of generalized extraneural skeletal metastases.

In the differential diagnosis of the neoplastic / carcinomatous/malignant meningitis, the other etiological factors must be carefully considered such as viral, bacterial, fungal, parasitic and chemical causes as well as chronic granulomatous disorder such as tuberculosis and sarcoidosis.

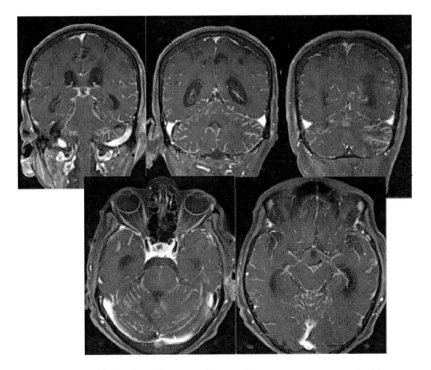

Figure 8. 52 year old female with a treated case of breast cancer, presented with headache. Post-contrast FAT SAT T1W coronal and axial images reveal-Leptomeningeal enhancement- which follows the pial surface of the brain and fills the subarachnoid spaces of the sulci, cisterns and between the cerebellar folia. These findings are very typical of carcinomatous meningitis.

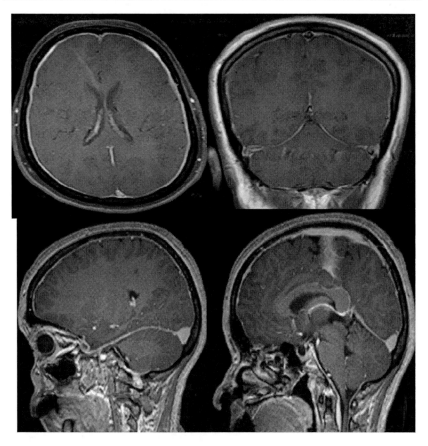

Figure 9. 50 years old lady presented with 3 months h/o orthostatic headache. Multiplanar MRI shows typical features of spontaneous intracranial hypotension-suggested by circumferential dural enhancement along the cerebral convexity, interhemispheric fissure and tentorium. Sagittal T1 3D image: shows sagging mid brain with buckling of medulla. Bilateral subdural hematomas [Not shown] were also present. This case shows a typical example of pachymeningeal enhancement- which occurs adjacent to the inner table of the skull; in the falx within the interhemispheric fissure; and also in the tentorium between the cerebellum, vermis, and occipital lobes. Pure dural enhancement, without pial or subarachnoid involvement, will not fill in the sulci or basilar cisterns.

Management and Prognosis [113,114]

The management modalities in cases of carcinomatous meningitis comprise of chemotherapy [115-116], radiotherapy and surgical therapies wherever indicated. [117] Neurosurgical procedures are primarily the insertion of a ventriculo-peritoneal shunt for the hydrocephalus, implantation of Ommayya reservoir with intraventricular catheter for the delivery of the chemotherapeutic medications and periodic lumbar punctures. More than one modalities of the management are usually needed. Chemotherapy remains the best modality of treatment for the entire neuraxis. Intrathecal drug therapy (via trans-ventricular route or trans-lumbar route) is used for the chemotherapeutic drug to reach all the corners of the subarachnoid spaces and the field radiotherapy for the significant focal intracranial mass lesions and subarachnoid blockages.. Among the chemotherapeutic agents (thio-TEPA, arabinoside, cytosine, methotrexate, etc), the methotrexate (intraventricular via reservoir) is frequently used with success in about 50% cases. Systemic chemotherapy may be needed either in addition or as a replacement of the intrathecal drug therapy. A course of radiotherapy (2400 rads) over 2 week's period is combined with chemotherapy for greater success especially in the secondaries from the breast cancer. However, whole neuraxis radiation is usually not given in solid tumors due to its severe myelo-suppressive effects. The clinical progress is mainly monitored with the CSF cytological studies but the low sensitivity of this test. The CSF flow dynamics and patency of the sub-arachnoid spaces can be assessed with radionuclide studies ([111]indium-diethylenetriamine pentaacetic acid or ^{99}Tc macroaggregated albumin). Patients with significant obliteration of the CSF spaces have poorer prognosis. Interestingly, field radiotherapy may help open these pathways in a significant number of patients (one in four at least) with little improvement in prognosis. Since the usual survival time in patient with untreated neoplastic meningitis ranges from six weeks (usually) to three or more (rarely) months. Combined multimodality therapy is offered to those patients, who are likely to live more than three months. The management including the supportive care facilities is mainly palliative to improve the quality of life, to maintain neurological status and to achieve some prolongation in survival period.

The available best multimodality of treatment in this serious condition of the carcinomatous meningitis is still far from being satisfactory. Intensive researches on the newer treatment modalities and strategies are needed to improve the morbidities and mortality associated with the carcinomatous meningitis. [118]

Pachymeningitis

The pachymeninges (thick meninges) are the dura mater. Pachymeningeal enhancement may be manifested up against the bone, or it may involve the dural reflections of the falx cerebri, tentorium cerebelli, falx cerebelli, and cavernous sinus [Figure 9]. Extraaxial pachymeningeal enhancement may arise from various benign or malignant processes, including transient postoperative changes, intracranial hypotension, neoplasms such as meningiomas, metastatic disease (from breast and prostate cancer), secondary CNS lymphoma, and granulomatous disease [Fungal/Tuberculous, sarcoid]. Linear pachymeningeal (dura-arachnoid) enhancement occurs after surgery and with spontaneous intracranial hypotension. Leptomeningeal (pia-arachnoid) enhancement is present in meningitis and meningoencephalitis.

CONCLUSIONS

The CNS infective lesions are serious threat to life. Each case need to be managed on its own basis and the therapeutic measures must be tailored according to the needs of these patients. The meningitis or meningoencephalitis is caused by a variety of etiological factors with differing demographical situations. Protean, diverse and perplexing clinical presentations pose special challenge for the clinicians to diagnose as to what form of meningitis and meningo-encephalitis is seriously life threatening (acute gram negative bacterial meningitis) from the one which can be managed on the out patient basis (mild aseptic viral meningitis). Diagnostic armamentarium comprises blood and the CSF analysis, neuro-imaging studies as well as microbiological and immunological tests. Medical therapies, intensive care management where indicated and various surgical procedures form the corner stone of their management. Timely management significantly improves morbidities and mortality associated with these high risk infections. The preventive measures are certainly having far reaching implications and can not be overemphasized.

ACKNOWLEDGEMENT

We are sincerely thankful to Dr. Abhishek Arora, Consultant Radiologist, Tata Memorial hospital, Mumbai for providing us the images for Figure 8.

REFERENCES

[1]   Sharma RR, Lad SD, Pawar SJ, Gurusinghe NT, Bhagwati SN, Mahapatra AK. Surgical Management of Fungal Infections of the Central Nervous System. In Schmidek HH, Roberts DW, (eds): *Schmidek & Sweet's Operative Neurosurgical Techniques, Indications, Methods and Results*, 5th ed, 2006, pp1633-71.

[2]   Canada Communicable Disease Report. *International Note: Global Advisory Committee on Vaccine Safety*, 11-12 june,2003.

[3]   CDC. Final 2008 West Nile Virus Activity in the United States. *Centers for Disease Control and Prevention.*http://bit.ly/fATcE1.

[4]   Desmond RA, Accortt NA, Talley L, Vilano SA, Song's, Whitley RJ. Enteroviral meningitis: natural history and outcome of plecoraril therapy. *Antimicrob Agents Chemother,* Jul2006:50(7): 2409-14.

[5]   Hviid A, Rubin S, Mulemann K. Mumps. *Lancet.* Mar15, 2008; 371(9616):932-44.

[6]   Jarhling PB, Peters CJ. Lymphocytic choriomeningitis virus: a neglected pathogen of man. *Arch Pathol Lab Med,* 1992;116:486-8.

[7]   King Rl, Lorch Sa, Cohen DM, Hodinka RL, Cohn KA, Shah SS. Routine cerebrospinal fluid enterovirus polymerase chain reaction testing reduces hospitalization and antibiotic use for infants 90 days of age or younger. *Paediatrics,* Sep 2009; 123(6):e967-71.

[8]   Landry ML, Greenwood J, Vikram HR. Herpes simplex type-2 menmingitis: presentation and lack of standardized therapy. *Am J Med,* Jul 2009:122(7):122(7):688-91.

[9]   Peters CJ. Arenaviruses. In:Richman DD, Whitley RJ, Hayden FG,EDS. *Clinical Virology.* New York: Churchill Livingstone, Inc 1997:973-96.

[10]   Peters CJ, Buchmeier M, Rollin PE, Ksiazek TG. Arenaviruses. In:Belshe RB, ed. *Textbook of Human Virology.*2nd ed. St.Louis: Mosby-Year Book, Inc. 1991:541-70.

[11]   Fleisher GR. Infectious disease emergencies. In: *Textbook of pediatric Emergency Medicine,* 5th ed, Fleisher GR, Ludwig S, Henretig FM, (Eds). 2006, pp783.

[12]   Swartz MN. Bacterial meningitis-a view of the past 90 years. *N Engl J Med*, 2004;351(18):1826-8.

[13]   Thigpen MC, Whitney CG, Messonnier NE, et al. Bacterial meningitis in the United States 1998-2007. *N Engl J Med,* 2011;364(21)2016-25.

[14]   Tunkel AR, Hartman BJ, Kaplan SL, etal. Practice guidelines for the management of bacterial meningitis. *Clin Infec Dis,* 2004;39:1267.

[15] Feigin RD, Cutrer WB. Bacterial meningitis beyond the neonatal period. In: *Textbook of Pediatric Infectious Diseases*, 6th ed, Feigin RD, Cherry JD, Demmler-Harrison GJ , Kaplan SL(eds).Saunders, Philadelphia, 2009 p.439.

[16] American Academy of Pediatrics. Meningococcal infections. In: Red Book:2009.*Report of the Committee on Infectious Diseases,* 28th ed, Pickering LK(Ed),American Academy of Pediatrics, Elk Grove Village, IL 2009, p.455.

[17] Brown EM, Fisman DN, Drews SJ, et al. Epidemiology of invasive meningococcal disease with decreased susceptibility to penicillin in Ontario, Canada,2000 to 2006. *Antimicrob Agents Chemother* 2010;54:1016.

[18] Ericson L, DeWals P. Complications and sequalae of meningococcal disease in Quebec, Canada 1990-1994. *Clin Inf Dis* 1998; 26: 1159-64.

[19] Kaplan SL, Schultze GE,Leake JA, et al. Multi-center surveillance of invasive meningococcal infections in children. *Pediatrics* 2006;118:e979.

[20] Kornelisse RF, Hazelzet JA, Hop WC, etal. Meningococcal septic shock in children: clinical and laboratory features, outcome and development of a prognostic score. *Clin Infect Dis* 1997;25(3):640-6.

[21] American Academy of Pediatrics. Haemophilus influenzae Infections. In: *Red Book: 2009 Report of the Committee on Infectious Diseases,* 28th ed, Pickering LK(Ed),American Academy of Pediatrics Elk Grove Village, IL 2009,p.455.

[22] Levin OS, Knoll MD, Jones A, Walker DG, Risko N, Gilani Z.Global status of Haemophilus influenzae type b and pneumococcal conjugate vaccines: evidence, policies and introductions. *Curr Opin Infect Dis,* 2010, 23(3):236-41.

[23] Peltola H. Worldwide Haemophilus influenzae type b disease at the beginning of the 21st century: global analysis of the disease burden 25 years after the use of the polysaccharide vaccine and a decade after the advent of conjugates. *Clin Microbiol Rev* 2000; 13:302.

[24] American Academy of Pediatrics. Pneumococcal infections.In:RedBook:2009, Report of the committee on the Infectious Diseases,28th ed, Pickering, LK (Ed),*American Academy of Pediatrics,* Elk Grove Village, IL 2009, P.524.

[25] Arditi M, Mason EO Jr, Bradley JS, etal. Three year multicenter surveillance of pneumococcal meningitis in Children: clinical

characteristics and outcome related to penicillin susceptibility and dexamethasone use. *Pediatrics* 1998;102:1087.

[26] Kornelisse RF, Westerbeek CM, Spoor AB, et al. Pneumococcal meningitis in children: prognostic indicators and outcome. *Clin Infect Dis* 1995;21:1390.

[27] Bridy-Pappas AE, Margolis MB, Center KJ. Isaacman DJ. Streptococcus pneumoniae: description of the pathogen, disease epidemiology, treatment, and prevention. *Pharmacotherapy* 2005;25(9):1193-212.

[28] Baraff LJ, Lee SI, Schriger DL. Outcomes of bacterial meningitis in children: a meta-analysis. *Pediatr Infect Dis J* 1993; 12:389.

[29] Beer R, Engelhardt KW, Pfausler B, et al. Pharmacokinetics of intravenous linezolid in cerebrospinal fluid and plasma in neuro-intensive care patients with staphylococcal ventriculitis associated with external ventricular drains. *Antimicrob Agents Chemother* 2007; 51: 379.

[30] Pong A, Bradlev JS. Bacterial meningitis and the newborn infant. *Infect Dis Clin North Am* 1999;13:711.

[31] Chavez-Bueno S, McCracken GH. Bacterial meningitis in children. *Pediatr Clin North Am* 2005;52(3):795-810.

[32] Kaplan SL, Fishman MA.Supportive therapy for bacterial meningitis. *Pediatr Infect Dis J* 1987;6(7): 670-7.

[33] Pomeroy SL,Holmes SJ, Dodge PR. Seizures and other neurological sequalae of bacterial meningitis in children. *N Engl J Med* 1990;323(24):1651-7.

[34] Segal S, Pollard AJ. The future of meningitis vaccines. *Hosp Med* 2003;64(3):161-7.

[35] Van de Beek D, de Gans J, Mc Intyre P, Prasad K. Corticosteroids for acute bacterial meningitis. *Cochrane Database Syst Rev* 2007;1:CD004405.

[36] Yogev R, Guzman-Cottril J. Bacterial meningitis in children: critical review of current concepts. *Drugs* 2005;65(8):1097-112.

[37] Nelson LJ, Schneider E, Wells CD, Moore M. Epidemiology of childhood tuberculosis in the united states, 1993-2001: the need for continued vigilance. *Paediatrics,* 2004;114(2):333-41.

[38] Shaw JE, Pasipanodya JG, Gumbo T. *Meningeal tuberculosis: high long term mortality despite standard therapy.* Medicine(Baltimore). 2010; 89(3):189-95.

[39] Schoeman JF, Van Zyl LE, Laubscher JA, Donald PR. Effects of
      corticosteroids on intracranial pressure, computed tomographic findings
      and clinical course in young children with tuberculous meningitis.
      Pediatrics 1997;99(2):226-31.
[40] Srikanth SG, Taly AB, Nagarajan K, Jayakumar PN, Patil S. Clinico-
      radiological features of tuberculous meningitis in patient over 50 years
      of age. *J Neurol Neurosurg Psychiatry*.2007;78(5):536-8.
[41] World   Health   Organization.   Tuberculosis:World   Health
      Organization.http://www.who.int/media centre/factsheets/fs104/en/.
[42] Dastur DK, Manghani DK, Udani PM. Pathology And pathogenetic
      mechanisms   in   neuro-tuberculosis.   *Radiol   Clin   North
      Am*1995:33(4):733-52.
[43] Hejazi N, Hassler W. Multiple intra cranial tuberculomas with atypical
      response to tuberculostatic chemotherapy: literature review and a case
      report. *Infection.* 1997:25(4):233-9.
[44] Kumar R, Dwivedi A, Kumar P, Kohli N. Tuberculous meningitis in
      BCG vaccinated and unvaccinated children. J Neurol Neurosurg
      Psychiatry 2005;76(11):1550-4.
[45] Kohli A, Kapoor R. Neurological picture. Embolic spread of
      tuberculomas in the brain in multidrug resistant tubercular meningitis. *J
      Neurol Neurosurg Psychiatry.* 2008;79(2):198.
[46] Misra UK, Kalita J, Srivastava M, et al. Prognosis of tuberculous
      meningitis: a multivariate analysis. *J Neurol Sci,*1996;137(1):57-61.
[47] Nicolls DJ, King M, Holland D, Bala J, del Rio C.Intracranial
      tuberculomas developing while on therapy for pulmonary tuberculosis.
      Lancet Infect Dis. Dec 2005; 5(12):795-801.
[48] Sharma RR. Fungal Infections of the Nervous System; Current
      Perspective and Controversies in Management. *IJS* 2010;8(8):591-601.
[49] Bazan C, Rinaldi MG, Rauch RR, Jinkins R. Fungal infections of the
      brain. *Neuroimag Clin N Am* 1991; 1:57-88.
[50] Bennett JE. Introduction to Mycoses. In Mandell GL, Bennett JE, Dolin
      R (eds). *Mandell, Douglas, and Bennett's Principles and Practice of
      Infectious Diseases,* 6th ed. Elsevier, Churchill Livingstone,2005, pp
      2935-38.
[51] Sharma RR, Lad SD, Desai AP, Lynch PG. Surgical Management of
      fungal infections of the Nervous System. In Schmidek HH (ed):
      Schmidek & Sweet's Operative Neurosurgical Techniques, Indications,
      Methods and Results, 4th ed 2000,pp1726-55.

[52] Edwards JE. Candida Species. In Mandell GL, Bennett JE, Dolin R (eds): Mandell, Douglas, and Bennett's Principles and Practice of Infectious Diseases, 6th ed. Elsevier, *Churchill Livingstone*,2005, pp 2939-57.

[53] Leenders AC, Reiss P, Portegies P, et al. Liposomal amphotericin B(Ambisome) compared with Amphotericin B followed by fluconazole in the treatment of AIDS-associated cryptococcal meningitis. *AIDS* 1997;11:1463-71.

[54] Miller DJ. Diagnosis and management of Candida and other fungal infections of the head and neck. *Current Infectious Disease Reports* 2002; 4(3):194-200.

[55] Azizirad O, Clifford DB, Groger RK, Prelutsky D, Schmidt RE. Histoplasmoma: Isolated central nervous system infection with histoplasma capsulatum in a patient with AIDS: case report and brief review of the literature. *Clin Neurol Neurosurg* 2007;109(2):176-181.

[56] Mathews M, Pare L, Hasso A. Intraventricular cryptococcal cysts masquerading as racemose neurocysticercosis. *Surg Neurol* 2007;67 (6):647-9.

[57] Nadkarni T, Goel A. Aspergilloma of the Brain: an overview. *JPGM* 2005;51(5):37-41.

[58] Saccente M. Central nervous system histoplasmosis. *Curr Treat Options Neurol* 2008;10(3):161-7.

[59] Sharma RR, Pawar SJ, Ravi RR, et al. A solitary primary Aspergillus Brain abscess in an immuno-competent host: CT guided stereotaxy with an excellent outcome. *Pan Arab J Neurosurg* 2002;6:62-5.

[60] Turgut M, Ozsunar Y, Oncu S, Akyuz O, Ertugrul MB,Tekin C, Gultekin B, Sakarya S. Invasive fungal granuloma of the brain caused by Aspergillus fumigatus: a case report and review of literature. *Surg Neurol* 2008; 69:169-74.

[61] Vieira MR, Milheiro A, Pacheco FA. Phaeohyphomycosis due to Cladosporium cladosporioides. *Medical Mycology* 2001;39(1):135-7.

[62] Akhaddar A, Gazzaz M, Albouzidi A, Lmimouni B, Elmostarchid B, Boucetta M. Invasive aspergillus terreus sinusitis with orbito-cranial extension: case report. *Surg Neurol* 2008; 69(5):490-5.

[63] Sharma RR, Pawar SJ, Delmendo A, et al. Fatal rhino-orbito-cerebral mucormycosis in an apparently normal host: case report and literature review. *J Clin Neurosci* 2001; 8:583-6.

[64] Sharma RR, Gurusinghe NT, Lynch PG. Cerebral infarction due to aspergillus arteritis following glioma surgery.*Br J Neurosurg* 1992:6:485-90.

[65] Gottileb JR, Eismont FJ. Nonoperative treatment of vertebral osteomyelitis associated with paraspinal abscess and cord compression. A case report. *JBJS Am* 2006; 88(4): 854-6.

[66] Khazim RM, Debnath UK, Fares Y. Candida albicans osteomyelitis of the spine: progressive clinical and radiological features and surgical management in three cases. *Eur Spine J* 2006; 15(9):1404-10.

[67] Mahiquez M, Bunton KL, Caney G, Weinstein MA, Small LM. Nonsurgical treatment of lumbosacral blastomycosis involving L2-S1: a case report. *Spine* (Phila Pa 1976) 2008; 33(13): E 442-6.

[68] Cross SA, Scott LJ. Micafungin. *Drugs* 2008;68:2225-55.

[69] DiNubile MJ, Strohmaier KM, Lupinacci RJ, Meibohm AR, Sable CA, Kartsonis NA. Efficacy and safety of caspofungin therapy in elderly patients with proven or suspected invasive fungal infections. *Eur J Clin Microbio Infect* Dis 2008;27(8):663-70.

[70] Dismukes WE. Guidelines from the infectious diseases society of America. Introduction to Antifungal Drugs. *Clin Infect Dis* 2000;30:653-7.

[71] Lai CC, Tan CK, Huang YT, Shao PL, Hsueh PR. Current challenges in the management of invasive fungal infection. *J Infection and Chemotherapy* 2008;14(2):77-85.

[72] Maschmeyer G, Haas A. Voriconazole: a broad spectrum triazole for the treatment of serious and invasive fungal infections. *Future Microbiology* 2007;1(4):365-85.

[73] Jain R, Prabhakar S, Modi M, Bhatia R, Sehgal R. Naegleria meningitis: a rare survival. *Neurol India* , 2002;50(4):470-2.

[74] Poungvarin N, Jariya P. The fifth nonlethal case of primary amoebic meningoencephalitis. *J Med Assoc Thai* 1991;74(2): 112-5.

[75] Cabanes PA, Wallet F, Pringuez E, Pernin P. Assessing the risk of primary amoebic meningoencephalitis from swimming in the presence of environmental Naegleria fowleri. Appl.Environ. *Microbiol* 2001;67:2927-31.

[76] Caruzo G, Cardozo J.Primary amoebic meningoencephalitis: a new case from Venezuela. *Trop Doct,* 2008;38(4):256-7.

[77] Cervantes-Sandoval I, Serranno-Luna Jde J, Garcia-Latorre E,Tsutsumi V, Shibayama m. Characterization of the brain inflammation during primary amoebic meningoencephalitis. *Parasitol Int* 2008;57(3):307-13.

[78] Vargas-Zepeda J, Gomez-Alcala AV, Vasquez-Morales JA, Licea-Amaya L, De Jonckheere JF, Lares-Villa F. Successful treatment of Naegleria fowleri meningoencephalitis by using intravenous amphotericin B, fluconazole and rifampicin. *Arch Med Res* 2005;36(1):83-6.

[79] Lo Re V, Gluckman SJ. Eosinophilic meningitis. *Am J Med* 2003;114:217-23.

[80] Slom TJ, Cortese MM, Gerber SI, etal. An outbreak of eosinophilic meningitis caused by angiostrongylus cantonensis in travelers returning from the Caribbean. *N Engl J Med* 2002;346:668-75.

[81] Rusnak JM, Lucey DR. Clinical gnathostomiasis: case report and review of the English language literature. *Clin Infect Dis* 1993;16:33-50.

[82] Scheld WM, Whitley RJ, Marra CM, Huang DB, Schantz Pewit CA. Helminthic infections. In: Scheld WM, Whitley RJ, Marra CM, editors. *Infections of the central nervous system.*3rd ed. Philadelphia, PA: Lippincott Williams &Wilkins:2004,p.797-828.

[83] Sarkar S, Bhattacharya P. Cerebral malaria caused by plasmodium vivax in adult subjects. *Indian J Crit Care Med* , 2008;12(4):204-5.

[84] Sachdev HP, Mohan M. Vivax cerebral malaria. *J Trop Pediatr* 1985; 31:213-5.

[85] Ozen M, Gungor S, Atambay M, Daldal N. Cerebral malaria owing to plasmodium vivax: case report. *Ann J Pediatr 2006*;26:141-4.

[86] Chotmongkol V, Wongjirat C, Sawadpanit K, Sawanyawisuth K. Treatment of eosinophilic meningitis with a combination of albendazole and corticosteroids. *Southeast Am J Trop Med Hyg* 2006;74:1122-4.

[87] Chotmongkol V, Sawadpanit K, Sawanyawisuth K. Treatment of eosinophilic meningitis with a combination of prednisolone and mebendazole. *Southeast Asian J Trop Med Public Health* 2004;35:172-4.

[88] Batmanian JJ, O'Neil JH. Eosinophilic meningo-encephalitis with permanent neurologic sequalae. *Intern Med J* 2004;34:214-9.

[89] Witoonpanich R, Chuhirun S, Soranastaporn S, Rojanasunan P. Eosinophilic myelo meningo-encephalitis caused by Angiostrongylus cantonensis report of three cases. *Southeast Asian J Trop Med Public Health* 1991;22:262-7.

[90] Corral I, Quereda C, Moreno A, et al. Intramedullary cysticercosis cured with drug treatment. *Spine* 1996;21:2284-7.

[91] Escobedo F, Garcia-Ramos G, Sotelo J.Parasitic disorders and epilepsy. In:Nistico G, Di Perri R, Meinardi H(Eds):Epilepsy: An update on Research and Therapy. *New York: Alan R Liss* 1983;p.227-33.

[92] Neal J. An endoscopic approach to cysticercosis cysts of the posterior third ventricle. *Neurosurgery,*1995;36:1040-43.

[93] Sotelo J, Flisser A. Neurocysticercosis: Practical treatment guidelines disease management.*CNS Drugs* 1997;7:17-25.

[94] Forgacs P, Geyer CA, Freidberg SR. Characterization of chemical meningitis after Neurological surgery. *Clinical Infectious Diseases,* 2001;32(2):179-185.

[95] Curtin JA. Pantopaque hypersensitivity meningitis. Annals of Internal *Medicine,* 1971;74:838.

[96] Obwegeser A, Seiwald M, Stockhammer G. Intraventricular chemotherapy. *Journal of Neurosurg,* 1998; 899(1):172-3.

[97] Mott MG, Stevenson P, Wood CB. Methotrexate meningitis. *Lancet,* 1972;ii:656.

[98] Thordarson H, Talstad I. Acute meningitis and cerebellar dysfunction complicating high dose cytosine arabinoside therapy. *Acta Medica Scan* 1986;220:493-5.

[99] Jolles S, Sewell WA, Leighton C. Drug induced aseptic meningitis: diagnosis and management. *Drug Safety* 2000;22(3):215-26.

[100] Eustace S, Buff B. Magnetic resonance imaging in drug induced meningitis. *Canadian   Association   of   Radiologists   Journal* 1994;4596:463-5.

[101] Worthington M, Callander N,Flynn R, Sulivan R. Acuter chemical meningitis after metrizamide-lumbar myelography. *Surg Neurol* 1983;19(5):456-8.

[102] Alexiou J, Deloffre D,Vandresse JH, Boucquey JP, Sintzoff S. Post myelographic meningeal irritation with iohexol. *Neuroradiology* 1991;33(1):85-6.

[103] Neveira FA, Speight KL, Rauck RL, Carpenter RL. Meningitis after injection of intrathecal baclofen. *Anesthesia & Analog* 1996;82(6):1297-9.

[104] Jackleg KA. Neoplastic meningitis from systemic malignancies: diagnosis, prognosis and treatment. *Seminars in Oncology,* 200; 33(3):312-23.

[105] Gleissner B, Chamberlain MC. Neoplastic meningitis. *Lancet neurology,*2006;5(5);443-52.

[106] Zachariah B, Zachariah SB,Varghese R, Balducci L. Carcinomatous meningitis: clinical manifestations and managements. *Int J Clin Pharm Therapeutics,*1995;33(1):7-12.

[107] Kaplan JG, De Souza TG, Farkash A, et al. Leptomeningeal metastases: Comparison of clinical features and laboratory data of solid tumors, lymphomas and leukemias. *J Neurooncol* 1990;9:225-9.

[108] Chamberlain MC. Carcinomatous meningitis. Arch Neurol 1997;54:16-7.

[109] Vinchon M, Ruchoux MM, Lejeune JP, Assaker R, Christiaens JL. Carcinomatous meningitis in a case of anaplastic meningioma. *Journal of neuro-oncology,* 1995;23(3):239-43.

[110] Jimenez Mateos A, Cabrera Naranjo F, Gonzalez Hernandez A, Fabre Pi O, Diaz Nicolas S, Lopez Fernandez JC. Neoplastic meningitis. Review of a clinical series. *Neurologia* (Barcelona, Spain) 2011;26(4):227-32.

[111] Wasserstrom WR, Glass JP, Posner JB. Diagnosis and treatment of leptomeningeal metastases from solid tumors. Experience with 90 patients. *Cancer* 1982;49:759-72.

[112] Siegal T, Lossos A, Pfeffer MR. Leptomeningeal metastases: Analysis of 31 patients with sustained off-therapy response following combined modality therapy. *Neurology* 1994;44:1463-9.

[113] Jayson GC, Howell A. Carcinomatous meningitis in solid tumours. *Annals of Oncology,*1996; 7(8): 773-80.

[114] Shapiro WR, Johanson CE, Boogerd W. Treatment modalities for leptomeningeal metastases. *Seminar in oncology* 2009;36(4 suppl 2):S 46-54.

[115] Beauchesne P. Intrathecal chemotherapy for treatment of leptomeningeal dissemination of metastatic tumours. *The Lancet oncology,*2010;11(9)871-9.

[116] Fukuhara T, Saijo Y, Sakakibara T, Inoue A, Morikawa N, Kanamori M, Nakashima I, Nukiwa T. Successful treatment of carcinomatous meningitis with gefitinib in a patient with lung adeno-carcinoma harboring. *The Tohoku journal of experimental medicine,* 2008;214(4):359-63.

[117] Chamberlain MC, Kormanik PA, Barba D. Complications associated with intraventricular chemotherapy in patients with leptomeningeal metastases. *Journal of Neurosurgery,*1997; 87(5): 694-9.

[118] Waki F, Ando M, Takashima A, Yonemori K, Nokihara H, Miyake M, Tateishi U, Tsuta K, Shimada Y, Fujiwara Y. Prognostic factors and

clinical outcomes in patients with leptomeningeal metastasis from solid tumours. *Journal of neuro-oncology* , 2009;9(2):205-12.

In: Meningitis: Causes, Diagnosis and Treatment   ISBN 978-1-62100-833-0
Editors: G. Houllis et al. pp. 83-140   ©2012 Nova Science Publishers, Inc.

Chapter 2

BACTERIAL MENINGITIS, MOLECULAR DIAGNOSIS AND EPIDEMIOLOGICAL TYPING: A REVIEW

*Ziad W. Jaradat**

Department of Biotechnology and Genetic Engineering,
Jordan University of Science and Technology,
Irbid, Jordan

ABSTRACT

Meningitis, an inflammation of the meninges is a medical emergency that requires prompt treatment to minimize or eliminate its devastating outcome. Its incidence is estimated at 0.6-4 cases per 100,000 adults in developed countries and might be far more than that in developing countries.Patients present to clinics with at least two of the following symptoms; headache, fever, neck stiffness and altered mental status.Proper and swift diagnosis is pivotal to attain a proper treatment and a successful outcome.Prior to the development of molecular diagnosis, traditional culture methods were used for the identification and confirmation of the etiologic agent. For example, bacterial meningitis was detected by culturing bacteria on specific media. Such methods needed several days to identify and confirm presence of the agent.In the last two

---

*Correspondence; Dr. Ziad W Jaradat; Tel; +962 2 7201000; Email; jaradatz@just.edu.jo. The author is currently spending a sabbatical leave at the Institute of Applied Technology, Al Ain, UAE; Tel; +971558331660. Email; ziad.jaradat@fchs.ac.ae.

decades, the development and use of molecular diagnostic techniques for the early detection of meningitis has revolutionized the management of the disease and has remarkably contributed to positive treatment outcomes which has resulted in a vast decrease in mortality and morbidity among cases. Nucleic acid based methods primarily polymerase chain reaction (PCR) targeting specific genes in the suspected agents have been used extensively for diagnosis of meningitis.PCR-based systems especially multiplex PCR enabled the detection of multiple etiologic agents from clinical samples with a degree of certainty and speed. In addition, PCR techniques are pivotal to diagnosis of fastidious and unculturable meningitis agents or detecting very low numbers which otherwise will not be detected by traditional methods.PCR diagnosis coupled with DNA sequencing is frequently used for confirmation of the etiologic agent or when there is ambiguity in the differential diagnosis of closely related agents.This review will give a comprehensive considerationof the major bacterial agents-causing meningitis with their diagnosis using molecular methods currently in practice.

1. INTRODUCTION

Meningitis is an inflammation of the three thin membranes covering the brain and the spinal cord which are collectively called the meninges. It is a serious and may be a fatal infection affecting the central nervous system and is caused by different bacterial or viral etiologic agents [30]. The subarachnoid space and its cerebral spinal fluid (CSF) are relatively defenseless against bacterial pathogens mainly due scarcity of phagocytic cells, complement system components and specific immunoglobulins because of their inability to cross the blood-brain barrier and enter this anatomical space [48]. When bacteria enter the CSF, their LPS, teichoic acids or other cell wall components provoke an overreaction of the immune system leading to over production of cytokines.Interleukin 1 along with tumor necrosis factor act synergistically to elicit the inflammatory response termed meningitis [48]. In addition to the high fatality rate inflected by the bacterial agent, between 10-20% of survivors develop permanent sequelae such as epilepsy, mental retardation, deafness or other neurological disabilities [110].

Bacterial meningitis is a medical emergency associated with sepsis or bacteremia that requires a multi-disciplinary approach in terms of diagnosis and therapy [107, 130, 144]. It is a life threatening disease which occurs at about 4-6 cases per 100,000 adults (older than 16 years of age) with *Streptococcus pneumoniae, Neisseria menigitidis, Haemophilus influenzae* type b, *S.agalactiae* (Group B streptococci; GBS),*Listeria monocytogenes, Mycobacterium tuberculosis* and other aerobic Gram-negative bacilli being the major bacterial causative agents with the first three pathogens incriminated in over 80% of the cases [144, 155].More rarely, *Escherichia coli, Staphylococci, Enterococci, Salmonella* groups B and D [24, 26, 94], *Acinetobacter* [108], *Rickettsia* [85] *and Brucella* have been identified as causative agents [150, 155].Fortunately, meningitis caused by *H. influenzae* type b has nearly been eliminated in many developed countries since the introduction of the conjugate vaccine against this pathogen in childhood vaccination programs [123]. In addition, meningitis cases caused *by S. pneumoniae* were substantially decreased due to introduction of the conjugated vaccine against seven different *S. pneumoniae* serotypes [40]. Nevertheless, infections by *S. pneumoniae* and *H. infleunzae* are still the leading causes of child mortality even more than deaths caused by HIV/AIDS, malaria and tuberculosis together in many parts of the world [120].

Meningitis can occur in sporadic cases or in the form of outbreaks characterized with severe sepsis and fatal outcomes [41].The definition of bacterial meningitis has changed throughout the years. Early definitions included: all compatible clinical syndromes with positive CSF cultures, positive bacterial antigen tests or positive blood cultures [107].Due to the inability to obtain positive cultures in blood or CSF in some cases, the definition of meningitis was revisited to include other diagnostic criteria such aselevated "opening pressure "upon lumbar puncture, as the presence of elevated CSF leukocyte counts (usually in bacterial meningitis neutrophils predominant), a low CSF glucose level due to its conversion to acid or elevated levels of CSF protein [107, 155]. Nonetheless, the more recent definitions of bacterial meningitis required the isolation of the organism from CSF or blood.Bacterial meningitis in children and infants more than 8 weeks old normally is defined if the child present with fever, irritability, impaired consciousness, vomiting, neck rigidity and other minor signs. In addition, a positive culture, positive Gram-stain or detection of the presence of bacterial antigens in CSF is considered confirmatory measures [107].

Meningitis is not only restricted to children or infants, it can affect adults as well. In fact, since the introduction of the conjugate vaccines against major bacteria causing meningitis to the children vaccination programs, meningitis become a disease of adults rather than of infants [123].Adults usually present to the clinics with at least 2 symptoms of the following; headache, fever, neck stiffness and altered mental status and photophobia [40].In adults, meningitis is mainly acquired as a nosocomial infection with different etiologic bacterial agents including *S. pneumoniae, S. aureus, H. influenzae, S. epidermidis, E. coli, Klebsiella pneumoniae, P. aeruginosa* and other bacterial agents [150]. The prevalence of particular etiologic agents for meningitis usually vary greatly depending on the geographical region, season of the year, ethnic background, age, sex, poverty and other demographic entities of patients [23, 48].

When bacterial meningitis is suspected, a lumbar puncture is mandatory for the proper diagnosis [144].Nevertheless, lumbar puncture is not a risk free, and thus there are certain precautions and procedures needed to be taken care of before it is performed. However, lumbar puncture should be given preference in immunocompromised patients especially if they present to clinics with impaired consciousness [144]. In all cases, lumbar puncture should not be done before neuroimaging of the brain is performed.Patients, who present to a clinic with signs of bacterial meningitis, should be put on antibiotic therapy as the delay of more than 4 hours of starting antibiotic therapy was associated with poor outcomes of the disease.Therefore, it was recommended that patients be put on an empirical antibiotic therapy before the imaging as the start of the therapy is critical and time sensitive [144].

Currently, bacterial culture is performed on CSF as a standard procedure for the isolation of bacterial agents in the sample.However, this technique usually takes 48-72 hours for confirming the presence of pathogen.In addition, not all the bacterial agents that cause meningitis can be cultured easily as some pathogens are fastidious and hard to grow such as *Mycoplasma* spp., *Brucella* spp. or *Tropheryma whipplei* [27, 45, 60]. In addition, CSF serology for the detection of bacterial antigens is not always used due to its lower sensitivity and specificity [19].Molecular diagnostic methods might provide the alternative for the use of inherently less sensitive methods especially when an antibiotic therapy protocol has been started.The use of nucleic acid based tests such as Polymerase Chain Reaction (PCR), nested PCR, real time PCR,16s rRNA sequencing and the several typing methodshave enabled more sensitive and rapid detection and typing of pathogens incriminated in meningitis [1].This review will focus on the molecular methods that are commonly used in the diagnosis and typing of major bacterial agents-causing meningitis.

2. MENINGITIS CAUSED BY MAJOR BACTERIAL AGENTS

2.1. *Neisseria Meningitidis*

Neisseria meningitidis, an exclusively human pathogen, colonizes the human naso-oro-pharyngeal mucosa in about 10% of normal individuals and is transferred from person to person by direct contact. The pathogen causes a broad spectrum of diseases ranging from mild fever to bacteremia and if not treated will cause septicemia and meningitis [155]. Once inside, the bacteria adheres to endothelial cells, and consequently crosses the Blood-CSF barrier and invade the brain causing meningitis and thus imparting the most damaging effect [55, 130, 154]. The annual incidence of meningococcal diseases in Europe in 1999-2000 ranged between 0.3 and 7.1 per 100,000 people [130].

Meningococcal diseases caused by *N. meningitidis*remains a major childhood infection worldwide. Meningitis and septicemia remain an important cause of morbidity and mortality among infected patients. Although major cases occur in children, other groups particularly young adults are infected by this pathogen and they too suffer from its damaging neurological effects [38, 55].The meningococcal capsule is a virulent factor that is critical for the pathogenesis of the disease [39, 55]. Several genes are responsible for capsular polysaccharide synthesis including *siaA, siaB, ciaC, ctrA, ctrB, ctrC* and *ctrD* [55].The uncapsulated serotypes of *Neisseria* are considered as commensals and associated with a carrier state but not disease causing especially in immunocompetent people [55].

There are 13 different recognized serogroups of *Neisseria* with only 5 serogroups(A, B, C, W135 and Y) are considered important as etiologic agents for meningitis with each serogroupprevalent in certain geographical areas of the world [118].For instance, serogroup C was a problem in UK in the 1990s, while serogroup B is more common in New Zealand [93] and serogroup A is more common in Sub Saharan Africaand recently serogroup W135 emerged as an epidemic meningitis agent in parts of Africa [39, 51, 130]. Nevertheless, the introduction of the conjugate meningococcal C vaccine to the adolescent, college-aged and elderly vaccination and booster programs decreased the incidence of meningitis caused by this serogorup dramatically in most of the affected countries [38].

Traditional laboratory diagnosis of bacterial meningitis might take up to 36 hours or even more. In addition, it is a common practice to start antibiotic therapy once patients present to emergency medicine personnel with meningitis symptoms thus complicating the isolation and identification of the pathogenic microorganism incriminated in the case. This decreases the ability of identifying the etiologic agent by culture methods in as much as 96% of the cases [30, 130].Classical non-culture methods of diagnosis of *N. meningitidis* are based on direct detection of the pathogen in a smear or antigen detection in CSF, blood or urine of the patient [130].However, the chances to detect the pathogen using this method are low and the high cross reactivity of the *N. meningitidis* antigen with other bacterial antigens further complicates the accuracy of the diagnosis [130]. Other methods were developed to detect antibodies against OMP of *N. meningitidis,* however, the sensitivity of the assay is low due to a lack of a robust immune response early in infection [10].

To address this problem, non-culturing diagnostic methods have been developed. PCR, nested PCR, real time PCR and 16S rRNA are among the most commonly used methods for diagnosis of meningococcal diseases.

2.2. *S. Pneumoniae* and other *Streptococcus*Species

S. pneumoniae (pneumococcus) is a Gram-positive, diplococcus, covered with a polysaccharide capsule and mainly colonizes the human nasopharynx canal with about 50 % of the carriers being children [91].It is frequently incriminated and considered a leader in causing, otitis media, pneumonia, and invasive diseases such as bacteremia and meningitis with meningitis being the most life-threatening pneumococcal illness [12, 18, 92]. It is the most common cause of community-acquired pneumonia, bacteremia and meningitis in adults as well as children and is responsible for killing 1.6 million people annually worldwide with about 1 million deaths are children [91, 92, 112, 136]. Due to the immaturity of their immune system, children below 2 years old are particularly susceptible to invasive pneumococcal diseases [16]. Sepsis, pneumonia and meningitis are responsible for considerable morbidity and mortality among neonates [5, 56]. The global incidence of pnemococcal meningitis in children was estimated at about 17 cases per 100,000 with the lowest incidence in Europe while highest incidence reported in Africa [105].

Along with *N. meningitidis, S. pneumoniae* is responsible for about 80% of the meningitis cases worldwide [96, 155].The pathogen produces a range of virulence and colonization factors including the capsule, choline-binding proteins and a pore-forming toxin called pneumolysin, which aids in its pathogenicity [57, 96]. Under certain circumstances, *S. pneumoniae* causes bacteremia by crossing the mucosa of the middle ear to the inner ear and enters the blood stream eventually leading to the meninges [149]. The threshold numbers of bacteria that are needed to cause meningitis has not been established; however the status of the immune system of the host plays a critical role in causing the disease [149]. Fortunately, the widespread use of the heptavalent pneumococcal conjugate vaccine against the seven major *S. pneumoniae* serotypes has resulted in a substantial decline in the invasive infections caused by antimicrobial resistant *S. pneumoniae* [18].

Virtually all serotypes of *S. pneumoniae* have a polysaccharide capsule which is used as the basis for serotyping [93]. As such, there are 91 recognized different serotypes of *S. pneumoniae* with only about 20 serotypes accounting for more than 80% of infections caused by this pathogen [57, 91].The dominant serotypes associated with pathogenic pnenumoccocal disease include 1, 3, 4, 6A, 6B, 7F, 8, 9V, 14, 18C, 19F, and 23F [91].Certain serotypes among those are highly invasive such as serotype 1 and 3 which could be due to the specific chemical composition of their capsule [57]. In addition, certain serotypes were found to be associated with increased resistance to penicillin [136]. Furthermore, infections by serotypes other than the dominant ones such as serotype 19A have recently emerged especially after the introduction of the heptavalent vaccine [58].

Other *Streptococcus*species: Group B *Streptococcus* (GBS) are a group of bacteria that normally colonizes the vaginal and rectal areas of women.This group has been recognized as the leading cause of meningitis in neonates worldwide with special emphasis in the developed parts of the world [47, 72]. In addition, this pathogen has been implicated in maternal morbidity and mortality [72].Heavily colonized women normally infect their babies while giving birth, thus, those neonates become more susceptible than babies of uncolonized mothers [72].Recent studies from some parts of Africa suggested that GBS are emerging as an important cause of neonatal meningitis [47].Interestingly, in a study conducted in Korea from 1996 to 2005, *S. agalactiae* (GBS) was the major causative agent of meningitis and was responsible for almost a quarter of the registered cases [25].

Other *Streptococcus* species have also been incriminated in meningitis. *Streptococcus suis* is an emerging zoonotic pathogen [90].It is an important pathogen associated with a wide range of infections in pigs and in humans especially those who have frequent exposure to pigs and their meat [90].Based on the type of the polysaccharide covering the surface of this pathogen, there are 35 serotypes of which only serotype 2 is mainly implicated in human meningitis and is the most frequent reported serotype-causing infections worldwide [90]. *Streptococcus bovis*, is a non Enterococcal group D *Streptococcus* and has also been identified as a causative agent of severe cases of both adult and neonatal meningitis [46].

The traditional biochemical diagnosis of *Streptococcus* spp.is mainly done by blood culture systems with *Streptococcus* spp. identified by β-hemolysis on blood agar, a test also used for detection of the non-hemolytic strains at the same time. Confirmation of the identity of GBS and other *Streptococcus* spp.Isnormally done using streptex agglutination tests.The Streptex® assay by Remel is recognized as the gold standard for Streptococcal serogrouping [47].

2.3. *Haemophilus Influenzae*

H. influenzae is a small pleomorphic Gram-negative cocobacilli classified into six serotypes (a, b, c, d, e and f) based on its polysaccharide capsule [77].It is an extremely common commensal microorganism that inhabits the human upper respiratory tract [100].Globally, *H. influenzae* serotype b causes approximately 3 million cases of serious illness in children less than 5 years old [12] with most of the cases (61%) occurring in developing countries in Asia and Africa [9, 148]. *H. influenzae* b was historically responsible for most of the meningitis outbreaks and causes approximately 95% of *H. influenzae* systemic infections [77]. This might be due to the presence of ribosyl-ribito phosphate in its capsule that imparts unusual virulence properties on this serotype [100].Meningitis caused by *H. influenzae* b is associated with high rates of mortality and long term morbidity, including hearing loss, seizures and motor and mental destruction [12].The rates of infections caused by *H. influenzae* b (Hib) have decreased dramatically since the introduction of the Hib vaccine in 1980s. However, despite the introduction of the Hib vaccine, *H. influenzae* is still one of the major causative agents of childhood as well as adult meningitis [25].Although the incidence of meningitis caused by *H. influenzae* b has dramatically decrease due to the introduction of the Hib vaccine, other serotypes particularly Hie are emerging and reported to cause invasive diseases such as bacteremia and meningitis resembles that of Hib meningitis [77].

Conventional isolation and identification of the organism is based on phenotypic characteristics and requires a lengthy time period with a low sensitivity especially when antibiotic treatment has been initiated prior to obtaining samples.Molecular methods offer quick and more accurate results in

CSF or other body secretions. In addition, real time PCR can actually quantitate the bacterial load in the tested samples [1].

3. MENINGITIS CAUSED BY LESS COMMON BACTERIAL PATHOGENS

Although most of the meningitis cases occurred due to the 3 major pathogens; *Neisseria, Streptococcus,* and *Haemophilus,* several other bacteria species can cause meningitis mainly in young children [94]. The following part briefly addresses meningitis caused by less frequently meningitis–associated bacterial agents.

3.1. *Mycobacterium Tuberculosis* Meningitis (TM)

Mycobacterium genera are ubiquitous in soil and water and can cause skin and soft tissue infections, pulmonary diseases and meningitis [136]. It is a non-motile, non-spore forming bacillus and is an obligate aerobic, acid-fast bacterium [75].According to WHO estimates, *M. tuberculosis* causes pulmonary tuberculosis, a debilitating disease with approximately 1.6 million deaths annually worldwide [50] and about 8.8 million new cases each year [75].While it is mainly a pulmonary disease, it causes one of the severe meningitis episodes with fatality rates reaching 100% in untreated patients [50].Virtually all forms of TB infections of central nervous system are caused by *M. tuberculosis* [75]. It gains entry into humans through the lungs by inhalation of aerosolized droplet nuclei and persists in the alveolar macrophages [85]. The pathogen then starts multiplication within the alveolar macrophages followed by hematogenous dissemination or by eruption of the pre-existing granuloma into the subarachnoid space or the ventricular regions [14, 75]. The release of *M. tuberculosis* into the subarachnoid space results in a local T-lymphocyte-dependent response, leading to the meningitis [75].Neurological abnormalities occur with the development of inflammatory exudates that affects mostly the Sylvain fissures, basal cisterns, brainstem, and cerebellum [75, 138].

Patients generally present to the clinic with sub-acute meningitis over a 1-3 week period [14].In developing countries, tuberculosis meningitis mainly occurs in children <3 years old; while in developed countries, it mainly occurs in adults with the highest percentage of cases occurring in elderly and immunocompromised individuals [14, 50]. Tuberculosis meningitis patients usually present to the clinic with progressively worsening malaise, drowsiness, low grade fever, headache, anorexia, mental confusion and a battery of other debilitating symptoms that might progress to a semicomatous state or progression into a deep coma due to hydrocephalus which is a common feature of TM [14, 15, 75].Advanced age was found to be associated with poor prognosis [109].

Other rapidly growing *Mycobacterium* species such as *M. abscessus, M. avium-intracellulare, M. bovis* and *M. fortuitum* were also reported to cause meningitis in addition to other skin and soft tissue infections in immunocompromised patients [75, 136].

*M. tuberculosis*are genetically diverse and some genotypes of *M. tuberculosis* may be more transmissible and thus more capable of causing diseases than other genotypes [139]. This difference in the virulence could be due to the production of glycolipids on the surface that tricks the host immune system thus, decreasing its ability to control the pathogen [139].

Tuberculous meningitis is difficult to diagnose as the clinical features are non-specific and can be misinterpreted [138]. In general, diagnosis of cerebral TB cannot be made or excluded on the grounds of clinical features only.It is rather made based on neurological symptoms and signs, CSF culture, and neuroimaging [75]. What complicates the diagnosis is that some times, clinical manifestations of TM might overlap with other CNS diseases such as viral and pyogenic meningitis [74]. Nevertheless, isolation of the pathogen from CSF or the presence of acid-fast bacilli in CSF or histological examination of specimens is useful diagnostic markers [15]. The numbers and types of white cells in the CSF also help differentiate TM from other meningitis agents [139]. The CSF usually has a high protein and low glucose levels and a raised number of lymphocytes. Acid-fast bacilli are sometimes seen on a CSF smear, but more commonly, *M. tuberculosis* is grown in culture. A spider web clot in the collected CSF is characteristic of TB meningitis, but is a rare finding. The enzyme-linked immunosorbent spot (ELISPOT) assay is a common method for monitoring immune responses in humans and animals. It was developed by Cecil Czerkinsky [17] and though not useful in the diagnosis of acute TB meningitis because it is often false negative but may paradoxically become positive after treatment has started, which helps to confirm the diagnosis.

Measuring adenosine deaminase levels was thought to be promising and may be another useful method in the diagnosis of TM. However, it was not proved to be specific for TM, as elevated amounts of this enzyme in CSF were also measured in other types of meningitisespecially illness caused by pyogenic organisms [74]. Nevertheless, the conventional diagnosis of the pathogen is widely regarded as either insensitive or very time consuming due to the lengthy growing period needed to isolate the organism [15, 138]. These lengthy procedures necessitated the development of new and improved methods of detection [15, 138]. Additionally, immediate antibiotic treatment upon seeking medical help limits the usefulness of culture methods by diminishing the ability to grow the pathogen. Furthermore, a large number of microorganisms (>100 CFU/ml) is normally needed to perform rapid tests like the latex agglutination tests [37]. PCR and other molecular methods provide alternative quick and more sensitive methods for detection of bacterial agents of meningitis.

3.2. *Salmonella*

Non-typhoidal *Salmonella* are a common cause of foodborne illness. The pathogen gains entry into the blood stream and causes infections that manifest into meningitis especially in children less than 5 years old. It is an important cause of meningitis in children especially in developing countries such as Brazil, Thailand and Africa [81, 95]. For instance, over an 11 year period, *Salmonella* was responsible for about 10% of meningitis cases reported in Bangkok, Thailand [95] while only 5% of meningitis cases were caused by *Salmonella* over 24 years in Malaysia [81]. In contrast, *Salmonella* is a rare cause of meningitis in developed countries [153]. Nevertheless, it is usually associated with a high case fatality and poor prognosis with mortality upwards to 37% [143, 153] whilea high percentage of survivors experiencing significant neurological sequelae and high relapse rates [81]. Although meningitis caused by *Salmonella* is mainly confined to children, meningitis caused by *Salmonella* in adults was reported in immunocompromised patients and normal patients as well [106]. The common *Salmonella* species isolated from CSF are the following in the order of their frequency; *Salmonella enterica* serovars; A*gona, Typhimurium, Heidelberg, Enteritidis, Typhi, St. Paul, Virchow* and *Panama* [21, 24, 26, 29, 44, 94, 95, 106].

Similar to meningitis caused by other bacterial agents,patients with meningitis caused by *Salmonella* present to the clinic with similar symptoms including high fever (39 °C) and seizures.The traditional diagnosis of these agents is done by culturing the CSF and biochemical identification of the etiologic agent and final serotyping or phage typing for confirmation [94].

3.3. *Cronobacter*

Cronobacter spp. (formerly *Enterobacter sakazakii*) is a non-spore forming, motile, facultative anaerobic Gram-negative bacillus belonging to family *Enterobacteriaceae* [61, 62].The genus *Cronobacter* is a heterogenic exhibiting a high degree of genetic and phenotypic diversity among species and comprises six species: *C. muytjensii, C. sakazakii, C. malonaticus, C. turicensis, C. dublinensis* and *C. genomospecies* I [63,64]. These bacteria are opportunistic pathogens, ubiquitous in nature and are incriminated in both meningitis and necrotizing enterocolitis in infants, while also causing septicemia and catheter-associated infections in elderly and immunocompromised individuals, with mortality rates ranging between 10 to 80% [43, 53]. Among meningitis cases, about half of the patients die within one week of onset of the infection and about 94% of the meningitis survivors exhibited severe neurological complications [43, 49, 84]. Fortunately, worldwide, only about 120-150 cases have been reported in high risk groups of people with the majority of them being neonatesless than 2 months old [42, 97].In USA, the frequency of the invasive diseases caused by *Cronobacter* was reported to be one in every 100,000 infants, and about 8.7 per 100,000 low birth neonates [42]. In United Kingdom, from1997 to 2007 only 18 cases of meningitis or bacteremia were reported due to this pathogen [42].Traditionally the microorganism is isolated using chromogenic media and undergoes biochemical tests for presumptive confirmation. However, due to the high heterogeneity of this genus, these methods are insufficient and thus necessitate the use of even more than one molecular method for final confirmation at the subspecies level [69].

3.4. *Staphylococcus Aureus* and other *Staphylococcus* Species

Staphylococcus aureus is a Gram-positive, coagulase positive coccus that mainly colonizes the skin and mucous membranes of the nares of humans [65]. Although it is one of the most common causative agents of blood stream infections, meningitis caused by this pathogen is still an uncommon disease accounting for only 1-9% of the bacterial meningitis [28, 109,114]. This could be attributed to the difficulty of *S. aureus* to cross the blood brain barrier [109]. In general, blood stream infections (bacteremia) are critical and if remained untreated will lead to deleterious complications such as meningitis and endocarditis. *S. aureus* can gain access to CNS through two pathways;

post neurosurgery procedures or due to head trauma or through Staphylococcal spontaneous infections secondary to Staphylococcal hematogenous infections outside the nervous system [3, 114]. The first type of meningitis is termed hospital-acquired or nosocomial and mainly affects young people while the spontaneous type is a community-acquired and mainly affects elderly people [114]. The mortality rate associated with spontaneous community-acquired S. aureus meningitis is very high and could reach up to 71% while that associated with postoperative meningitis is far lower which could be up to 28%. This large difference in mortality rates might be due to the nature of the people affected by each type [13, 114]. Meningitis caused by methicillin resistant S. aureus (MRSA) has recently emerged as a cause of nosocomial infections of CNS [87]. However, both MRSA and methicillin sensitive S. aureus (MSSA) are incriminated in causing meningitis with meningitis caused by MRSA presenting a therapeutic challenge [3].

In a study of nosocomial bacterial meningitis, Weisfelt et al. [150] reported the S. aureus as the second causative agent of nosocomial bacterial meningitis cases among patients with a history of neurosurgery [150]. For instance, in Spain, about 63% of meningitis caused by S. aureus over 20 years occurred in postoperative patients [114].In contrast, S. aureus was not a significant cause of community-acquired bacterial meningitis cases reported over 14 years in Taiwan [88]. Similar results were reported in New Zealand where only 24% of the meningitis cases caused by S. aureus were community-acquired [117].

Other Staphylococcusspecies: Since 1980s coagulase-negative Staphylococcus (CoNS) has been responsible for half of Staphylococcus infections especially in infants and premature babies [65]. Meningitis caused by CoNS is considered rare compared to that of coagulase-positive Staphylococcus, however, there are some sporadic cases reported in medical literature. In Australia for instance, from 1991 to 2000 there were 5 reported cases of CoNS meningitis in neonates [65]. CoNS meningitis is not only confined to neonates, cases of adult meningitis have also been reported in the literature [59]. In addition, the severity and the mortality rate are low for these infections compared to that of the coagulase-positive S. aureus [65]. S. epidermidis and S.haemolyticus, both CoNS were incriminated in 14 adult nosocomial meningitis cases in Taiwan between 1999 and2003 [65].S. intermedius, another CoNS strain was incriminated in a child meningitis case in Slovak Republic [36].

Traditional diagnosis of S. aureus meningitis is based on microbial culturing of CSF.In addition to direct detection of the pathogen in the culture, typical findings would be low glucose level, increased lactate and protein concentrations, and the predominance of polymorphonuclear cells [87].However, in contrast to other types of bacterial meningitis, *S. aureus* is not detected in high numbers in the CSF when examined by Gram-stain [114]. The classical symptoms of meningitis; the fever and theconsciousness disturbances normally help in the final decision in diagnosis [87].

3.5. *Listeria Monocytogenes*

*Listeria monocytogenes*is a Gram-positive bacilli, facultative anaerobe, displays tumbling motility on wet-drop slide preparations and produces hemolysis around its colonies when grown on blood agar [31, 67].Although infections by *L. monocytogenes* are not common, nearly all cases of listeriosis are foodborne [66].The pathogen particularly infects elderly patients, those with impaired cellular immunity, infants and pregnant women. *L. monocytogenes* cause what is called community –acquired meningitis, a severe type of meningitis that might lead to a poor prognosis when appropriate therapy is not initiated on time [34]. In a three year multicenter surveillance study reported by Amaya-Villar et al. [4],*L. monocytogenes* was found to be the third most common cause of community-acquired meningitis only to *S. pneumonia* and *N. meningitidis* [4].Nevertheless, *L. monocytogenes* was reported to cause nosocomial meningitis at least in patients with long stay at hospitals [111].In a survey for the causative agents of 248 meningitis cases in USA in 1995, *L. monocytogenes* was responsible for about 8% of the cases but the case fatality rate was 15% which was second only to the fatality rate of meningitis caused by *S. pneumoniae* [123].In developing countries, the estimated frequency of the community-acquired meningitis is about 0.2 cases per 100,000 people [4]. Serotypes 4b and 1/2b were the two most incriminated serotypes responsible about 78% of meningitis cases caused by *L. monocytogenes* [123]. Interestingly, *L. monocytogenes* and *S. agalactiae* are the more prevalent pathogens causing meningitis in infants less than 3 months and elderly patients more than 50 years old [151]. Early diagnosis of *L. monocytogenes* meningitis is difficult as CSF Gram-stains are negative in about 50% of the time [31]. *Listeria* infections in infants usually cause meningoencephalitis by invading the brain stem rather than supratentorial areas, a condition that is accompanied by complications such as hydrocephalus [80]. Similar to other meningitis symptoms, meningitis caused by *Listeria* induces vomiting, fever, headache, and altered mental status [80]. Traditional diagnosis of the pathogen like any other pathogens need long time and several steps for confirmation leaving the door wide open for molecular techniques.

Other Less Common Meningitis-Causing Agents

Several other infectious agents have been reported in the literature causing sporadic cases of meningitis. *Pseudomonas fulva* [2], *P. aeruginosa* [150], *S. epidermidis* [150], *Brucella*, and *K. pneumoniae* [150] are among those agents that occasionally cause meningitis. Due to the rarity of the meningitis cases caused by these bacteria they will not be discussed further in this review.

4. MOLECULAR DETECTION OF BACTERIAL MENINGITIS

4.1. Universal Detection of Major Bacterial Pathogens Causing Meningitis Using PCR, Nested PCR, Multiplex PCR and Real Time PCR

When an infectious agent other than the common meningitis agents is detected in CSF samples by Gram-staining or by culture, it is pivotal to identify the causative agent. Molecular methods in this case can help in identifying the pathogen.PCR assays are now routinely utilized in the molecular diagnosis of human, veterinary and food pathogens.Due to the nature of the method which involves the DNA amplification, it is utilized for the detection of low or trace amounts of pathogens.The application of the method for testing the presence of pathogens in CSF has revolutionized the diagnosis of meningitis and definitely has great contribution in minimizing the deleterious effects of the bacterial meningitis [103]. Depending on the set of primers usedand the target gene, the detection of meningitis etiologic agents in CSF by PCR [20] can be of two types; universal detection of pathogens based on the detection of universal genes such as the 16S rRNA gene, or the specific detection of certain pathogens by using primers targeting specific genes for particular pathogens.Collectively, these methods would enhance the sensitivity of the detection particularly when the culture results are negative.For instance, Chen et al, [20], designed a set of universal PCR primers targeting the 16S rRNA gene (Table 1) and used them in a quantitative real time PCR assay for detection of general bacterial pathogens in CSF and found a rate of detection that was significantly higher than that of a culture method.More specific PCR assays detecting a specific number of bacteria have also been designed.Pingle et al. [113] reported the development of a novel high-throughput PCR-ligase detection reaction-capillary electrophoresis (PCR-LDR-CE) assay for the detection of 20 blood borne pathogens at the same time. Their assay detects the following; *S. epidermidis, S. aureus, Bacillus cereus, Enterococcus faecium, L. monocytogenes, S. pneumoniae, S. pyogenes, S. agalactiae, E. coli, K. pneumoniae, H. influenzae, P. aeruginosa, Acinetobacter baumanii, N. meningitis, Bacteriodes fragilis, Bacillus anthracis, Yersinia pestis, Francisella tularensis* and *Brucella abortus.*This detection method relied on amplification of the 16S rRNA gene in these bacteria using a universal PCR primers set giving amplicon size range between 375 and 415 bp (Table 1). Within each amplicon, SNPs common to specific groups of organisms were detected.In the same fashion, Lu et al. [89] developed a PCR method using universal pairs of primers targeting the 16S rRNA gene of *Eubacteria*including the following; *S. aureus, S. epidermidis, S. pyogenes, S. agalactiae, S. pneumoniae, Enterococcus faecium, Enterococcus faecalis, M. tuberculosis, Legionella pneumophila, E. coli, K. pneumoniae, Serratia marcescens, Enterobacter cloacae, P. aeruginosa, Acinetobacter baumannii, H. influenzae* and *N.* meningitidis. The amplified DNA from all these bacteria was a 996 bp amplicon. However, when digested with the restriction enzymes *Hae*II, *Mnl*I, *Dde*I or *Bst*BI these bacteria gave different patterns thus were differentiated based on restriction fragment length polymorphism (RFLP) pattern differences. The sensitivity of these universal primers was 92.3 %.Table 1 shows the primers and the running conditions for this PCR assay.A multiplex PCR assay based on the Luminex bead technology was developed by Boving et al. [11] for the detection of both bacterial and viral meningitis agents. In this assay, these authors used a multiplex PCR design with 8 sets of primers (Table 2) recognizing *N. meningitidis, S. pneumoniae, E. coli, S. aureus, L. monocytogenes, S. agalactiae* and two sets of primers detecting herpes simplex virus I &II and varicella-zoster virus.The sensitivity for the most two important pathogens (*S. pneumoniae and N. meningitidis*) was 95% and 100% respectively.

Backman et al. [8] developed a semi-nested PCR assay for the simultaneous detection of *N. meningitidis, H. influenzae, S. pneumoniae, S. agalactiae,* and *L. monocytogenes* in CSF with a universal 16S rRNA primer in the first step followed by amplification of species–specific regions in the second step. Table 3 shows the primers used in this study and the running conditions for the PCR.The test was specific for the bacteria in general by 97% while specificity for detecting specific bacteria ranged from 87 to 94%.

Real time PCR assays were also developed and reported in several studies.Rothman et al. [119] have developed a quantitative broad-basedreal time PCR assay for the detection and identification of the most common bacterial species that cause meningitis (*N. meningitidis, H. influenzae, S. pneumoniae, S. aureus,S. epidermidis, E. coli* and *L. monocytogenes*).

Table 1. Showing the primers used for the universal amplification of the 16S rRNA sequencing according to Chen et al. [20]

Oligonu-cleotide	Tar-get gene	Primer sequences (5'-3')	Amplicon size (bp)	Ref
PCR1 BFN[1]	16s	CGCTGCCAACTACCGCACAT CACTGAGACACGGYCCARA CTCCTAC	Variable	[113]
PCR2RN[1]	16s	CGCTGCCAACTACCGCACAT CBATMTCTRCGCATTTCACY GCTAC	Variable	
PCR3FN[1]		CGCTGCCAACTACCGCACAT CCAAACAGGATTAGATACC CTGGTAGTC	Variable	
PCR4RN[1]		CGCTGCCAACTACCGCACAT CAYTTGACGTCRTCCCCRCC TTC	Variable	
U1 (518-537)[2]	16s RNA	CCAGCAGCCGCGGTAATAC G	996	[89]
U2 (1513-1491)		ATCGG(C/T)TACCTTGTTACG ACTTC		
P690F[3]	16s RNA	TGTGTAGCGGTGAAATGCG CATCGTTTACGGCGTGGAC		[20]
P829R[3]		TCTAATCCTGTTTGATCCCC		
UnProbe[3]		ACG		

[1] Samples were amplified using the following protocol; 10 min @ 95 °C, followed by 35 cycles(95 °C for 15 s, 60 °CC for 1 min, and 72 °C for 1 min) and final extension at 72 °C for 7 min followed by 99.9 °C for 30 min to destroy polymerase. [2] initial denaturation at 94 °C for 10 min, followed by 35 cycles of denaturation for 1 min at 94 C, annealing for 1 min at 55 °C and extension for 2 min at 72 °C followed by incubation for 10 at 72 °C C. [3] initial denaturation for 4 min at 94 °C and then 40 cycles of 94 C for 20 s and 60 C for 60 s.

Table 2. Primers and probes designed for use in a multiplex PCR Luminex-based assay as adapted from Boving et al. [11]

Species	Primer name	Primer sequence (5'-3')	Target gene	Position
N. meningitidis	Nme-s	GTGATGGTGCGTTTGGTGCAGAATA-biotin	*ctrA*	504-528
	Nme-as	CACATTTGCCGTTGAACCACCTACC		644-620
	Nme-Pas	C$_{12}$- CAACACACGCTCACCGGCTGCCGTCAGCGGCATAC		605-571
S. pneumoniae	Spn-s	CGCAATCTAGCAGATGAAGCAGGTT-biotin	*lytA*	911-935
	Spn-as	AAGGGTCAACGTGGTCTGAGTGGTT		1034-1010
	Spn-Pas	C$_{12}$-ACTCGTGCGTTTTAATTCCAGCTAAACTCCCTGTA		986-952
S. aureus	Sau-s	AGCTGCACCCATGCCGACAC	*coa*	2681-2700
	Sau-as	GAATGTGAATGGTGGCGCTATTGCT-biotin		2831-2807
	Sau-Ps	C$_{12}$-CAATACACATCGTAACCATGCCGTAACGGCTAT		2701-2733
E. coli	Eco-s	CGTGGTGGTCGCTTTTACCACAGAT	*metH*	133-157
	Eco-as	TCCACTTTGCTGCTCACACTTGCTC-biotin		239-215
	Eco-Ps	C$_{12}$-GCGTTTATGCCAGTATGGTTTGTTGAATTTTATT		158-192
L. monocyto-genes	Lmo-s	TGTAAACTTCGGGCGCAATCAGTGAA	*hly*	712-736
	Lmo-as	GCTTTGCCGAAAAATCTGGAAGGTC-biotin		831-807
	Lmo-Ps	C$_{12}$-GGGAAAATGCAAGAAGAAGTCATTAGTTTTAAACA		737-771
S. agalactiae	Sag-s	GCCCAGCAAATGGCTCAAAAGC	*cfp*	449-470
	Sag-as	TCAGGGTTGGCACGCAATGAA-biotin		579-577
	Sag-Ps1	C$_{12}$-TATCAAAGATAATGTTCAGGGAACAGATTATGAAAAAACGG		499-535
	Sag-Ps2	C$_{12}$-TATCAAAGATAATGTTCAGGGAACAGATTATGAAAACCGC		449-535

Running conditions; initial denaturation at 95 °C for 15 min, 14 cycles of 94 °C for 30 s, 65 °C, -1/2 °C for 3 min and 60 °C for 30 s; 36 cycles of 94 °C for 10 s, 58 °C for 30 s, and 60 °C for 30 s and 1 cycle of 72 °C for 5 min for final extension.

Table 3. Primers used for the general and specific detection of the major bacterial meningitis causing agents as adapted from Backman et al. [8]

Step	Primer name and specificity	Primer sequence(5´-3´)	Programme
I	U3, ru8 (bacteria in general)	U3-AACT(C/A)CGTGCCAGCAGCCGCGGTAA	94 °C for 10 min
		RU8- AAGGAGGTGATCCA(G/A)CCGCA(G/C)(G/C)TTC	94 °C for 30 s
			64-54 C^a for 30s
			51 cycles
			7 °C for 1 min^b
IIA	*N. meningitidis*	NM-TGTTGGGCAACCTGATTG	94 °C for 30 s
	H. influenzae	HI-CCTAAGAAGAGCTCAGAG	54 °C for 30 s
	STREP in general	STREP-GTACAACGAGTCCAAGC	5 cycles
	Ru8	RU8- AAGGAGGTGATCCA(G/A)CCGCA(G/C)(G/C)TTC	7 °C for 1 min^b
IIB	*S. pneumoniae*	SP-GCTGTGGCTTAACCATAGTAG	
	S. agalactiae	SA-ACCGGCCTAGAGATAGGC	
	L. monocytogenes	LM-GGAGCTAATCCCATAAACTA	
	Ru8	RU8- AAGGAGGTGATCCA(G/A)CCGCA(G/C)(G/C)TTC	

^{a} Touchdown PCR by decreasing annealing temperature by 1 C/cycle from 64-59 °C followed by 58 °C for 15 cycles and 54 °C for other 30 cycles.

^{b} PCR synthesis, extension for 7 min in the final cycle before lowering to 4 °C.

Table 4. Primers and probes used for the detection of the five meningitis causing-agents as adapted from Hedberg et al. [54]

Species/target	Primer/probe	Sequence 5'-3'	Amplicon size (bp)
Sp/ *lytA*	*lytA* F	CAGCGGTTGAACTGATTGA	173
	lytA R	TGGTTGGTTATTCGTGCAA	
	lytA P1	GAAAACGCTTGATACAGGGGAGTT-FL	
	lytA P2	LCRed640-AGCTGGAATTAAAACGCACGAG-PH	
Hi/ p6	P6 F	CCAGCTGCTAAAGTATTAGTAGAAG	156
	P6 R	TTCACCGTAAGATACTGTGCC	
	P6 P1	ACGTCGTGCAGATGCAGT-FL	
	P6 P2	LCRed705-AAGGTTATTTAGCWGGTAAAGGTGTTGATG-PH	
GBS/ *cfb*	*cfb* F	CTGGAACTCTAGTGGCTG	122
	cfb R	CATTTGCTGGGCTTGATTATTAC	
	cfb P1	ACCAGCTGTATTAGAAGTACATGCTGATCA-FLLCRed640-	
	cfb P2	TGACAACTCCACAAGTGGTAAATCATGT-PH	
Lm/ *hly*	*hly* F	CTGCAAGTCCTAAGACGC	131
	hly R	ACCTTTCTTGGCGGCA	
	hly P1	ATGAAATCGATAAGTATATACAAGGATTGGATTA-FL	
	hly P2	LCRed705-	
		ATAAAAACAATGTATTAGTATACCACGGAGATGCA-PH	
Nm/ *ctrA*	*ctrA* F	GCTGCGGTAGGTGGTTCAA	111
	ctrA R	TTGTCGCGGATTTGCAACTA	
	ctrA P	6-FAM-CATTGCCACGTGTCAGCTGCACAT-TAMRA	
All/ 16S	16S U2 F	CTACGGGAGGCAGCAGT	200
	16S U3 R	CCGTATTACCGCGGCT	
	16SFAM	6-FAM-GGCTAACTMCGTGCCAGC-TAMRA	
	Seq-19b	GCTGGCACGTAGTTAGCCG	
	Seq-31b	GTTAGCCGGTGCTTCTTCTG	

Running conditions; initial denaturation at 95 °C for 10 min, 45 cycles; 95 °C for 5 s, 60 °C for 20 s, 72 °C for 8 s.

Table 5. Primers and probes for the real time PCR assay as described by Chiba et al. [23] and Morozumi et al. [99] for detection of 8 different meningitis causative agents

Species primer and probe	Primer or probe sequence	Target gene	Amplicon size (bp)	Ref
s. pneumoniae	F- 5'-CAACCGTACAGAATGAAGCGG-3' R- 5'-TTATTCGTGCAATACTCGTGCG-3' Probe; HEX- *GCGATC*AGGTCTCAGCATTCCAACCGCC *GATCGCG*-BHQ1	*lytA*	319	[99]
H. influenzae	F- 5'-TTGACATCCTAAGAAGAGCTC-3' R- 5'-TCTCCTTTGAGTTCCCGACCG-3' Probe: FAM-*CGCGATC*CTGACGACAGCCATGCAGCAC *GATCGCG*-BHQ1	16S rRNA	167	[99]
E. coli	F-5'-GGGGAGTAAAGTTAATACCTTTGC-3' R-5'-CTCAAGCTTGCCAGTATCAG-3' Probe: HEX-*CGCGATC*ACTCCGTGCCAGCAGCCGCG *GATCGCG*-BHQ1	16S rRNA	204	[23]
S.agalactiae	F-5'-AGGAATACCAGGCGATGAAC-3' R-5'-AGGCCCTACGATAAATCGAG-3' Probe: FAM-*CGCGATC* ATTTGGCTAGTTATGAAGTCCCTTATGC *GATCGCG*-BHQ1	*dltS*	331	[23]

Table 5. Continued

Species primer and probe	Primer or probe sequence	Target gene	Amplicon size (bp)	Ref
N.meningitidis	F- 5'-CATATCGGAACGTACCGAGT-3' R- 5'-GCCGCTGATATTAGCAACAG-3' Probe: HEX-*CGCGATC*CTATTCGAGCGGCCGATATC *GATCGCG*-BHQ1	16S rRNA	356	[23]
L.monocytogenes	F- 5'-CGCTTTTGAAAGATGGTTTCG-3' R- 5'-CTTCCAGTTTCCAATGACCC-3' Probe: FAM- *CGCGATC*GCGGCGGTTGCTCCGTCAGACTT *GATCGCG*-BHQ1	16S rRNA	457	[23]
M.pneumoniae	F-5'-GTAATACTTTAGAGGCGAACG-3' R-5'-TACTTCTCAGCATAGCTACAC-3' Probe: HEX- *CGCGATA*CCAACTAGCTGATATGGCGCA *ATCGCG*-BHQ1	16S rRNA	225	[99]
S.aureus	F- 5'-TACATGTCGTTAAACCTGGTG-3' R- 5'-TACAGTTGTACCGATGAATGG-3' Probe: FAM- *CGCGATC*CAAGAACTTGTTGTTGATAAGAAGCAA CC *GATCGCG*-BHQ1	*spa*	224	[23]

PCR conditions: initial denaturation step of 95 °C for 30 s, followed by 40 cycles of 95 °C for 15 s, 50 °C for 30 s, and 75 °C for 20 s, and at 75 °C for 30 s successively.

The 16S rRNA gene which contains both conserved and variable regions was used for the PCR and gave an 88% sensitivity of identifying the target bacteria after proper optimization of the assay.Similarly, Hedberg et al. [54] developed a rapid and efficient real time PCR assay for the rapid detection of *N. meningitidis, H. influenzae, S. pneumonia, S. agalactiae, L. monocytogenes* also using a primer pair derived from the conserved 16S rRNA sequence that detected all bacterial agents (Table 4).This method was proven to be rapid and efficient in detecting all these bacteria in about 3 hours. In addition to the detection of the three major meningitis etiologic agents, a real time PCR was developed for the detection of a total of 8 etiologic agents simultaneously [23]. The PCR assay detected the following agents; *S. pneumoniae, H. influenzae, Mycoplasma pneumoniae, N. meningitidis, E. coli, S. agalactiae, S. aureus,* and *L. monocytogenes* with significantly better rates of detection than culture methods. The limit of detection for these pathogens ranged from 5 copies to 28 copies per tube. All the primers used in this study are listed in Table 5.

4.2. Simultaneous Detection of the Major Bacterial Agents of Meningitis; *N. Meningitidis, H. Influenzae*and *S. Pneumoniae*by Using Multiplex PCR

Multiplex PCR is an amplification reaction in which two or more sets of primers are added in the same reaction tube to amplify genes of different organisms. The annealing temperature of the primers and the other conditions should be the same; otherwise, some of the primers will not anneal and thus cannot be amplified [137].Tuyama et al. [141] reported a multiplex PCR assay that detects *N. meningitidis* (*crgA*), *S. pneumoniae* (*ply*) and *H. influenzae* (*bexA*) in CSF of patients who presented to emergency medical personnel with meningitis symptoms. Table 6 shows the PCR primers and the running conditions used for the simultaneous detection of these three major pathogens.Tzanakaki et el. [142] designed a multiplex PCR assay for the detection of these three major pathogens using the *ctrA, ply* and *bexA*genetargets for *N. meningitidis, S. pneumoniae* and *H. influenzae,* respectively (Table 6).The authors reported the detection of as low as 5-10 pg of DNA with sensitivities of 94%, 92% and 88% for the *N. meningitidis, S. pneumoniae* and *H. influenzae,* respectively, with an overall specificity of 100% [142]. Similarly, Failace et al. [37] and Saruta et al. [122], utilized semi-nested multiplex PCR assays for the detection of the three pathogensby amplifying a region of bacterial gene 16S rRNA in one stage of amplifications while they applied species-specific primers (one for each pathogen) for the second stage.

Table 6. PCR primers and reaction parameters used in the multiplex PCR assays as described by Tuyama et al. (141) and Tzanakai et al. (142) to identify the three main microorganisms that cause > 90% of bacterial meningitis

Microorganism	Gene amplified	Sequence 5'-3'	Amplicon size (bp)	Ref
H. influenzae type b[*]	*bexA* F	TATCACACAAATAGCGGTTGG	181	
	bexA R	GGCCAAGAGATACTCATAGAACGTT		[142]
N. meningitidis[*]	*CtrA* F	GCTGCGGTAGGTGGTTCAA	110	
	CtrA R	TTGTCGCGGATTTGCAACTA		[142]
				[141]
	CrgA F	GCTGGCGCCGCTGGCAACAAAATTC	230	
				[129]
	CrgA R	CTTCTGCAGATTGCGGCGTGCCGT		
S. pneumonia[*]	*Ply* F	TGCAGAGCGTCCTTTGGTCTAT	80	
				[142]
	Ply R	CTCTTACTCGTGGTTTCCAACTTGA		
N. meningitidis[$]	*nspA* F	AGCACTTGCCACACTGATTG GGAACGGACGTTTTTGACAG	481	[33]

[*] Running conditions;95 °C for 5 min, followed by 35 cycles of 95 °C for 25 s, 57 °C for 40 sand 72 °C for 1 min.

$ 5 min 94 °C, 35 cycles of 1 min at 94 °C,1 min at 60 °C, 2 min at 72 °C and a final extension of 7 min at 72 °C.

Radstrom et al. [115] designed a semi-nested PCR assay for the detection of *N. meningitidis, H. influenzae* and *Streptococcus* spp. The PCR assay was first performed using primers for the general detection of these bacteria while a second set of PCR primers were used for the specific detection of each pathogen [115]. Both sets of primers were deduced from the sequence of 16S rRNA genes of *N. meningitidis, H. influenzae, S. pneumoniae, S. agalactiae*, and *S. epidermidis* (Table 7). In contrast to Radstorm et al. [115] who performed a two-step multiplex PCR assay for the detection of the three major meningitis etiologic agents (*N. meningtitidis, H. influenzae*, and *S. pneumoniae*), Chakrabarti et al. [19] used theuniversal 16S rRNA primers (u3 and u8) and three species-specific primers pairsto detectthe three major meningitis causative agents in a one-stepmultiplex PCRassay (Table8). The reported overall sensitivity and specificity of detection of the meningitis agents were 80 and 97%, respectively.

Table 7.PCR primer sequences used for general detection, specific detection, cloning and sequencing of *N. meningitidis* (NM), *H. influenzae* (HI) and *S. pneumoniae* (SP) as Adapted from Radstrom et al. [115]

Primer[a]	Position in 16S rRNA sequence of *E. coli*[b] (region)	Primer sequence (5'-3')	Specificity and use of the primers
u3'	515-534 (U3)	GTGCCTGCAGCCGCGGTAAT	PCR (*Pst*I site), cloning
u3	509-533 (U3)	AACT(C/A) CGTGCCAGCAGCCGCGGTAA	PCR, detection of eubacteria
u4	793-810 (U4)	CTCGGTACCCTGGTAGTCCACGC	PCR (*Kpn*I site), cloning
NM	831-847 (V8)	TGTTGGGCAACCTGATTG	PCR, detection of NM
u5'	907-926 (U5)	AAACTCAAATGAATTGACGG	Sequencing
ru5'	926-907 (U5)	CCGTCAATTCATTTGAGTTT	Sequencing
HI	998-1015 (V3)	CCTAAGAAGAGCTCAGAG	PCR, detection of HI
rs5'	1099-1083 (S5a)	CTCGTCGACGGGACTTAACCCAACA	PCR (*Sal*I site), cloning
u6'	1220-1240 (U6)	GGGCTACACACGTGCTACAAT	Sequencing
ru6'	1240-1220 (U6)	ATTGTAGCACGTGTGTAGCCC	Sequencing
SP	1246-1263 (V9)	GTACAACGAAGTCGCAAGC	PCR, detection of SP spp.
ru7'	1406-1392 (U7)	ACGGGCGGTGTGTAC	Sequencing
ru8'	1541-1522 (U8)	AAGGAGGGGATCCAACCGCA	PCR, (*Bam*HI site), cloning
ru8	1541-1517 (U8)	AAGGAGGTGATCCA(G/A) CCGCA (G/C) (G/C)TTC	PCR, detection of eubacteria

[A] primes denote primers used for cloning and sequencing.

[B] numbering is based on the corresponding position in the secondary structure of the 16S rRNA from E. coli defined by Woese et al. [155].

Running conditions; the assay used a semi-nested multiplex PCR strategy where two independent PCR reactions were performed;

First step consisted of amplification of primers u3 and ru8; denaturation for 6 min at 94 °C, 28 cycles with denaturation for 1 min at 94 °C, annealing for 1 min at 54 °C, and DNA extension at 72 °C for 2 min and final extension for 7 min at 72 °C.

Second step consisted of amplification with primers NM, HI,SP and ru8 under same conditions used in the first step but annealing was 1 min at 55 °C and the number of cycles was 25.

Ziad W. Jaradat

Table 8. PCR primer sequences and product sizes of the multiplex PCR assay that detects the major three meningitis causing agents, as described by Chakrabartiet al. [19]

Primer name	Primer sequence 5'-3'	Amplicon size (bp)
U3	GTGCCTGCAGCCGCCGTAAT	1000
Ru8	AAGGAGGGGTGTGTAC	
S. pneumoniae	GTACAACGAGTCGCAAGC	293
H. influenzae	CCTAAGAAGAGCTCGAG	543
N. meningitidis	TGTTGGGCAACCTGATTG	710

Running conditions; initial denaturation of 5 min at 94 °C, then the reaction was runfor 35 cycles of denaturation for 30 s at 94 °C annealing for 30 s at 55 °C and extension for 30 s at 72 °C and a final extension period of 15 min at 72 °C.

Table 9. Sequences and positions of the oligonucleotide primers used in a real time PCR assay for the detection of *N. meningitidis*, *H. influenzae* and *S. pneumoniae* as described by Corless et al. [30]

Oligonucleotide position	Target Gene	Primers	Dye labeled probe
617-63	*ctrA* F	GCTGCGGTAGGTGGTT CAA	6 FAM-CATTGCCACGTGTCAGCTGC ACAT
727-708	*ctrA* R	TTGTCGCGGATTTGCA ACTA	
142-160	*bexA* F	GGCGAAATGGTGCTGG TAA	TET-CACCACTCATCAAACGAATG AGCGTGG
241-217	*bexA* R	GGCCAAGAGATACTCA TAGAACGTT	
894-915	*Ply* F	TGCAGAGCGTCCTTTG GTCTAT	VIC-TGGCGCCCATAAGCAACACT CGAA
975-950	*Ply* R	CTCTTACTCGTGGTTTC CAACTTGA	

Heating at 95 °C 10 min followed by 45 cycles of two stage temperature profile of 95 °C for 15 s and 60 °Cfor 1 min. TaqMan machine was used for the detection.

Similarly, Smith et al. [124] developed a fluorescence-based multiplex PCR assay using the *ctrA*, *ply*, and *bexA* genes from *N. meningitis*, *S. pneumoniae* and *H. influenzae*, respectively as described by Corless et al. [30] (Table 9).A 100 % specificity for the detection of these pathogens was reported.A PCR assay targeting the 16S rRNA genes of the three major meningitis causative agents coupled with sequencing was developed by Arosio et al. [6]. It was reported, that this assay, in addition to, traditional culture methods improved the diagnosis and detection of pathogens in CSF especially after the beginning of antibiotic treatment and negative culture results.

4.2.1. Real Time PCR Detection and Serotyping of the Three Major Meningitis Agents

In addition to the specific primers that are used for the detection of meningitis agents separately, real time PCR protocols were developed that enable the detection of the three major meningitis agents simultaneously. Corless et al. [30] developed a real time PCR assay with primers detecting genes encoding for capsular transport (*ctrA*) gene, capsulation (*bexA*) gene and pneumolysin (*ply*) gene in *N. meningitidis*, *H. influenzae* and *S. pneumoniae*, respectively (Table 9).The primers were 100% specific and their sensitivities were 88.4%, 100% and 91.8% for *N. meningitidis*, *H. influenzae* and *S. pneumoniae*, respectively. Furthermore, the *ctrA* primers amplified serotypes A, B, C, 29E, W135, X, Y and Z, while the *ply* primers amplified pneumococcal serotypes 1-9, 10A, 11A, 12, 14, 15B, 17F, 18C, 19, 20, 22, 23,24, 31 and 33 and the *bexA* primers amplified both *H. influenzae* serotypes b and c.

Table 10. Oligonucleotide PCR primers and probesfor the detection and quantitation of *S. pneumoniae*, *H. influenzae* and *N. meningitidis* using real time PCR, as described by Abdeldaim et al. [1]

Target gene	Oligomer sequence 5'-3'	Position in the target gene
S. pneumoniae		
*spn*9802 F	AGTCGTTCCAAGGTAACAAGTC	3370-3392
*spn*9802 R	ACCAACTCGACCACCTCTTT	3525-3506
*spn*9802 FAM	FAM-aTcAGaTTgCTgATaAAaCgA-BHQ1	
H. influenzae		
*hiP*6 F	CCAGCTGCTAAAGTATTAGTAGAAG	302-326
*hiP*6 R	TTCACCGTAAGATACTGTGCC	477-457
*hiP*6 JOE	JOE-CAgATgCAgTTgAAgGTtAtttAG-BHQ1	
N. meningitidis		
ctrA F	GCTGCGGTAGGTGGTTCAA	
ctrA R	TTGTCGCGGATTTGCAACTA	
ctrA ROX	ROX-CATTGCCACGTGTCAGCTGCACAT-BHQ1	

The lower case letters indicate locked nucleic acids. Running conditions were as following; 15 min of enzyme activation at 95 °C, followed by 45 cycles of 95 °C for 15 s and 60 °C for 40 s.

Van Gastel, [145] evaluated the performance of a real time PCR for the detection of *N. meningitidis* and *S. pneumoniae* and compared that to Gram-staining and culture methods using the *ctr*A and *ply* primers published by Corless et al. [30] (Table 9). The real time PCR assay was superior to both Gram-stain and the culture methods in detecting both pathogens.

Recently, Abdeldaim et al. [1] developed a quantitative real time PCR for the detection of the three major meningitis causing bacteria. Table 10, shows the primers used for the study and the running conditions. The assay was specific, sensitive and quantitative enabling the detection of meningitis agents even after the initiation of antibiotic therapy.

Similarly, Azzari et al. [7] also developed a real time PCR protocol for the detection of the three major meningitis agents (*N. meningitidis, S. pneumoniae* and *H. influenzae*) directly from the clinical samples (Table 11).This test gave significantly higher detection sensitivities than culture methods used for these pathogens.

Table 11. Primers and probes used for the RT-PCR for detection of *N. meningitidis, S. pneumoniae* and *H. influenzae,* as described by Azzari et al. [7]

Gene	Primer sequence 5'-3'	Probe sequence 5'-3'
ctrA	F-GCTGCGGTAGGTGGTTCAA	6-FAM-
(*N. meningitidis*)	R-TTGTCGCGGATTTGCAACTA	CATTGCCACGTGTCAGCT GCA-CAT-TAMRA
lytA	F- ACGCAATCTAGCAGATGAAGC	(JOE)-
(*S. pneumoniae*)	R-TGTTTGGTTGGTTATTCGTGC	TTTGCCGAAAACGCTTGA TACAGGG-(TAMRA)
bexA	F-GGCGAAATGGTGCTGGTAA	NED-
(*H. influenzae*)	R-GGCCAAGAGATACTCATAGAACGTT	CACCACTCATCAAACGA ATGAGCGTGG-TAMRA

Running conditions; 95 °C for 10 min followed by 45 cycles of a two–stage temperature profile of 95 °C for 15 s and 60 °C for 1 min.

Although general detection of meningitis causative agents is vital as a first step in diagnosing meningitis cases, the precise identification of the causative agent should not be underestimated. The following section will address the detection of the major and minor meningitis bacterial agents.

4.3. Specific Detection of Meningetic Pathogens and the Serotype Identification byRegular PCR, Multiplex or Real Time PCR)

In this part of the review, the detection of the major bacterial pathogens in CSF using species–specific PCR assays will be discussed. Simple PCR, nested PCR and real time PCR formats will be discussed.

4.3.1. Detection of Neisseria Meningitidis

General detection by PCR: PCR strategies to amplify specific *N. meningitidis* genes of different chromosomal loci are widely used.Multicopy insertion sequence IS 1106 PCR was used for detection of *N. meningitis* with 91% sensitivity and specificity for the detection of meningococcal meningitis [104, 139]. However, due to the occurrenceof some false-positive reactions with the IS 1106, other target genes were used including the gene coding for dihydropteroate synthase (*dbps*), the gene coding for a major porin protein PorB (*porB*), and the *ctrA*gene that encodes an outer membrane protein and other genes [130, 131]. Filippis et al. [33] utilized the published genome sequence of the *N. meningitidis* and designed specific primers that detected the sequence of the *nspA* gene of the *N. meningitidis* and *N. gonorrhoeae* in a nested PCR assay (Table 12).However, it appeared that not all the *N. meningitidis* strains contain *ctrA* gene whichleadsto misdiagnosis of uncapsulated pathogens.As a solution for this problem, Thomas et al. [35] developed a real time PCR assay targeting the cu-zn-superoxide dismutase gene (*osdC*) with a 99.7% efficiency of identifying *N. meningitidis*. Table 13 shows the primers and probes used in their study.

Table 12. PCR Primers used for the nested PCR assay for the amplification of the *nep*A gene of *N. meningitidis* and *N. gonorrhoeae*, as described by Filippis et al. [33]

Primer name	Primer sequence 5'-3'	Amplicon size (bp)
*nsp*A-1	F- AGCACTTGCCACACTGATTG	481
*nsp*A-2	R-GGAACGGACGTTTTTGACAG	
*nsp*A-Nest-1	F-TAGGTTCTGCCAAAGGCTTC	
*nsp*A-Nest-2	R-CAGTGTTGACTTTGCCGATC	

Reaction conditions; initial denaturation for 5 min at 94 °C, 35 cycles of 1 min at 94 °C, 1 min at 60 °C, 2 min at 72 °C, and final extension of 7 min at 72 °C.

Table13. PCR Primers and probes used for the real time PCR amplification of *sodC* genes specific for *N. meningitidis* as described by Thomas et al. [35]

Target gene	Use of the primers	5'-3' nucleotide sequence	Amplicon size (bp)
sodC	PCR sequencing	F-CCTTATTAGCACTAGCGGTTAG R-CCGGTCATCTTTTATGCTCCAA	537
sodC	rt-PCR rt-PCR rt-PCR	F-GCACACTTAGGTGATTTACCTGCAT R-CCACCCGTGTGGATCATAATAGA FAM-CATGATGGCACAGCAACAAATCCTGTTT-(BHQI)	127

Running conditions; 2 min at 50 °C, 10 min at 95 °C,and then 50 cycles (15 s, at 95 °C,plus 1 min at 60 °C).

Table 14. PCR Oligonucleotides used for serotyping of *N. meningitidis*, as described by Fraisier et al. [41]

Oligonu-cleotide	Sequence (5'-3')	Gene amplified (serogroup)	Amplicon size (bp)	Ref
98-28	GCAATAGGTGTATATATTCTTCC	*orf-2* (A)	400	154
98-29	CGTAATAGTTTCGTATGCCTTCTT	*orf-2* (A)		
98-19	GGATCATTTCAGTGTTTTCCACCA	*synB* (B)	450	154
98-20	GCATGCTGGAGGAATAAGCATTAA	*synB* (B)		
98-17	TCAAATGAGTTTGCGAATAGAAGGT	*synE* (C)	250	154
98-18	CAATCACGATTTGCCCAATTGAC	*synE* (C)		
98-32	CAGAAAGTGAGGGATTTCCATA	*synG* (W135)	120	154
98-33	CACAACCATTTTCATTATAGTTACTGT	*synG* (W135)		
98-36	ACGATATCCCTATCCTTGCCTA	*synF* (Y)	75	36
98-35	CTGAAGCGTTTTCATTATAATTGCTAA	*synF* (Y)		
XF	AATGCAAATTCAATTGGTTG	*ctrA* (X)	190	36
XR	CTTGGGCCTTATACAAAGAC	*ctrA* (X)		
98-6	GCTGGCGCCGCTGGCAACAAAATTC	*crg A*	230	154
98-10	CTTCTGCAGATTGCGGCGTGCCGT	*ceg A*		

Amplification conditions; initial denaturation at 94 °C for 3 min, annealing at 55 °C for 30 s and polymerization at 72 °C for 20 s. the conditions were repeated for 35 cycles as following; 92 °C for 40 s, annealing at 55 °C for 30 s and extension at 72 °C for 20 s and a final extension step at 72 °C for 10 min [129].

Serogroup detection of N. meningitidis; once the species has been identified, serotype- specific primers can be used to identify the serotype and has been useful when a particular serotype is frequently incriminated in meningitis [130]. Fraisier et al. [41] described a standard multiplex PCR assay for the simultaneous detection of the six *N. meningitidis* serogroups (A, B, C, W135, Y and X).The PCR assay targeted a specific gene for each serotype (Table 14). Likewise, Taha [129] used the primers described by Fraisier et al. [41] in a multiplex PCR assay except that Taha used primers targeting *crgA* instead of the *ctrA*gene for detecting serogtop X (Table 14). The assay was specific and discriminated between the serotypes with high accuracy comparable to that of the serological agglutination assay [41, 129]. Further, Taha [129] reported performing a single PCR assay for each of the serotypes after the completion of the multiplex PCR as a double check for the identity of the serotypes. An accurate serotype identification of 32 out of 33 serotypes was attained [129]. Other methods were also used for strain subtyping of the *N. meningitidis*. Killoran et al. [78] used MLVA for subtyping of *N. meningitis* C.Their method gave comparable results to PFGE, the gold standard. Table 15 shows the MLVA primers used in their study and the reaction conditions and the amplicon size of each product.

Table 15.Genome location and characteristics of VNTRs amplified in MLVA for subtyping group C of *N. meningitidis*, as adapted from Killoran et al. [78]

VNTR	Genome	Genome location	Primer sequences (5'-3')	Amplicon Size (bp)
2	C	1844470	F-GATGTCGAGGGCTGTACCGTATT R-ATGCCTGCCGCTCATATAAAGAAC	104
3	C	1043724	F-CCCCGATAGGCCCCGAAATACCTG R-AAGCGGCGGGAATGACGAAGAGTG	532
4	B	863508	F-GGTGTACGCCGATAAAGGGTTTTT R-TCGGTTACGCGTTTTGAAGTTTTG	165
8	B	1572486	F-GTTTGCCGCTGCTTTGTTGTCTTT R-AAGGGAATCTGATGCCGTCTGAAA	361
12	C	1408985	F-TGGCGGCATCTTTCATTTTGTCTG R-GCCGAGTCTGCCGCTTCTGC	232

Running conditions of VNTR; 95 °C for 15 min, 30 cycles of 94 °C for 30 s, 55 °C for 90 °C, and 72 °C for 3 min followed by a final extension of 10 min at 72 °C.

4.3.2. Detection of S. pneumoniae

Although culture assay is the gold standard for detection of pneumococcus, culturing body fluids is not always the preferred method due to the low detection of the pathogen especially after the initiation of antibiotic treatment [91, 92]. Common diagnosis of *S. pneumoniae* is performed by an immunochromatographic method (Binax, Portland, USA) which detects pneumococcal antigens in urine or CSF of suspected patients or using immunoassays for detecting antibodies against the pathogen in blood [92].PCR detection of S. *pneumoniae*specific genes were developed and tested on samples from patients and controls as well. Dagan et al. [32] developed a PCR assay that detected the pneumolysin gene of the *S. pneumoniae*. However, the test gave a high proportion of false-positives, a result that contradicts reports from Toikka et al. [140] who reported no false positives among the blood samples from healthy subjects tested for pneumolysin. The reason for the differences in the results although both researchers tested for pneumolysin gene was probably due to little modification in the primer sequencesand the addition of the extra pair of primers that amplified an inner part of the pneumolysin gene (nested PCR) as described by Toikka et al. [140] study (Table 16).

Table 16. PCR Primer sequences and reaction running conditions, used in the studies described by Dagan et al. [32] and Toikka et al. [140]

Oligonucleotide	Gene	Primer sequence 5'-3'	Amplicon size (bp)	Ref
	Pneumolysin	GTAGATATTTCTGTAACAGCTACC GAGAATTCCCTGTCTTTTCAAAG	355	[32][1]
Outer primer Ia Ib	Pneumolysin	ATTTCTGTAACAGCTACCAACGA GAATTCCCTGTCTTTTCAAAGTC	348	[140][2]
Inner primer IIa IIb	Pneumolysin	CCCACTTCTTCTTGCGGTTGA TGAGCCGTTATTTTTTCATACTG	208	[140][2]

[1] 30 cycles denaturation at 94 °C, annealing at 60 °C for 1 min and synthesis at 72 °C for 1 min.

[2]Amplifications were done for 40 cycles as following; 30 s at 94 °C for denaturation, 30 s at 56 °C for annealing and 30 s at 72 °C for extension. Nested amplifications were carried out as for the first round PCR.

Cherian et al. [22] developed a nested PCR-enzyme immunoassay assay for the detection of all serotypes of *S. pneumoniae* in CSF samples without any false-negative reactions.In their test they targeted a 413 bp fragment of the autolysin (*lytA*) gene of *S. pneumoniae* (Table 17).

Other primers derived from the *lytA* gene were also used in a PCR assay that was designed by Saha et al. [121] to validate the results obtained by an immunochromatographic test for the detection of *S. pneumoniae* in CSF. The following primers were used; F-5'-TGAAGCGGATTATCACTGGC -3' and

R-5'-GCTAAACTCCCTGTATCAAGCG-3' that amplify a 273 bp Amplicon size. The reaction conditions were as following; denaturation was at 94 °C for 2 min, followed by 30 s at 94 °C, 55 °C and 72 °C per cycle for 30 cycles. Afinal extension step was done for 10 min at 72 °C. The primers were excellent in validating the immunochromatographic test with 100% matching between the two methods.

Table 17. PCR Primers and nested primers developed for the detection of *S. pneumoniae* serotypes, as described by Cherian et al. [22]

Name of the primer	Sequence 5'-3'
lytA	F-GTCGGCGTGCAACCATATAGGCAA
	R-GGATAAGGGTCAACGTGGTCTGAG
Nested primer	A3-T7-
	TTAATACGACTCACTATAGGTGAAGCGGATTATCACTGG
	A4-AGCGTTTTCGGCAAACCTGCTT
Detection probe	Biotin-
	TGCATCATGCAGGTAGGACCTGTTGATAATGGTGCCTGGGA
	CGTT

The target DNA was amplified by running PCR cycler for 30 cycles at 94 °C, 55 °C and 72 °C for 1 min at each temperature.

Table 18. Real time PCR primers and probes used for the detection and quantification of GBS in CSF, as adapted from Ke et al. [76]

Primer	Primer sequence 5'-3'	Gene location	Amplicon size (bp)
GBS-specific primers	Sag59- TTTCACCAGCTGTATTAGAAGTA	369-391	153
	Sag190- GTTCCCTGAACATTATCTTTGAT	500-522	
Probes for GBS	STB-F AAGCCCAGCAAATGGCTCAAA[*]		
	STB-C CY5-		
	GCTTGATCAAGATAGCATTCAGTTGA[$]		
Probes for internal control	ICF- TTATTGCAGCTTCGCCACAGGAA[*]		
	CY5-GGTCCAGCAATGTGAAGAGGCAT[$]		

Running conditions for conventional PCR; denaturation at 94 °C for 3 min, 40 cycles (1 s at 95 °C, 30 s at 55 °C, hold 2 min at 72 °C).

Running conditions for rt-PCR; initial denaturation at 94 °C for 3 min, 45 cycles (0 s at 95 °C, 14 s at 55 °C and 5 s at 72 °C).

[*] Fluorescein labeled.

[$] Phosphate labeled.

Group B *Streptococcus* (GBS, *S. agalactiae*) are considered major meningitis causing agents especially in extremely young infants 3 < months old, or elderly people [76]. The detection of this pathogen is as important as the detection of the *S. pneumoniae*, therefore, a real time PCR assay specific for this pathogen was developed.KE et al. [76] designed a real time PCR assay for the rapid detection of *S. agalactiae* (GBS), the leading cause of sepsis in newborn infants.The *cfb* gene encoding the Christie-Atkins-Munch-Petersen (CAMP) factor was selected for this method [76]. The assay enabled the detection of as little as one genome copy and the assay was comparable to the conventional PCR assay and was faster in amplification (Table 18).

4.3.3. Molecular Diagnosis of H. influenzae

H. influenzae b is one of the major causative agents of infant and childhood meningitis.However, after the introduction of the Hib vaccine, the incidence of meningitis by this pathogen has declined significantly. Nevertheless, it is still considered to be one of the major pathogens of concern and the need for its detection in CSF of suspected patients is important especially in geographic areas where the vaccine cannot be given.Primers derived from the published sequence of the *bexA* gene as well as primers derived from the sequence of the outer membrane protein P6 gene were used for this purpose [146].Table 19 shows the primer sets and the running conditions used in the assay.The assay detected all the different serotypes of the *H. influenzae* as well as the non-capsulated strains and some closely related species yielding results comparable to those obtained by culture conditions.

Table19. PCR primers and probes used for the detection of *H. influenzae* DNA in CSF samples as adapted from van Ketel et al. [146]

Primer origin	Primer/Probe sequence 5'-3'	Amplicon size (bp)	Running conditions
bexA protein	F-5'-CGTTTGTATGATGTTGATCCAGACT-3' R-5'-TGTCCATGTCTTCAAAATGATG-3' Probe; 5'- GTGATTGCAGTAGGGGATTCGCGCTTTGCAG- 3'	343	35-40 cycles 1 min at 95 °C 1 min at 55 °C 2 min at 72 °C Final extension 8 min at 72 °C
P6 protein	F-5'-ACTTTTGGCGGTTACTCTGT-3' R-5'-TGTGCCTAATTTACCAGCAT-3' Probe; 5'- GCATATTTAAATGCAACACCAGCTGCT-3'	273	35-40 cycles 1 min at 95 °C 1 min at 55 °C 2 min at 72 °C Final extension 8 min at 72 °C

Recently, a real time PCR was also developed for the specific detection and quantitation of both typable and non typable *H. influenzae* by Wang et al. [147].This RT-PCR identified more cases than culture or latex agglutination kits.The two RT-PCR assays detected 97% and 99% of the *H. influenzae*isolatesand were superior for detecting both typeable and untypeable *H. influenzae* isolates as compared to theRT-PCRassay that utilized the *bexA* and *ompP2* genes.Table 20 shows the RT-PCR assay developed by Wang et al. [147] for the detection of *H. influenzae* and could even distinguish *H. influenzae* from other *Haemophilus*spp..

Table 20.PCR primers and probes used in the real time PCR assay for the detection of the *H. influenzae*, as adapted from Wang et al. [147]

Target gene	Primer designation	5'-3' Primer sequence	Amplicon size (bp)
hpd assay 1	hpdF729	AGATTGGAAAGAAACACAAGAAAAAGA	113
	hpdR819	CACCATCGGCATATTTAACCACT	
	hpdPbr762i[b]	AAAACATCCAACG"T"AATTATAGTTTACC CAATAACCC	
hpd assay 2	hpdF822	GGTTAAATATGCCGATGGTGTTG	151
	hpdR952	TGCATCTTTACGCACGGTGTA	
	hpdPbr896i[b]	TTGTGTACACTCCGT"T"GGTAAAAGAACTT GCAC	

PCR mixtures were first incubated for 10 min at 50°C, and then, 40 cycles of 1 min at 95°C and 1 min at 60°C were performed.

4.3.4. Molecular Diagnosis of L. Monocytogenes

The traditional diagnosis of *L. monocytogenes* meningitis normally is based on culturing the CSF after lumbar puncture and the direct Gram-staining of CSF smears.However, viewing the microorganism is not always feasible especially following the initiation of the antibiotic treatment. PCR techniques offer the detection of relatively low number of *L. monocytogenes*. Several genes were used as targets for the detection and differentiation of *L. monocytogenes*.A gene that encodes the invasion association protein (*iap*) is one of the genes used for detection of *L. monocytogenes* [71]. Table 21 shows two sets of primers that detect this gene [70, 71]. In addition, other genes are used for the detection of *L. monocytogenes* in foods and clinical samples. Hemolysin A and B genes, internalin and other genes are used for this purpose [70]. These primers were used for the detection of the pathogen in clinical samples as well as food and environmental samples with accuracy and specificity.

Table 21. PCR primers specific for different *L. monocytogenes* virulence genes, as adapted from Jaradat[2] et al. [70] and Jaton[1] et al. [71]

Name of gene	Primer sequence 5'-3'	Gene location	Amplicon size (bp)
iap-A[1]	CAAAGGTGGATCCAAACTAACTGT	760-783	486
iap-B	TGGAGCTTCCGAATTCACTTCTG	1228-1206	
iap-1[1]	CGAATCTAACGGCTGGCACA	793-812	287
iap-3	GCCCAAATAGTGTCACCGCT	1080-1061	
inlA-F[2]	CCTAGCAGGTCTAACCGCAC	936-1190	255
inlB-R	TCGCTAATTTGGTTATGCCC		
inlB-F[2]	AAAGCACGATTTCATGGGAG	922-1067	146
inlB-R	ACATAGCCTTGTTTGGTCGG		
actA-F[2]	GACGAAAATCCCGAAGTGAA	691-958	268
actA-R	CTAGCGAAGGTGCTGTTTCC		
hlyA-F[2]	CGGAGGTTCCGCAAAAGATG	1044-1277	234
hlyA-R	CCTCCAGAGTGATCGATGTT		
plcA-F[2]	CGAGCAAAACAGCAACGATA	447-575	129
plcA-R	CCGCGGACATCTTTTAATGT		
plcB-F[2]	GGGAAATTTGACACAGCGTT	463-723	261
plcB-R	ATTTTCGGGTAGTCCGCTTT		

[1] Cycling conditions; precycling was done at 97 °C for 5 min,and 74 °C for 1 min and annealing at 50 °C for 1 min and extension at 74 °C for 2 min. For cycles 1-30, denaturation was done at 94 °C for 30 s, annealing at 50 °C for 1 min, extension at 74 °C for 1 min and final extension at 74 °C for additional 5 min.

[2] Running conditions; initial denaturation at 94 °C for 3 min, followed by 35 cycles [denaturation at 94 °C for 1 min, annealing at 60 °C for 2 min and extension at 72 °C for 1 min].

4.3.5. Molecular Detection of Mycobacterium Tuberculosis

Mycobacterium tuberculosis meningitis is considered the most devastating form of meningitis [50].A rapid diagnosis therefore, is pivotal for a better patient prognosis [50].Unfortunately, the diagnosis of tuberculosis meningitis remains a complex issue due to the inability to detect the pathogen in the CSF smears and culture methods are time consuming.Any delay in the diagnosis might lead to detrimental consequences.The detection of *M. tuberculosis* DNA in the CSF by PCR has been used as a rapid and more sensitive method for the detection of the pathogen. Takahashi et al. [135] developed a nested real time PCR for the detection and quantification of *M. tuberculosis* in CSF samples.The assay was sensitive enough to identify the pathogen in 24 out 43 CSF samples. In addition, the numbers of detected pathogen in the positive samples were decreasing during the course of the treatment indicating the usefulness of the method for assessing the clinical course of therapy. The primers and the running conditions for the PCR assay are listed in Table 22.

Table 22. PCR Primers and probes used for the nested real-time PCR assay used in the detection of *M. tuberculosis* in CSF and other biological fluids as adapted from Takahashi et al. [135]

Objective	Type	Sequence 5'-3'	Amplicon Size (bp)
Conventional nested PCR Step 1	Outer forward primer Outer revers primer	ATCCGCTGCCAGTCGTCTTCC CTCGCGAGTCTAGGCCAGCAT	239
Conventional nested PCR Step 2	Inner forward primer Inner reverse primer	CATTGTGCAAGGTGAACTGAGC AGCATCGAGTCGATCGCGGAA	194
Internal control	Human beta globin forward Human beta globin reverse	GGCAGACTTCTCCTCAGGAGTC CTTAGACCTCACCCTGTGGAGC	196
Quantitative nested real time PCR	TaqMan forward primer TaqMan reveres primer TaqMan probe – wild-VIC TaqMan probe-mutation-FAM	GTGAACTGAGCAAGCAGACCG GTTCTGATAATTCACCGGGTCC VIC-TATCGATAGCGCCGAATGCCGG-TAMRA FAM-ATGGGACGGCTAGCAATCCGTC-TAMRA	77

Running conditions; as per Takahashi et al. 2005; 2006 [132, 133].

Latter, Takahashi et al. [134] developed a wide range quantitative nested real time PCR assay for the detection of *M. tuberculosis* in which they obtained more accurate quantitation of the numbers of *M. tuberculosis* and thus widened the detection limit of the pathogen. Haldar et al. [50] also developed a quantitative real time PCR and a conventional gel based PCR assay (IS6110 primers)for the detection of *M. tuberculosis*DNA in CSF pellet and supernatant using the following pair of primers; devRf3- 5'-ATCTGTTGTCCCGCATGCC-3' and devRr3-5'GTCCAGCGCCC ACATC TTT-3' with running conditions as per the Haldar et al. [50]. The assay yielded 92% specificity for both pellet and supernatant samples.In addition, the sensitivity of detection was 87.6% and 53% in supernatant and pellets respectively thus highlighting the possibility of using the supernatant as reliable method for the detection of this peculiar pathogen [50]. Similarly, Huang et al. [60] developed a nested PCR assay for the detection of *M. tuberculosis* meningitis targeting the *ropB* gene (Table 23).

Table 23.PCR primer sequences and the running conditions for detection of *M. tuberculosis* in CSF, as adapted from Huang et al. [60]

Primer	Sequence	conditions	Amplicon size (bp)
Outer primers for the *ropB* gene	F-1-5-CGTGGAGGCGATCACACCGCAGACGTTG-3' R-1-5'-GACCTCCAGCCCGGCACGCTCACG-3'	5min 94 °C 30 cycles of 30 s at 95 °C 40s at 72 °C 5min at 72 °C	193
Inner primers for the *ropB* gene	F-2-5'-CGCCGCGATCAAGGAGTTCT-3' R-2-5'-TCACGTGACAGACCGCCGGG-3'	5min 95 °C 35 cycles of 20 s at 95 °C 30s at 65 °C 30s at 72 °C 5min at 72 °C	126

The assay had 86% sensitivity and 100% specificity for detection of *M. tuberculosis* DNA in CSF samples.

4.3.6. Detection of Cronobacter spp.

Cronobacter, a newly emerging bacterial genus comprises six different species that were incriminated in infant meningitis through the consumption of temperature-abused contaminated powdered infant formula.The detection and confirmation of this genus is peculiar as there was no one single method that proved to be sufficient. Jaradat et al. [69] used 8 different PCR primers that were designed to detect *Cronobacter* spp. and none of them was free of either false positives or false negatives.

In their study, Jaradat et al. [69] used eight sets of primers to ascertain the identities of 29 food isolates. Only 13 isolates were positive with all the primers while the other 16 isolates did not give the predicted PCR product with at least one set of primers although they were identified as *Cronobacter* spp. by other biochemical and/or chromogenic methods. In addition none of the 8 primers confirmed the identity of all the isolates with the highest sensitivity (93.3%) was obtained with the primers recognizing an outer membrane protein (OMP) in *Cronobacter* spp.

Table 24 shows all these primers that were used for the detection of *Cronobacter* and the running conditions.It is note worth to mention that these primers were used for detection of *Cronobacter* in foods and infant formula and none of them was used for the detection of the pathogen in CSF.

Table 24. Oligonucleotide primer pairs and PCR running conditions used for detection and identification of *Cronobacter* as adapted from Jaradat et al. [69]

Primer	Sequence	Targeted site	Amplicon size (bp)	Ref.
SG-F	GGGTTGTCTGCGAAAGCGAA[a]	ITS-G	282	Liu et al
SG-R	GTCTTCGTGCTGCGAGTTTG	ITS-G and IA		[86]
SI-F	CAGGAGTTGAAGAGGTTTAACT[b]	ITS-IA	251	Liu et al
SI-R	GTGCTGCGAGTTTGAGAGACTC	ITS-G and IA		[86]
Saka 1a	ACAGGGAGCAGCTTGCTGC[c]	V1[g]	952	Hassan et
Saka 2b	TCCCGCATCTCTGCAGGA	V3[h]		al., [52]
Zpx F	GAAAGCGTATAAGCGCGATTC[d]	zpx	94	Kothary
Zpx R	GTTCCAGAAGGCGTTCTGGT			et al., [79]
BAM122	AWATCTATGACGCGCAGAACCG[e]	zpx	350	Kothary
BAM123	AAAATAGATAAGCCCGGCTTCG			et al., [79]
EsgluAf	TGAAAGCAATCGACAAGAAG[f]	gluA	1680	Lehner et
EsgluAr	ACTCATTACCCCTCCTGATG			al., [82]
EsgluBf	TGAGTGAAGCACCGACGCAG[f]	gluB	1720	Lehner et
EsgluBr	GTTACGTCACAGGTTTTGAT			al., [83]
ESSF	GGATTTAACCGTGAACTTTTCC[i]	ompA	469	Nair and
ESSR	CGCCAGCGATGTTAGAAGA			Venkitan arayanan [102]

[a]&[b]Running conditions;94 °C for 10 min; 30 cycles of 94 °C for 30 s each; 57 °C for 1 min; 72 °C for 1 min;a final extension period of 5 min at 72 °C.

[c]Running conditions;95 °C for 4 min;30 cycles of 95 °C for 60 sec each;50 °C for 1 min;72°C for 90 s ; final extension period of 4 min at 72 °C.

[d]&[e]Running conditions;The hot start polymerase was activated by incubation for 15 min at 95 °C; followed by 35 cycles of 1 min at 95 °C; 62 °C for *zpx* primers (50.5 °C was used for 8 isolates) or 50 °C for BAM primers for 1 min; 72 °C for 1 min; final extension period of 10 min at 72 °C for *zpx* and 7 min for BAM primers.

Running conditions; The hot start polymerase was activated by incubation for 15 min at 95 °C;followed by 30 cycles of 30s at 94° C;56 (*gluA*) or 58 °C (*gluB*)for 1 min;72°C for 1.5 min; finalextension period of 5 min at 72 °C.

[g]&[h]Variable regions of the 16S rRNA gene.

[i]Running conditions: 94 °C for 2 min; 30 cycles 94 °C for 15sec each ; 60 °C for15 sec; 72 °C for 30 s; final extension period of 5 min at 72 °C.

A real time PCR assay was developed to detect *Cronobacter* in powdered infant formula using a TaqMan Probe predicted from the sequence of the 16S rRNA gene in addition to other 4 sets of primers designed to detect all the species of *Cronobacter* [73] (Table 25).The detection limits of the developed Rt-PCR for *Cronobacter* and purified DNA were about 2.3 CFU/assay and 100 fg/assay, respectively [71].

Taking advantage of gene targets such as the metalloprotease gene, *zpx* described by Kothary et al. [79]or the macro-molecular synthesis (MMS) operon gene dnaG described by Seo and Bracket [126]lead to the development of a species-specific detection method for *Enterobacter sakazakii* [79, 126].Seo and Bracket [126] reported a detection limit of 100 CFU/ml andthe assay was specific enough to differentiate *E. sakazakii* from other *Enterobacter* spp.

Furthermore, Stoop et al. [127] developed a species-specific PCR assay scheme that takes advantage of species-specific single nucleotide polymorphisms associated with the *rpoB* gene. The assay was too specific giving 100% specificity in differentiating the different *Cronobacter* species.

Table 25. PCR Primers and probe sequences for the detection and identification of *Cronobacter sakazakii*, as adapted from Kang et al. [73] and Seo and Brackett. [126]

Primers and probe	Primer sequence 5'-3'	Amplicon size (bp)
sF1	TAACAGGGAGCAGCTTGCTGCTCTG	426
sR3	CGGGTAACGTCAATTGCTGCGGT	
sF1	TAACAGGGAGCAGCTTGCTGCTCTG	960
sR5	AAGGCACTCCCGCATCTCTGCA	
sF1	TAACAGGGAGCAGCTTGCTGCTCTG	1031
sR6	AGTCTCCTTTGAGTTCCCGGCCGA	
sF4	CAATTGACGTTACCCGCAGAAGAA	560
sR5	AAGGCACTCCCGCATCTCTGCA	
Probe	CCGCATAACGTCTACGGACCAAA	
rpsU*	GGGATATTGTCCCCTGAAACAG	
dnaG*	CGAGAATAAGCCGCGCATT	
MMS probe*	6FAM-AGAGTAGTAGTTGTAGAAGCCGTGCTTCCGAAAG-TAMRA**	

The PCR reactions were run using the following program; 1 cycle of 2 min at 50 °C and 10 min at 94 °C, 40 cycles of 15 s at 94 °C and 1 min at 60 °C.

* these primers were used by Seo and Brackett [126]; reactions were as following; The reaction was run at 50°C for 2 min and then 95 °C for 10 min, followed by 50 cycles of 95 °C for 15 s and 60 °C for 60 s.

** FAM, 6-carboxyfluorescein (the reporter dye); TAMRA, 6-carboxytetramethylrhodamine (the quencher dye).

Molecular serotyping determination in *Cronobacter* species based on the O-antigen genes was initially reported by Mullane et al. [98] and has been furthered by the work of Jarvis et al. [68] who used the MobII restriction fragment length polymorphism (RFLP) of the O-antigen gene clusters. There are now 5 LPS types (O1-O5) that can be determined by a PCR scheme targeting various genes associated with the LPS biosynthesis operon.A serological scheme has also been proposed by Sun et al. [128]which correlate well with the molecular schemes proposed by Mullane and Jarvis [68, 98].

Nevertheless, as this bacterium is new, and despite its incrimination in infant meningitis, no methods have been developed for the detection of this pathogen in CSF. However, I do believe that these assays can be easily adapted to detect the pathogen in CSF and other body fluids.

4.3.7. Diagnosis of Salmonella by PCR

Similar to the diagnosis of most meningitis agents, diagnosis of *Salmonella* is divided into two parts; species-specific diagnosis of *Salmonella* where universal *Salmonella* primers from conserved regions are used followed by strain-specific primers that differentiates among the different strains. Stone et al. [125] have developed a PCR assay for the general detection of *Salmonella* species by detecting parts of two virulence genes; *invE* and *invA*.

Table 26. PCR primer sequences and running conditions used for the general detection of *Salmonella* in clinical samples and other biological samples as adapted from Rahn et al. [116], Stone et al. [125], and Myint et al. [101]

Primers	Primer sequence 5'-3'	Amplicon size (bp)	Ref
invA[1]	GTGAAATTATCGCCACGTTCGGGCAA TCATCGCACCGTCAAAGGAACC	248	[116]
invE[2]	TGCCTACAAGCATGAAATGG AAACTGGACCACGGTGACAA	457	[125]
ST11[3] ST 15	AGCCAACCATTGCTAAATTGGCGCA GGTAGAAATTCCCAGCGGGTACTG	429	[101]

[1] Running conditions; initial denaturation at 94 °C for 5 min then 35 cycles with 94 °C for 30 s, 55 °C for 45s and 72 °C for 45s and a final extension at 72 °C for 10 min.

[2] PCR was performed for 35 cycles (each cycle contains 94 °C for 15 s, 52 °C for 15 s and 72 °C for 15s) and a final extension step at 72 °C for 2.5 min.

[3] initial denaturation for 2 min at 94 °C,followed by 35 cycles of amplification at 95 °C for 30 s, 60 °C for 30 s and 72 °C for 30 s and a final extension period for 10 min at 72 °C.

The assay detected as low as 9 CFU of *Salmonella* in pure culture or as little as 30 fg of purified DNA. Similarly, Rahn et al. [116] designed primers from the *invA* gene that detects *Salmonella*. In addition, Myint et al. [101] designed a set of PCR primers that also detects all *Salmonella* species with a detection limit of about 100 CFU/ ml.Nevertheless, all these primers gave false-positives, especially with *Citrobacter freundii* which is used as a surrogate for *Salmonella*. However, when these primers are used for the detection of bacteria in CSF, the indication of the presence of any microbial agent necessitate an immediate therapeutic protocol.Table 26 describes the PCR primers and reaction conditions used in this universal PCR assay.

CONCLUSION

In acute meningitis, reliable and rapid diagnosis is pivotal for good patient management and prognosis of meningitis cases. Detection of the pathogen by culture from CSF and/or blood is considered to be the gold standard to initiate a therapeutic protocol if it was not initiated merely based on symptoms. However, culturing or detection of a pathogen in Gram-stains is not always feasible especially if an antibiotic regimen has been initiated. It is therefore, important for the clinician to be aware of the presence of other alternative techniques that can help in rapid and proper diagnosis. PCR assays in both phases; general or specific, provide a multi-pathogen detection ability where more than one agent can be tested for in CSF or other biological fluids or can target a specific pathogen. Furthermore, real time PCR assays can provide not only a quantitation approach for detection of pathogens but can also be used for monitoring the progress of the therapeutic protocol. In general molecular techniques, along with other newly emerging biotechnological methods, will improve the detection of pathogens and provide successful prognoses of meningitis cases regardless of the causative agent.

ACKNOWLEDGMENTS

The author would like to acknowledge the document delivery system personnel in the library of the Jordan University of Science and Technology.

REFERENCES

[1]   Abdeldaim, G.M., Strålin, K., Korsgaard, J., Blomberg, J., Welinder-Olsson, C., Herrmann, B. (2010) Multiplex quantitative PCR for detection of lower respiratory tract infection and meningitis caused by *Streptococcus pneumoniae, Haemophilus influenzae* and *Neisseria meningitidis. BMC Microbiol.*,10,310.

[2]   Almuzara, M.N., Vazquez, M., Tanaka, N., Turco, M., Ramirez, M.S., Lopez, E.L., Pasteran, F., Rapoport, M., Procopio, A., Vay, CA.(2010) First case of human infection due to *Pseudomonas fulva*, an environmental bacterium isolated from cerebrospinal fluid. *J. Clin.Microbiol.*, 48, 660-664.

[3]   Al Kandari, M., Jamal, W., Udo, E.E., El Sayed, A., Al Shammri, S., Rotimi, V.O. (2010) A case of community-onset meningitis caused by hospital methicillin-resistant *Staphylococcus aureus* successfully treated with linezolid and rifampicin. *Med. Princ.Pract.*, 19, 235-239.

[4]   Amaya–villar, R., Carcia-cabrera, E., Sullerio-lgual, E., Fernandez-viladrich, P., Catalan-alonso, P., Rodrigo-gonzalo de liria, C., Coloma-conde, A., Grill-diaz, F., Guerreo-espejo, A., Pachon, G., Prats-pastor, G. (2010)Three-year multicenter survillance of community-acquired *Listeria monocytogenes* meningitis in adults. *BMC infect. Dis.*, 10, 2-8.

[5]   Arda, B., Sipahi, O.R., Atalay, S., Ulusoy, S. (2008) Pooled analysis of 2,408 cases of acute adult purulent meningitis from Turkey. *Med. Princ.Pract.*, 17, 76-79.

[6]   Arosio, M., Nozza, F., Rizzi, M., Ruggeri, M., Casella, P., Beretta, G., Raglio, A., Goglio, A. (2008) Evaluation of the MicroSeq 500 16S rDNA-based gene sequencing for the diagnosis of culture-negative bacterial meningitis. *New Microbiol.*, 31, 343-349.

[7]   Azzar, I. C., Moriondo, M., Indolfi, G., Massai, C., Becciolini, L., de Martino, M., Resti, M. (2008)Molecular detection methods and serotyping performed directly on clinical samples improve diagnostic sensitivity and reveal increased incidence of invasive disease by *Streptococcuspneumoniae* in Italian children. *J. Med. Microbiol.*, 57(Pt 10), 1205-1212.

[8]   Backman, A., Lantz, P. G., Radstrom, P. and Olcen, P. (1999) Evaluation of an extended diagnostic PCR assay for detection and verification of the common causes of bacterial meningitis in CSF and other biological samples. *Mol. Cell Probes*, 13, 49-60.

[9]   Batuwanthudawe, R., Rajapakse, L., Somaratne, P., Dassanayake, M., Abeysinghe, N. (2010) Incidence of childhood *Haemophilus influenzae* type b meningitis in Sri Lanka. *Int. J. Infect. Dis.*, 14, e372-6.

[10] Belo, E.F., Farhat, C.K., Gaspari, E.N. (2010) Comparison of dot-ELISA and standard ELISA for detection of *Neisseria meningitidis* outer membrane complex-specific antibodies. *Braz. J. Infect. Dis.*, 14, 35-40.

[11] Bøving, M.K., Pedersen, L.N., Møller, J.K. (2009) Eight-plex PCR and liquid-array detection of bacterial and viral pathogens in cerebrospinal fluid from patients with suspected meningitis. *J. Clin.Microbiol.*, 47, 908-13.

[12] Bröker, M. (2009) Burden of invasive disease caused by *Haemophilus influenzae*type b in Asia. *Jpn. J. Infect. Dis.*, 62, 87-92.

[13] Brouwer, M.C., Keizerweerd, G.D., De Gans, J., Spanjaard, L., Van De Beek, D. (2009) Community acquired *Staphylococcus aureus* meningitis in adults. *Scand. J. Infect. Dis.*, 41, 375-377.

[14] Byrd, T.F., Davis, L. E., (2007) Multidrug-resistant tuberculous meningitis. *Curr. Neurol. Neurosci. Rep.* 7, 470-475.

[15] Carbonnelle, E. (2009). Laboratory diagnosis of bacterial meningitis: usefulness of various tests for the determination of the etiological agent. *Med. Mal. Infect.*, 39, 581-605.

[16] Cartwright, K. (2002) Pneumococcal disease in Western Europe: burden of disease, antibiotic resistance and management. *Eur. J. Pediatr.*, 161, 188–195.

[17] Czerkinsky, C., Nilsson, L., Nygren, H., Ouchterlony, O., Tarkowski, A. (1983) A solid-phase enzyme-linked immunospot (ELISPOT) assay for enumeration of specific antibody-secreting cells. *J. Immunol. Methods* 65, 109-121.

[18] Centers for Disease Control and Prevention (CDC) (2007) Emergence of antimicrobial-resistant serotype 19A *Streptococcus pneumoniae*-Massachusetts, 2001-2006. *MMWR Morb. Mortal. Wkly. Rep.*, 56, 1077-1080.

[19] Chakrabarti, P., Das, B.K., Kapil, A. (2009)Application of 16S rDNA based seminested PCR for diagnosis of acute bacterial meningitis. *Indian J. Med. Res.*, 129, 182-8.

[20] Chen, L.H., Duan, Q.J., Cai, M.T., Wu, Y.D., Shang, S.Q. (2009)Rapid diagnosis of sepsis and Rbacterial meningitis in children with real-time fluorescent quantitative polymerase chain reaction amplification in the bacterial 16S rRNA gene. *Clin. Pediatr. (Phila)*, 48, 641-647.

[21] Chen, T.L., Thien, P.F., Liaw, S.C., Fung, C.P., Siu, L.K. (2005) First report of *Salmonella enterica* serotype Panama meningitis associated with consumption of contaminated breast milk by a neonate, *J. Clin.Microbiol.*, 43, 5400-5402.

[22] Cherian, T., Lalitha, M.K., Manoharan, A., Thomas, K., Yolken, R.H., Steinhoff, M.C. (1998) PCR-Enzyme immunoassay for detection of *Streptococcus pneumoniae* DNA in cerebrospinal fluid samples from patients with culture-negative meningitis. *J. Clin.Microbiol.*, 36, 3605-3608.

[23] Chiba, N., Murayama, S.Y., Morozumi, M., Nakayama, E., Okada, T., Iwata, S., Sunakawa, K., Ubukata, K. (2009) Rapid detection of eight causative pathogens for the diagnosis of bacterial meningitis by real-time PCR. *J. Infect.Chemother.*, 15, 92-98.

[24] Chiu, C. H., Chu, C., Su, L. H., Wu, W. Y., Wu, T. L. (2002) Characterization of a laboratory-derived high-level ampicillin-resistant *Salmonella enterica* serovar Typhimurium starin that caused meningitis in an infant. *Antimicrob.Agents chemother.*, 46,1604-1606.

[25] Cho, H.K., Lee, H., Kang, J.H., Kim, K.N., Kim, D.S., Kim, Y.K., Kim, J.S., Kim, J.H., Kim, C.H., Kim, H.M., Park, S.E., Oh, S.H., Chung, E.H., Cha, S.H., Choi, Y.Y., Hur, J.K., Hong, Y.J., Lee, H.J., Kim, K.H. (2010) The causative organisms of bacterial meningitis in Korean children in 1996-2005. *J. Korean Med. Sci.*, 25, 895-899.

[26] Choudhury, S.A., Berthaud, V., Weitkamp, J.H. (2006) Meningitis caused by *Salmonella panama* in infants. *J. Natl. Med. Assoc.*, 98, 219-22.

[27] Christie, L. J., Honarmand, S., Talkington, D. F., Gavali, S. S., Preas, C., Pan, C. Y., Yagi, S., Glaster, C. A. (2007) Pediatric encephalitis: what is the role of *Mycoplasma pneumoniae*? *Pediatrics,* 120, 305-313.

[28] Chua, T., Moore, C.L., Perri, M.B., Donabedian, S.M., Masch, W., Vager, D., Davis, S.L., Lulek, K., Zimnicki, B., Zervos, M.J. (2008)Molecular epidemiology of methicillin-resistant *Staphylococcus aureus* bloodstream isolates in urban Detroit. *J. Clin.Microbiol.,*46, 2345-2352.

[29] Cooke, F.J., Ginwalla, S., Hampton, M.D., Wain, J., Ross-Russell, R., Lever, A., Farrington, M. (2009) Report of neonatal meningitis due to *Salmonella enterica* serotype Agona and review of breast milk-associated neonatal *Salmonella* infections. *J.Clin.Microbiol.*, 47, 3045-3049.

[30] Corless, C.E., Guiver, M., Borrow, R., Edwards-Jones, V., Fox, A.J., Kaczmarski, E.B. (2001)Simultaneous detection of *Neisseria meningitidis, Haemophilus influenzae*, and *Streptococcus pneumoniae* in suspected cases of meningitis and septicemia using real-time PCR. *J. Clin.Microbiol.,*39, 1553-1558.

[31] Cunha, B. A., Fatehpuria, R. and Eisentein, L. E. (2007) *Listeria monocytogenes* encephalitis mimicking Herpes simplex virus encephalistis: the defferential diagnositc improtances of cerbrsopinal fluid lactic acid levels. *Heart and Lung*, 36, 226-231.

[32] Dagan, R., Shriker, O., Hazan, I., Leibovitz, E., Greenberg, D., Schlaeffer, F., Levy, R. (1998) Prospective study to determine clinical relevance of detection of pneumococcal DNA in sera of children by PCR. *J. Clin.Microbiol.*, 36, 669-73.

[33] de Filippis, I., do Nascimento, C.R., Clementino, M.B., Sereno, A.B., Rebelo, C., Souza, N.N., Riley, L.W. (2005) Rapid detection of *Neisseria meningitidis* in cerebrospinal fluid by one-step polymerase chain reaction of the nspA gene. *Diagn. Microbiol. Infect. Dis.*, 51, 85-90.

[34] Deutch, S., Møller, J.K., Ostergaard, L. (2008) Combined assay for two-hour identification of *Streptococcus pneumoniae* and *Neisseria meningitidis* and concomitant detection of 16S ribosomal DNA in cerebrospinal fluid by real-time PCR. *Scand. J. Infect. Dis.*, 40, 607-14.

[35] Dolan Thomas, J., Hatcher, C.P., Satterfield, D.A., Theodore, M.J., Bach, M.C., Linscott, K.B., Zhao, X., Wang, X., Mair, R., Schmink, S., Arnold, K.E., Stephens, D.S., Harrison, L.H., Hollick, R.A., Andrade, A.L., Lamaro-Cardoso, J., de Lemos, A.P., Gritzfeld, J., Gordon, S., Soysal, A., Bakir, M., Sharma, D., Jain, S., Satola, S.W., Messonnier, N.E., Mayer, L.W. (2011) SodC-Based Real-Time PCR for Detection of *Neisseria meningitidis. PLoS One*, 6,e19361.

[36] Durdik, P., Fedor, M., Jesenak, M., Hamzikova, J., Knotkova, H., Banovcin, P. (2010)*Staphylococcus intermedius*; rare pathogen of acute meningitis. *Int. J. Infect. Dis.*, 14 Suppl 3, e236-238.

[37] Failace, L., Wagner, M., Chesky, M.,Scalco, R.,Jobim, L.F .(2005) Simultaneous detection of *Neisseria meningitidis, Haemophilus influenzae* and *Streptococcus*spp. by polymerase chain reaction for the diagnosis of bacterial meningitis. *Arq. Neuropsiquiatr.*, 63, 920-924.

[38] Fazio, C., Neri, A., Tonino, S., Carannante, A., Caporali, M.G., Salmaso, S., Mastrantonio, P., Stefanelli, P. (2009) Characterisation of

Neisseria meningitidis C strains causing two clusters in the north of Italy in 2007 and 2008. *Euro Surveill,* 14 pii: 19179.

[39]   Findlow, H., Vogel, U., Mueller, J.E., Curry, A., Njanpop-Lafourcade, B.M., Claus, H., Gray, S.J., Yaro, S., Traoré, Y., Sangaré, L., Nicolas, P., Gessner, B.D., Borrow, R., (2007) Three cases of invasive meningococcal disease caused by a capsule null locus strain circulating among healthy carriers in Burkina Faso. *J. Infect. Dis.,* 195, 1071-1077.

[40]   Fitch, M. T., van de Beek, D. (2007) Emergency diagnosis and treatment of adult meningitis. *Lancet infect. Dis.,* 7, 191-200.

[41]   Fraisier, C., Stor, R., Tenebray, B., Sanson, Y., Nicolas, P., (2009)Use of a new single multiplex PCR-based assay for direct simultaneous characterization of six *Neisseria meningitidis* serogroups. *J. Clin.Microbiol.,* 47, 2662-6.

[42]   Friedemann, M. (2009) Epidemiology of invasive neonatal *Cronobacter* (*Enterobacter sakazakii*) infections. *Eur. J. Clin. Microbiol. Infect. Dis.,* 28, 1297-1304.

[43]   Gallagher, P. G (1990) *Enterobacter* bacteremia in pediatric patients. *Rev. Infect. Dis.* 12, 808-812.

[44]   Gille-Johnson, P., Kövamees, J., Lindgren, V., Aufwerber, E., Struve, J. (2000) *Salmonella virchow* meningitis in an adult. *Scand. J. Infect. Dis.,* 32, 431-433.

[45]   Goyo, D., Camacho, A., Gómez, C., de Las Heras, R.S., Otero, J,R., Chaves, F. (2009)False-positive PCR detection of *Tropheryma whipplei* in cerebrospinal fluid and biopsy samples from a child with chronic lymphocytic meningitis. *J. Clin.Microbiol.,* 47,3783-3784.

[46]   Grant, R.J., Whitehead, T.R., Orr, J.E. (2000) *Streptococcus bovis* meningitis in an infant. *J. Clin.Microbiol.,* 38, 462-463.

[47]   Gray, K.J., Bennett, S.L., French, N., Phiri, A.J., Graham, S.M. (2007) Invasive group B streptococcal infection in infants, Malawi. *Emerg. Infect. Dis.,* 13, 223-229.

[48]   Gray, L. D., Fedorko, D. P. (1992) Laboratory diagnosis of bacterial meningitis. *Clin. Microbiol. Rev.,* 5, 130-145.

[49]   Gurtler, J.B., Kornacki, J.L., Beuchat, L. (2005) *Enterobacter sakazakii*: A coliform of increased concern to infant health. *Int. J. Food Microbiol.,* 104, 1-34.

[50]   Haldar, S., Sharma, N., Gupta, V.K., Tyagi, J.S. (2009)Efficient diagnosis of tuberculous meningitis by detection of *Mycobacterium tuberculosis* DNA in cerebrospinal fluid filtrates using PCR.*J. Med. Microbiol.,* 58(Pt 5), 616-624.

[51] Hart, C. A., Cuevas, L. E. (1997) Meningococcal diseases in Africa. *Ann. Trop. Med. Parasitol.*, 91, 777-785.

[52] Hassan, A. A., Akineden, O., Kress, C., Estuningsih, S., Schneider, E., Usleber, E. (2007) Characterization of the gene encoding the 16S rRNA of *Enterobacter sakazakii* and development of a species-specific PCR method. *Int. J. Food Microbiol.*, 116, 214-220.

[53] Healy, B., Cooney, S., O'Brien, S., Iversen, C., Whyte, P., Nally, J., Callanan, J.J., Fanning, S. (2010) *Cronobacter* (*Enterobacter sakazakii*): an opportunistic foodborne pathogen.*Foodborne Pathog. Dis.*, 339-350.

[54] Hedberg, S.T., Olcén, P., Fredlund, H., Mölling, P. (2009) Real-time PCR detection of five prevalent bacteria causing acute meningitis. *APMIS*, 117, 856-860.

[55] Hoang. L.M., Thomas, E., Tyler, S., Pollard, A.J., Stephens, G., Gustafson, L., Mc, Nabb, A., Pococ,. I., Tsang, R., Tan, R. (2005). Rapid and fatal meningococcal disease due to a strain of *Neisseria meningitidis* containing the capsule null locus. *Clin. Infect. Dis.*, 40, e38-42.

[56] Hoffman, J.A., Mason, E.O., Schutze, G.E., Tan, T.Q., Barson, W.J., Givner. L.B., Wald, E.R., Bradley, J.S., Yogev, R., Kaplan, S.L. (2003) *Streptococcus pneumoniae* infections in the neonate. *Pediatrics,* 112, 1095-1102.

[57] Hsieh, Y.C., Lee, W.S., Shao, P.L., Chang, L.Y., Huang, L.M. (2008) The transforming *Streptococcus pneumoniae* in the 21st century. *Chang. Gung. Med. J.,* 31, 117-24.

[58] Hsu, K.K., Shea, K.M., Stevenson, A.E., Pelton, SI.; Massachusetts Department of Public Health. (2010) Changing serotypes causing childhood invasive pneumococcal disease: Massachusetts, 2001-2007. *Pediatr. Infect. Dis. J.,* 29, 289-293.

[59] Huang, C. R., Lu, C. H., Wu, J. J., Chang, H. W., Chien, C. C., Lei, C. B., Chang, W. N. (2005)Coagulase-negative Staphylococcal meningitis in adults; Clinical characteristics and therapeutic outcomes. *Infection,* 33, 56-60.

[60] Huang, H.J., Xiang, D.R., Sheng, J.F., Li, J., Pan, X.P., Yu, H.Y., Sheng, G.P., Li, L.J. (1999) rpoB nested PCR and sequencing for the early diagnosis of tuberculous meningitis and rifampicin resistance. *J. Hosp. Infect.,* 42, 205-212.

[61] Iversen, C., Druggan, P. Forsythe, S. J. (2004) A selective differential medium for *Enterobacter sakazakii*; a prelimianry study. *Int. J. Food Microbiol.* 96, 133-139.

[62] Iversen, C. Forsythe, S. J. (2007) Comparison of media for the isolation of *Enterobacter sakazakii*. *Appl. Environ.Micrbiol.*, 73, 48-52.

[63] Iversen, C., Lehner, A., Mullane, N., Bidlas, E., Cleenwerck, I., Marugg, J., Fanning, S., Stephan, R., Joosten, H. (2007) The taxonomy of *Enterobacter sakazakii*: proposal of a new genus *Cronobacter* gen. nov. and descriptions of *Cronobacter sakazakii* comb. no. *Cronobacter sakazakii* subsp. *sakazakii*, comb.nov.,*Cronobacter sakazakii* subsp.*malonaticus* subsp. Nov., *Cronobacter dublinensis* sp. Nov. and *Cronobactergenomospecies* I. *BMC Evolut. Biol.*, 7, 46.

[64] Iversen, C., Mullane, M., McCardell, B., Tall, B.D., Lehner, A., Fanning, S., Stephan, R., Joosten, H. (2008) *Cronobacter*gen. nov., a new genus to accommodate the biogroups of *Enterobacter sakazakii*, and proposal of *Cronobacter sakazakii* gen. nov., comb. nov., C. *malonaticus* sp. nov., C. *turicensis*, sp. nov., C. *muytjensii* sp. nov., C. *dublinensis* sp. nov., *Cronobacter genomospecies* I, and of three subspecies. C. *dublinensis* sp. nov. subsp. *dublinensis* subsp. nov. C. *dublinensis* sp. nov. subsp. *Lausannensis* subsp. nov., and C. *dublinensis* sp. nov. subsp. *lactaridi* subsp. Nov. *Int. J. Sys. Evol. Microbiol.* 58, 1442-1447.

[65] Isaacs, D. (2003) Australasian Study Group for Neonatal Infections. A ten year, multicentre study of coagulase negative staphylococcal infections in Australasian neonatal units.*Arch. Dis. Child. Fetal. Neonatal. Ed.,* 88, F89-93.

[66] Jackson, K.A., Iwamoto,M. and swerdlow,D. (2010) Pregnancy-associated listeriosos. *Epidemiol.Infect.,* 138, 1503-1509.

[67] Jamal, W.Y., Al_shomari, S. , Boland, F., Rotimi, V.O .(2005) *Listeria monocytogenes* meningitis in an immunocompetent adult patient. *Med.Princ.Pract.,* 14, 55-57.

[68] Jarvis, K. G., Grim, C. J., Franco, A. A., Gopinath, G., Sathyamoorthy, V., Hu, L., Sadowski, J., Lee, C., Tall, B. D (2011) Molecular Chcterization of *Cronobacter*lipopolysaccharide O-Antigen gene clusters and development of serotype-specific PCR assays. *Appl. Environ. Microbiol.* 77, 4017-4026.

[69] Jaradat, Z. W., Ababneh, Q. O. Saadoun, I. M., Samara, N. A., Rashdan, A.M. (2009) Isolation of *Cronobacter*spp. (Formerly *Enterobacter sakazakii*) from infant food, herbs and environmental samples and the subsequent identification and confirmation of the isolates using biochemical, chromogenic assays, PCR and 16S rRNA sequencing. *BMC Microbiol.* 9, 225.

[70] Jaradat, Z. W., Schutze, G. E., Bhuni, A. K. (2000) Genetic homogeneity among *Listeria monocytogenes* strains from infected patients and meat products from two geographic locations determined by phenotyping, ribotyping and PCR analysis of virulence genes. *Int. J. Food Microbiol.*, 76, 1-10.

[71] Jaton, K., Sahli, R., Bille, J. (1992) Development of polymerase chain reaction assays for detection of *Listeria monocytogenes* in clinical cerebrospinal fluid samples. *J. Clin.Microbiol.*, 30,1931-1936.

[72] Joachim, A., Matee, M.I., Massawe, F.A., Lyamuya,E.F.(2009) Maternal and neonatal 132eningitidis of group B *Streptococcus* at Muhimbili National Hospital in Dar es Salaam, Tanzania: prevalence, risk factors and antimicrobial resistance. *BMC Public Health* 9,437.

[73] Kang, Sil, E., Nam, Y. S. and Hong, K. W. (2007) Rapid detection of *Enterobacter sakazakii* using TaqMan real-time PCR assay. *J. Microbiol.Biotechnol.,*17, 516-519.

[74] Kashyap, R.S., Kainthla, R.P., Mudaliar, A.V., Purohit, H.J., Taori, G.M., Daginawala, H.F. (2006)Cerebrospinal fluid adenosine deaminase activity: a complimentary tool in the early diagnosis of tuberculous meningitis. *Cerebrospinal Fluid Res.*, 3, 1-6.

[75] Katti, M.K. (2004) Pathogenesis, diagnosis, treatment and outcome aspects of cerebral tuberculosis. *Med. Sc. Monit.*, 10, RA215-RA229.

[76] Ke, D., Ménard, C., Picard, F.J., Boissinot, M., Ouellette, M., Roy, P.H., Bergeron, M.G. (2000) Development of conventional and real-time PCR assays for the rapid detection of group B Streptococci. *Clin. Chem.*, 46, 324-31.

[77] Kiliç, A.U., Altay, F.A., Gürbüz, Y., Otgun, S.N., Sencan, I. (2010) *Haemophilus influenzae* serotype e meningitis in an adult. *J. Infect.Dev.Ctries.*, 4,253-5.

[78] Killoran, P.B., O'Connell, J., Mothershed, E.A., Probert, W.S. (2006) Rapid laboratory detection of meningococcal disease outbreaks caused by serogroup C *Neisseria meningitidis. J. Microbiol. Methods*, 67, 330-8./fr1

[79] Kothary, M. H., McCardell, B. A., Frazar, C. D., Deer, D., Tall, B. D. (2007) Characterization of the zinc-containing metalloprotease encoded by zpx and development of a species-specific detection method for *Enterobacter sakazakii. Appl. Environ.Microbiol.*,73, 4142-4151.

[80] Lee, J. E., Cho, W. K., Nam, C. H., Jung, M. H., Kang, J. H. and Suh, B. K.(2010) A case of meningoencephalitis caused by *Listeria monocytogenes* in ahealthy child, 53, 653-656.

[81] Lee, W.S., Puthucheary, S.D., Omar, A. (1999) *Salmonella* meningitis and its complications in infants.*J. Paediatr. Child Health*, 35, 379-82.

[82] Lehner, A., Nitzsche, S., Breeuwer, P., Diep, B., Thelen, K., Stephan, R. (2006) Comparison of two chromogenic media and evaluation of two molecular based identification systems for *Enterobacter sakazakii*detection. *BMC Microbiol.* 6,15.

[83] Lehner, A., Riedel, K., Rattei, T., Ruepp, A., Frishman, D., Breeuwer, P., Diep, B., Eberl, L., Stephan, R. (2006) Molecular characterization of the glucosidaseactivity in *Enterobacter sakazakii* reveals the presence of a putative gene cluster for palatinose metabolism. *Syst. Appl. Microbiol.* 29, 609-625.

[84] Lehner, A., Stephan, R. (2004) Microbiological, epidemiological, and food safety aspects of *Enterobacter sakazakii. J. Food Prot.,* 67, 2850-2857.

[85] Lindblom, A., Severinson, K., Nilsson, K. (2010) Rickettsia felis infection in Sweden: report of two cases with subacute meningitis and review of the literature. *Scand. J. Infect. Dis.*, 42, 906-909.

[86] Liu, Y., Gao, Q., Zhang, X., Hou ,Y., Yang, J., Huang, X. (2006) PCR and oligonucleotide array for detection of *Enterobacter sakazakii* in infant formula. *Mol.Cell Probe.*, 20, 11-17.

[87] Lu, CH., Chang, W.N. (2000)Adults with meningitis caused by oxacillin-resistant *Staphylococcus aureus. Clin. Infect. Dis.*, 31, 723-727.

[88] Lu, C.H., Huang, C.R., Chang, W.N., Chang, C.J., Cheng, B.C., Lee, P.Y., Lin, M.W., Chang, H.W. (2002) Community-acquired bacterial meningitis in adults: the epidemiology, timing of appropriate antimicrobial therapy, and prognostic factors. *Clin. Neurol. Surg.*, 104, 352-358.

[89] Lu, J.J., Perng, C.L., Lee, S.Y., Wan, C.C. (2000) Use of PCR with universal primers and restriction endonuclease digestions for detection and identification of common bacterial pathogens in cerebrospinal fluid. *J. Clin.Microbiol.*, 38, 2076-80.

[90] Lun, Z.R., Wang, Q.P., Chen, X.G., Li, A.X., Zhu, X.Q. (2007) *Streptococcus suis*: an emerging zoonotic pathogen. *Lancet Infect. Dis.,* 7, 201-209.

[91] Lynch, J.P. 3rd, Zhanel, G.G. (2010) *Streptococcus pneumoniae*: epidemiology and risk factors, evolution of antimicrobial resistance, and impact of vaccines. *Curr. Opin. Pulm Med.*, 16, 217-25.

[92] Maestro, B., Sanz, J.M. (2007) Novel approaches to fight *Streptococcus pneumoniae.Recent Pat Antiinfect. Drug Discov.*, 2, 188-196.

[93] Martin, D. R., Walker, S. J., Baker, M. G., Lennon, D. R. (1998) New Zealand epidemic of meningococcal disease identified by a strain with phenotype B:4:P1. *A. J. Infect. Dis.,* 177, 497-500.

[94] Menezes, G.A., Harish, B.N., Parija, SC. (2008) A case of fatal acute pyogenic meningitis in a neonate caused by extended-spectrum beta-lactamase producing *Salmonella* group B. *Jpn. J. Infect. Dis.*, 61, 234-235.

[95] Messer, R.D., Warnock, T.H., Heazlewood, R.J., Hanna, J.N. (1997)*Salmonella* meningitis in children in far north Queensland. *J. Paediatr. Child Health,* 33, 535-8.

[96] Mitchell, A.M., Mitchell, T.J. (2010) *Streptococcus pneumonia*: virulence factors and variation. *Clin.Microbiol.Infect.*, 16, 411-418.

[97] MMWR Morb Mortal Wkly Rep. (2009)*Cronobacter* species isolation in two infants-New Mexico.*CDC*, 58, 1179-1183.

[98] Mullane, N., O'Gaora, P., Nally, J. E., Iversen, C., Whyte, P., Wall, P. G., Fanning, S. (2008) Molecular analysis of the *Enterobacter sakazakii* O-antigen gene locus. *Appl. Environ. Microbiol.*, 74, 3783-3794.

[99] Morozumi, M., Nakayama, E., Iwata, S., Aoki, Y., Hasegawa, K., Kobayashi, R., Chiba, N., Tajima, T., Ubukata, K and the acute respiratory diseases study group. (2006) Simultaneous detection of pathogens in clinical samples from patients with community-acquired pneumonia by real-time PCR with pathogen-specific molecular beacon probes. *J. Clin.Microbiol.*, 44, 1440-1446.

[100] Moxon, E.R. (2009) Bacterial variation, virulence and vaccines. *Microbiology,* 155, 997-1003.

[101] Myint, M. S., Johnson, Y.J., Tablante, N. L., Heckert, R. A. (2006) The effect of pre-enrichment protocol on the sensitivity and specificity of PCR for detection of naturally contaminated *Salmonella* in raw poultry compared to conventional culture. *Food Microbiol.,* 23, 599-604.

[102] Nair, M. K. M., Venkitanarayanan, K. S. (2006) Cloning and Sequencing of theompA Gene of *Enterobacter sakazakii* and development of an ompA-targeted PCR for rapid detection of *Enterobacter sakazakii* in infant formula. *Appl. Environ.Microbiol.*, 72, 2539-2546.

[103] Nghiem, P.P., Schatzberg, S.J. (2010) Conventional and molecular diagnostic testing for the acute neurologic patient. *J. Vet. Emerg. Crit. Care (San Antonio),*20, 46-61.

[104] Ni, H., Knight, A.I., Cartwright, K., Palmer, W.H., McFadden, J. (1992) Polymerase chain reaction for diagnosis of meningococcal meningitis.*Lancet,* 340, 1432-1434.

[105] O'Brien, K.L., Wolfson, L.J., Watt, J.P., Henkle, E., Deloria-Knoll, M., McCall, N., Lee, E., Mulholland, K., Levine, O.S., Cherian, T.; Hib and Pneumococcal Global Burden of Disease Study Team (2009) Burden of disease caused by *Streptococcus pneumoniae* in children younger than 5 years: global estimates. *Lancet,* 374, 893-902.

[106] OhAiseadha, C.O., Dunne, O.M., Desmond, F., O'Connor, M. (2010) *Salmonella* meningitis and septicaemia in an non-immunocompromised adult, associated with a cluster of *Salmonella Enteritidis* PT 14b, Ireland, November 2009. *Euro Surveill,* 15(7). pii: 19489.

[107] Overturf, G.D.(2005) Defining bacterial meningitis and other infections of the central nervous system. *Pediatr. Crit. Care Med.,* 6(3 Suppl), S14-18.

[108] Ozaki, T., Nishimura, N., Arakawa, Y., Suzuki, M., Narita, A., Yamamoto, Y., Koyama, N., Nakane, K., Yasuda, N., Funahashi, K.(2009) Community-acquired *Acinetobacter baumannii* meningitis in a previously healthy 14-month-old boy. *J. Infect.Chemother.,* 15, 322-324.

[109] Pedersen, M., Benfield, T.L., Skinhoej, P., Jensen, A.G. (2006) Haematogenous *Staphylococcus aureus* meningitis. A 10-year nationwide study of 96 consecutive cases. *BMC Infect. Dis.,* 16, 49.

[110] Perez A. E., Dickinson F. E. and Rodríguez, M. (2010) Community acquired bacterial meningitis in Cuba: a follow up of a decade. *BMC Infect. Dis.,* 10,130.

[111] Perez, J. M. H., Hernandez, R. L. and Gil, P. U. (2008) Nosocomial infection caused by *Listeria monocytogenes* in a patient with a lung transplant. *Online Archivos DE Bronconeumologia,* 44,1.

[112] Pilishvili, T., Lexau, C., Farley, M. M., Hadler, J., Harrison, L. H., Bennett, N. M., Reingold, A., Thomas, A., Schaffner, W., Craig, A. S., Smith, P. J., Beall, B. W., Whitney, C. G. Moore, M. R. (2010) Sustained reductions in invasive pneumococcal disease in the era of conjugate vaccine. *J. Infect. Dis.,* 201, 32-41.

[113] Pingle, M.R., Granger, K., Feinberg, P., Shatsky, R., Sterling, B., Rundell, M., Spitzer, E., Larone, D., Golightly, L., Barany, F. (2007) Multiplexed identification of blood-borne bacterial pathogens by use of a novel 16S rRNA gene PCR-ligase detection reaction-capillary electrophoresis assay. *J. Clin.Microbiol.,* 45, 1927-1935.

[114] Pintado, V., Meseguer, M., Fortún, J., Cobo, J., Navas, E., Quereda, C., Corral I., Moreno, S. (2002) Clinical study of 44 cases of *Staphylococcus aureus* meningitis. *Eur. J. Clin. Microbiol. Infect. Dis.* 21, 864-868.

[115] Rådström, P., Bäckman, A., Qian, N., Kragsbjerg, P., Påhlson, C., Olcén, P. (1994) Detection of bacterial DNA in cerebrospinal fluid by an assay for simultaneous detection of *Neisseria meningitidis, Haemophilus influenzae*, and Streptococci using a seminested PCR strategy.*J.Clin.Microbiol.*, 32, 2738-2744.

[116] Rahn, K., De Grandis, S. A., Clarke, R. C., McEwen, S. A., Galan, J. E., Ginocchio, C., Curtiss III, R., Gyles, C. L. (1992) Amplification of an *invA* gene sequence of *Salmonella typhimurium* by polymerase chain reaction as a specific method of detection of *Salmonella. Mol. Cell Probes,* 6, 271-279.

[117] Ritchie, S.R., Rupali, P., Roberts, S.A., Thomas, M.G. (2007) Flucloxacillin treatment of *Staphylococcus aureus* meningitis.*Eur. J. Clin. Microbiol. Infect. Dis.*, 26, 501-504.

[118] Rosenstein, N. E., Perkins, B. A., Stephens, D. S., Popovic, T., Hughes, J.M. (2001) Meningococcal disease. *N. Eng. J. Me*d., 344, 1378-1388.

[119] Rothman, R., Ramachandran, P., Yang, S., Hardick, A., Won, H., Kecojevic, A., Quianzon, C., Hsieh, Y.H., Gaydos, C. (2010) Use of quantitative broad-based polymerase chain reaction for detection and identification of common bacterial pathogens in cerebrospinal fluid. *Acad. Emerg. Med.*, 17, 741-747.

[120] Rudan, I., Campbell, H. (2009) The deadly toll of *S.pneumoniae* and *H. influenzae* type b. *Lancet,* 374, 854-856.

[121] Saha, SK., Darmstadt, G.L., Yamanaka, N., Billal, D.S., Nasreen, T., Islam, M., Hamer, D.H. (2005) Rapid diagnosis of pneumococcal meningitis: implications for treatment and measuring disease burden. *Pediatr. Infect. Dis. J.,* 24, 1093-8.

[122] Saruta, K., Matsunaga, T., Kono, M., Hoshina, S., Kanemoto, S., Sakai, O., Machida, K. (1997) Simultaneous detection of *Streptococcus pneumoniae* and *Haemophilus influenzae* by nested PCR amplification from cerebrospinal fluid samples. *FEMS Immunol. Med. Microbiol.*, 19, 151-157.

[123] Schuchat. A., Robinson, K., Wenger .J, Harrison .L, Farley. M,Reingold ,A. , Lefkowitz, L., Perkins, B. (1997) Bacterial Meningitis in the united states in 1995, *N. Eng. J. Med.*, 33 , 970-976.

[124] Smith, K., Diggle, M.A., Clarke, S.C. (2004) Automation of a fluorescence-based multiplex PCR for the laboratory confirmation of common bacterial pathogens. *J. Med. Microbiol.*, 53, 115-7.

[125] Stone, G. G., Oberst, R. D., Hays, M. P., Mcvey, S., Chengappa, M. M. (1994) Detection of *Salmonella* serovars from clinical samples by enrichment broth cultivation-PCR procedure. *J. Clin.Microbiol.*, 32, 1742-1749.

[126] Seo, K. H., Brackett, R. E. (2005) Rapid, Specific Detection of *Enterobacter sakazakii* in Infant Formula Using a Real-Time PCR Assay. *J. Food Prot.*, 68, 59-63.

[127] Stoop, B., Lehner, A., Iversen, C., Fanning, S., Stephan, R. (2009) Development and evaluation of rpoB based PCR systems to differentiate the six proposed species within the genus *Cronobacter. Int. J. Food Microbiol.*136, 165-168.

[128] Sun, Y., Wang, M., Liu, H., Wang, J., He, X., Zeng, J., Guo, X., Li, K., Cao, B. Wang, L. (2011) Development of an O-Antigen Serotyping Scheme for *Cronobacter sakazakii. Appl. Environ.Microbiol.*, 77, 2209-2214.

[129] Taha, M. K. (2000) Simultaneous approach for nonculture PCR-based identification and serogroup prediction of *Neisseria meningitidis. J. Clin.Microbiol.*, 38,855-857.

[130] Taha, M.K., (2002) Molecular detection and characterization of *Neisseria meningitidis. Expert. Rev. Mol. Diagn.*, 2, 143-150.

[131] Taha, M.K., Olcén, P. (2004) Molecular genetics methods in diagnosis and direct characterization of acute bacterial central nervous system infections. *APMIS,* 112, 753-770.

[132] Takahashi, T., Nakayama, T. (2006) Novel technique of quantitative nested real time polymerase chain reaction assay for *Mycobacterium tuberculosis*DNA. *J. Clin.Microbiol.*, 44, 1029-1039.

[133] Takahashi, T., Nakayama, T., Tamura, M., Ogawa, K., Tsuda, H., Morita, A. (2005) Nested polymerase chain reaction for assessing the clinical course of tuberculous meningitis. *Neurology,* 64, 1789-1793.

[134] Takahashi, T., Tamura, M., Asami, Y., Kitamura, E., Saito, K., Suzuki, T., Takahashi, S.N., Matsumoto, K., Sawada, S., Yokoyama, E., Takasu, T. (2008) Novel wide-range quantitative nested real-time PCR assay for *Mycobacterium tuberculosis* DNA: development and methodology. *J. Clin.Microbiol.*, 46, 1708-1715.

[135] Takahashi, T., Tamura, M., Takahashi, S.N., Matsumoto, K., Sawada, S., Yokoyama, E., Nakayama, T., Mizutani, T., Takasu, T., Nagase, H.

(2007) Quantitative nested real-time PCR assay for assessing the clinical course of tuberculous meningitis. *J. Neurol. Sci.*, 255, 69-76.

[136] Talati, N.J., Rouphael, N., Kuppalli, K., Franco-Paredes, C. (2007) Spectrum of CNS disease caused by rapidly growing *Mycobacteria. Lancet Infect. Dis.*, 8, 390-398.

[137] Tang, Y. W., Procop, G. W., Persing, D. H. (1997) Molecular diagnosis of infectious diseases. *Clin. Chem.*, 43, 2021-2038.

[138] Thwaites, G. E., Hien, T. T. (2005) Tuberculous meningitis: many questions, too few answers. *Lancet Neurol.*, 4, 160-170.

[139] Thwaites, G., Caws, M., Chau, T.T., D'Sa, A., Lan, N.T., Huyen, M.N., Gagneux, Anh, P.T., Tho, D.Q., Torok, E., Nhu, N.T., Duyen, N.T., Duy, P.M., Richenberg, J., Simmons, C., Hien, T.T., Farrar, J. (2008) Relationship between *Mycobacterium tuberculosis* genotype and the clinical phenotype of pulmonary and meningeal tuberculosis. *J. Clin.Microbio.*, 46, 1363-1368.

[140] Toikka, P., Nikkari, S., Ruuskanen, O., Leinonen, M., Mertsola, J. (1999) Pneumolysin PCR-based diagnosis of invasive pneumococcal infection in children. *J. Clin.Microbiol.*, 37, 633-637.

[141] Tuyama, M., Boente, R.F., Rebelo, M.C., Igreja, R.P., Barroso, D.E. (2008) The utility of the polymerase chain reaction assay for aetiologic definition of unspecified bacterial meningitis cases. *Mem. Inst. Oswaldo Cruz.*, 103, 138-142.

[142] Tzanakaki, G., Tsopanomichalou, M., Kesanopoulos, K., Matzourani, R., Sioumala, M., Tabaki, A., Kremastinou, J. (2005) Simultaneous single-tube PCR assay for the detection of *Neisseria meningitidis, Haemophilus influenzae* type b and *Streptococcus pneumoniae. Clin. Microbiol. Infect.*, 11, 386-390.

[143] Vaagland, H., Blomberg, B., Krüger, C., Naman, N., Jureen, R., Langeland, N.(2004) Nosocomial outbreak of neonatal *Salmonellaenterica* serotype Enteritidis meningitis in a rural hospital in northern Tanzania. *BMC Infect. Dis.*, 14, 4,35.

[144] van de Beek, D., de Gans, J., Tunkel, A. R., Wijdicks, E. F. M. (2006) Community-acquired bacterial meningitis in adults. *N. Eng. J. Med.*, 354, 44-53.

[145] van Gastel, E., Bruynseels, P., Verstrepen, W., Mertens, A. (2007) Evaluation of real-time polymerase chain reaction assay for the diagnosis of pneumoccal and meningococcal meningitis in a tertiary care hospital. *Eur. J. Clin. Mmicrobial. Infect. Dis.*, 26, 651-653.

[146] van Ketel, R. J., DE Wever, B., van Alphen, L. (1990) Detection of *Haemophilus influenzae* in cerebrospinal fluids by polymerase chain reaction DNA amplification. *J. Med. Microbiol.*, 33, 271-276.

[147] Wang, X., Mair, R., Hatcher, C., Theodore, M.J., Edmond, K., Wu, H.M., Harcourt, B.H., Carvalho Mda, G., Pimenta, F., Nymadawa, P., Altantsetseg, D., Kirsch, M., Satola, S.W., Cohn, A., Messonnier, N.E., Mayer, L.W. (2011) Detection of bacterial pathogens in Mongolia meningitis surveillance with a new real-time PCR assay to detect *Haemophilus influenzae*. *Int. J. Med. Microbiol.*, 301, 303-309.

[148] Watt, J.P., Wolfson, L.J., O'Brien, K.L., Henkle, E., Deloria-Knoll, M., McCall, N., Lee, E., Levine, O.S., Hajjeh, R., Mulholland, K., Cherian, T.; Hib and Pneumococcal Global Burden of Disease Study Team (2009) Burden of disease caused by *Haemophilus influenzae* type b in children younger than 5 years: global estimates. *Lancet*, 374, 903-911.

[149] Wei, B.P., Shepherd, R.K., Robins-Browne, R.M., Clark, G.M., O'Leary, S.J. (2010) Pneumococcal meningitis post-cochlear implantation: potential routes of infection and pathophysiology. *Otolaryngol. Head Neck Surg.*, 143 (5 Suppl 3), S15-S23.

[150] Weisfelt, M., van de Beek, D., Spanjaard, L., de Gans, J. (2007) Nosocomial bacterial meningitis in adults: a prospective series of 50 cases. *J. Hosp. Infect.*, 66, 71-78.

[151] Williams, A.J., Nadel, S. (2001) Bacterial meningitis: current controversies in approaches to treatment.CNS Drugs, 15, 909-919.

[152] 152. Woese, C. R., Gutell, R., Gupta, R., Noller, H. F. (1983) Detailed analysis of the higher-order structure of 16S-like ribosomal ribonucleic acids. *Microbiol. Rev.*, 47, 621-669.

[153] Workman, M. R., Price, E. H., Bullock, P. (1999) *Salmonella* meningitis and multiple cerebral abscesses in an infant. *Int. J. antimicrob.Agents,* 13, 131-132.

[154] Yakubu, D.E., Abadi, F,J., Pennington, T.H., (1999) Molecular typing methods for *Neisseria meningitidis*. *J. Med. Microbiol.*, 48, 1055-1064.

[155] Zaia, A., Griffith, J, M., Hogan, T.R., Tapsall, J.W., Bainbridge, P., Neill, R., Tribe, D. (2005) Molecular tests can allow confirmation of invasive meningococcal disease when isolates yield atypical maltose, glucose or gamma-glutamyl peptidase test results. *Pathology,* 37, 378-379.

Reviewed By: Dr. Ben Davies Tall - Virulence Mechanisms Branch, Division of Virulence Assessment, Center for Food Safety and Applied Nutrition, U. S. Food and Drug Administration, 8301 Muirkirk Road, Laurel, Maryland 20708. Tel; 301-2107880; Fax; 301-2107976. Email; ben.tall@fda.hhs.gov.

In: Meningitis: Causes, Diagnosis and Treatment   ISBN 978-1-62100-833-0
Editors: G. Houllis et al. pp. 141-173   ©2012 Nova Science Publishers, Inc.

Chapter 3

TUBERCULOUS MENINGITIS: NEW APPROACH FOR AN OLD DISEASE

Fernando Alarcon[1,] and Gonzalo Dueñas[2]*
[1]Neurology Department, Hospital Eugenio Espejo,
[2]Radiology Department, Hospital Metropolitano, Quito-Ecuador

ABSTRACT

Tuberculous meningitis (TBM) is the most severe form of tuberculosis. It is an important cause of death and disease among both children and adults throughout the world, especially in developing countries.

The prognosis is worse in patients with HIV, in patients with severe neurological impairment, in chronic cases, and in patients with a resistance to drugs. The disease's pathogenesis has not as yet been sufficiently understood. Despite progress achieved over the past decades, a diagnosis of TBM is difficult to reach in many cases, because there is not as yet any diagnostic test sufficiently sensitive, targeted and timely. The percentage of patients where a definitive diagnosis of TBM can be established is low. TBM diagnosis and treatment are a challenge for neurologists. There is no characteristic medical profile, which makes it difficult to reach a diagnosis. Systemic symptoms of infection by Mycobacterium tuberculosis (MT), along with meningeal signs, may be suggestive of tuberculous meningitis. HIV infection does not change how tuberculous meningitis is presented.

---
[*] E-mail: falarcn2000@hotmail.com; Phones: 593 2 2221 202; 593 2 2503 296.

In 80% of patients with TBM, symptoms appear at least one week before diagnosis. The time profile for the onset of TBM symptoms could be used to differentiate tuberculous meningitis from bacterial meningitis. The percentage of patients diagnosed as having tuberculous meningitis might increase if a molecular diagnostic test were applied. Hydrocephalus, pre-contrast hyperdensity-hyperintensity, basal leptomeningeal enhancement, obliteration of the basal cisterns, infarcts and tuberculomas are highly frequent findingson CT and MRI studies. The diagnostic approach is based on clinical criteria, laboratory test results, and image findings.

TBM prognosis depends on the presence of HIV, resistance to drugs, abnormal CT or MRI, substantial rise of proteins in CSF and onset of antituberculosis treatment three days after admission to hospital. The need to reach a diagnosis and administer early antituberculosis treatment is very important to reduce death and improve the prognosis. Recently, a consensus in terms of clinical diagnostic, laboratory and imaging criteria have been defined and recommended for tuberculous meningitis to be used in future clinical research.

INTRODUCTION

One third of the world's population is infected by the tubercle bacillus. Autopsy series have revealed that 5-15% of people exposed to MT develop symptomatic pulmonary disease, and 5-10% of these individuals eventually develop CNS disease, most commonly meningitis [1]. HIV infection is the most important risk factor for the development of tuberculosis and carries a poor prognosis [2]. TBM is the most severe form of tuberculosis and is a major cause of disease and death among adults and children. TBM primarily affecting brain and spinal cord meninges, along with the adjacent brain parenchyma, tends to predominate in children from developing countries and adults from developed countries. TBM characterized by slow progressive granulomatous inflammation of the basal meninges, leading to hydrocephalus, cerebral infarct or death if the patient is not treated, is the most frequent form of tuberculous CNS [1, 3]. Formation of tuberculomas and abscesses, as well as affectation of the spinal cord, may also occur [2, 3]. Although anti-tubercular treatment is increasingly effective, disease and death rates continue to be high, making CNS tuberculosis a potentially devastating disease. Clinical, laboratory and imaging findings are not very sensitive or specific for the diagnosis. Diagnosing CNS tuberculosis is, in many cases, a true challenge, owing to the wide variability of clinical signs and symptoms and the absence of sensitivity of acid-fast bacillus (AFB) smear and culture of CSF [4]. A better prognosis can be ensured when treatment starts early in the disease [5]. Recent reviews have been published on the pathogenesis, diagnosis and treatment of tuberculous meningitis, highlighting major controversial issues that have been overturned or mistakenly accepted in the literature [6].

EPIDEMIOLOGY

MT infection´s incidence has risen drastically over recent years, not only in areas that were traditionally endemic but also in areas where the incidence of tuberculosis has been declining [7]. Although the lungs are the primary target of the infection, many organs are potentially affected and it is estimated that 10% of immunocompetent patients who have tuberculosis develop the disease in the CNS. In United States, 5 to 9% of AIDS patients have pulmonary or extrapulmonary tuberculosis. Tuberculosis is the most common opportunistic infection in persons infected with HIV. The main way of contagion is person-to-person transmission by inhalation of droplet nuclei that have aerosolized. These nuclei have few bacilli, but it is estimated that only 1 to 10 organisms are need to trigger the infection. The tubercles consist of mononuclear cells surrounding a caseous necrotic center that can be formed in the lung as well as in secondary sites [7]. The exact incidence and prevalence of TBM in HIV-infected patients is not known. Tuberculosis is a major cause of death among HIV-infected persons [8]. In 2008, WHO estimated that there were 33.4 million HIV-infected cases. That same year, there were about 1.4 million new cases of tuberculosis among HIV-infected persons and tuberculosis accounted for 23% of AIDS-related deaths. Worldwide, 14 million people are currently co-infected with tuberculosis and HIV [8]. In 2007, the estimated number of tuberculosis prevalent cases amounted to 13.7 million (206 per 100,000 inhabitants). During this period, 9.27 million new cases of tuberculosis were recorded worldwide and about 1.3 million died. Out of the new cases of tuberculosis, 1.37 million were HIV-positive [9].

PATHOGENESIS

TBM is caused by MT bacteria which is a gram-positive, aerobic, non-spore-forming, non-motile, pleomorphic rod and a acid-fast bacterium. This organism is an obligate aerobic bacillus whose entire genome has been sequenced. The genome has provided a wealth of information that may result in much-needed improvements in treatment, diagnosis and prevention. The most widely used acid-fast smear method for MT is the Ziehl-Neelsen stain. The Lowenstein-Jensen medium is the most popular and widely available culture medium to grow MT [7, 9]. TBM, which usually occurs as an immediate or remote complication of a primary infection or can develop over the course of chronic tuberculosis, can appear without any other evidence of associated pulmonary or extrapulmonary tuberculosis. In children miliary tuberculosis is directly involved in the pathogenesis of TBM, whereas in adults it is part of a widely disseminated tubercular process [3]. MB transmission to a healthy person is primarily by airborne droplet nuclei. In the lungs, MT bacteria multiplies in alveolar macrophages. Within two to four weeks, through blood circulation, bacilli spread to extrapulmonary sites and produce small granulomas in the meninges and adjacent brain parenchyma [9]. These small granulomas, now called Rich foci, are found predominantly within the brain parenchyma, but also in the meninges and in the subpial or subependymal surface of the brain [6, 9]. Rich foci remain dormant for years. Meningitis occurs when mycobacteria contained within these lesions are released into the subarachnoid space, and that might happen even months or years after the initial bacteremia [3, 6, 9]. There is no precise knowledge about the exact trigger for the rupture of Rich foci. Brain trauma, HIV infection and other factors that reduce immunity are believed to play a role [3, 9].

The ability of MT to spread in the blood seems to be the key component of the pathogenesis of tuberculosis [6]; however, it is not well understood how the bacteria pass from the lungs to the blood stream. Pulmonary alveolar macrophages represents the most plausible vehicle to transport MT from alveolar lumen to blood. Bacillemia associated with miliary dissemination enhances the probability of the formation of a meningeal or subcortical tuberculous focus, which may eventually caseate and give rise to TBM [9]. The bacillus passes into the CNS traversing the blood brain barrier. Persons infected with Koch bacillus experience a period of usually asymptomatic lymphohematogenous spread, which is the interval between infection and development of the tissue's specific hypersensitivity, manifested by a positive tuberculin reaction. This pre-allergic bacillemic phase usually establishes metastatic foci of infection that can remain inactive or become active after variable periods of clinical latency, which may be immediate or may last for months or years. It is likely that, in some cases, the foci of chronic tuberculosis become sources of secondary hematogenous spread, usually abortive by themselves, but capable of establishing other metastatic foci, including some adjacent to the subarachnoid space with a potential subsequent rupture. This mechanism could explain episodes of intermittent fever and general discomfort that are not well understood and that appear in some patients weeks or months before the development of TBM. This intermittent chronic form of presentation is associated with severe symptoms and is potentially disabling in patients with TBM [3].

Some strains of MT are considered to be highly virulent and are capable of causing more disseminated and meningeal forms of tuberculosis than others [9]. The different genotypes of MT may appear with variable clinical manifestations in the host. It has been suggested that some genotypes of MT are associated with drug-resistant tuberculosis and with a high incidence of co-infection with HIV [9]. MT is an intracellular pathogen that survives withinthe phagosome of host macrophages. Apoptosis of infected macrophages is an effective mechanism used by the host against tubercle bacilli. Virulent strains of MT have evolved several genetic mechanisms to subvert host immune responses, leading to their prolonged survival and growth in the host's macrophages [9].

CLINICAL FEATURES OF TUBERCULOUS MENINGITIS

The clinical manifestations of TBM are related to the pathological changes seenin this neuro-infection [3]. TBM has a non-specific clinical history. Its clinical presentation may differ, depending on whether it is occurring in adults or in children and whether or not it is occurring in HIV-infected patients [7]. Typically, a prodromal period has been recognized between the second and fourth week, which may extend from a few days to several months before its presentation [3-5, 7].

In our series [3], we have been able to identify three presentations in the prodromal period: an acute prodromal period, with signs and symptoms lasting up to one week from the onset of symptoms, accounting for 13% of cases; a subacute presentation lasting two to eight weeks, accounting for 80% of cases; and a chronic presentation lasting for eight weeks up to various months, accounting for 7% of cases [3]. In patients with a subacute presentation, three stages can be recognized [3]. The first stage, of general manifestations, courses with nonspecific symptoms, general discomfort, hyporexia, fever, intermittent headache and muscle aches. In this stage, infants may show irritability, abdominal pain and tense fontanelle. Children show meningism and gastro-intestinal symptoms. Elderly patients may shows states of confusion and absence of fever. This stage would be associated with the presence and initial spread of the tubercle bacillus in the subarachnoid space. The second stage courses especially with meningeal manifestations, neck pain and nuchal rigidity, fever, especially at night, continuous and severe headache, irritability, vomiting, cranial nerve palsy, somnolence, delirium and impaired consciousness. This second stage could be associated with the allergic reaction to the tuberculoprotein, which leads to changes in the CSF and basal exudate development . The third stage courses especially with cerebral or spinal parenchymatous manifestations, characterized by the presentation of papilledema, impaired consciousness, focal neurological deficit secondary to ischemia or cerebral infarct and compromise of the brain stem and the spinal cord or its roots. In this stage, patients may present with paraparesis or paraplegia and movement disorders that include chorea, ballism, tremor, parkinsonism, dystonia and myoclonus. Chorea-ballistic movements prevail in children [3, 10]. The third stage is associated with the progressive increase of brain and spinal meningeal exudate, vasculitis and vascular occlusion, cerebral edema, pressure distortion secondary to tuberculomas, hydrocephalus and intracranial hypertension [3, 11, 12]. Convulsions are present in 10 to 15% of cases [3].

In the acute presentation before admission, symptoms last for less than one week and can manifest as acute meningitis, clinically undifferentiated from pyogenic meningitis with fever, headache, nuchal rigidity and impaired consciousness, also capable of simulating viral encephalitis with unilateral focal deficit, convulsions, impaired consciousness and intracranial hypertension, especially in children. It is highly unlikely that there might be myeloradiculitis or myelopathy. Children can present movements disorders such as chorea and dystonia. The acute presentation could be related to a sudden discharge of a large amount of tuberculoprotein in the CSF [3].

In the chronic presentation, there might be symptoms that last more than eight weeks before admission.The patient has intermittent fever, progressive headache, apathy, cognitive impairment, irritability, gait ataxia, urinary incontinence, impairment of cranial pairs, delirium, tremor, myoclonus or other abnormal movements, motor impairment, with progressive hemiparesis, tetraparesis or paraparesis affecting the sphincter and, in some cases, radicular impairment. Paraplegia may be caused by tuberculousradiculomyelitis, arachnoiditis, intramedullary tuberculomas, or syringomyelia. This form of presentation, which is especially frequent in adults, corresponds to a late chronic form of neurotuberculosis, associated with reinfection or resurgence of tuberculous infection in the CNS with abortive episodes of spreading of the bacillus or with intermittent discharges of bacilli or tuberculous antigens from a caseous juxtaependymal focus in the subarachnoid space. The CSF in these cases can show a moderate to severe rise in proteins, up to four grams, with the response depending on the immunological reaction of the host [3].

In our series of 310 patients with TBM, the average age was 34.5 years (range from 0.5 to 80 years). The most frequent signs and symptoms were asthenia in 79.6% of patients, irritability in 79.5%, fever in 79%, headache in 78.4%, meningeal signs in 77.5%, altered mental state in 70%, weight loss in 64.9%, motor deficit in 54.7%, cranial nerve compromise in 25.4%, papilledema in 20.3%, abnormal movements in 18.4%, convulsions in 13.9%, disconjugate eye movements in 9.7%, nystagmus in 4.2%, and aphasia in 3.2%. Sixth cranial nerve was the most commonly affected. Third and fourth cranial nerves were less frequently affected [13].

Atypical clinical manifestations in the elderly may contribute to delay the diagnosis of TBM. In both elderly patients and children, meningeal signs are less frequent. In a study carried out in patients over 50 years of age [14], the main clinical manifestations were fever in 81% of cases, abnormal mental state in 72%, headaches in 47%, vomiting in 34%, rigidity in 51%, altered sensory in 64%, crises in 28%, and focal neurological deficit in 24%. TBM may appear in elderly patients or HIV patients with subacute dementia, personality changes and frontal lobe signs. In pediatric patients, prevailing clinical manifestations are coma, rise in intracranial pressure, crises, and focal neurological deficit [9].

Movement disorders may occur over the course of TBM [10]. Dystonia, chorea-ballism, tremor, myoclonus and parkinsonism have been found in 16.6% of patients with TBM [10]. Movement disorders are more common in children and young people. Chorea is most frequent in children under five years of age. Tremor is the most frequent abnormal movement. In patients with movement disorders because of TBM, there is a poor correlation between the type, distribution or severity of the abnormal movement and CT or MRI findings. In 60%, hydrocephalus was found and in 46.6% cerebral infarcts were found. The patients showed a high frequency of ischemic or hemorrhagic infarcts and exceptionally deep hematomas affecting the internal capsule, mesencephalus, basal ganglia and diencephalus. Vasculitis of the vessels surrounded by the purulent exudate, has been proposed as the cause of cerebral infarcts in patients with TBM. Ischemic infarcts in the basal ganglia, including the subthalamic nucleus as a consequence of vasculitis, is a probable mechanism for patients who show movement disorders. Hydrocephalus may play an important role in some cases. Multifactor mechanisms have been deemed responsible for the abnormal involuntary movements (AIMs) in patients with TBM [10].

One third of patients with brain tuberculomas (32.6%) may be associated with movement disorders [11, 12]. In patients with tuberculomas, chorea, which predominates in children, is the most frequent abnormal movement. Chorea and dystonia are usually associated with deep tuberculomas and tremor with superficial lesions. In patients with movement disorders, multiple tuberculomas were found in 68.7% of cases, with a predominant deep supratentorial location. In patients with chorea, there is a high correlation between motor deficit and abnormal movements (87.5%), suggesting that when patients have this association and show, in the image, one or various expansive lesions, especially in the basal ganglia, it is highly probable that its etiology is tuberculosis. The pathogenesis of movement disorders caused by intracranial tuberculomas has been related with a pressure-distortion mechanism that can be aggravated by edema, ischemia, toxic bacterial factors and hydrocephalus [12].

Dastur and Udani [15,16] were the first to describe children with disseminated tuberculosis a variant that they called "tuberculous encephalopathy." These children have a cerebral disorder characterized by rapid and diffuse cerebral affectation with convulsions, involuntary movements, stupor or coma with absence of significant meningeal signs. CSF may show pleocytosis and normal or discreetly augmented proteins. Dastur has argued that the pathogenesis of tuberculous encephalopathy may differ from TBM. In post-mortem studies, diffuse cerebral edema has been found along with demyelinization and sometimes traces of hemorrhage, which may be more typical of post-infectious allergic encephalomyelitis [16On brain CT , there is extensive hypodensity of brain white matter [3]. Improvement has been reported when steroids were administered [3,17].

TBM with spinal affectation, which commonly appears as paraplegia, is a severe complication in TBM, occurring in 10 to 15% of cases [3, 14]. It may be caused by vertebral tuberculosis (Pott's disease), which can be associated with fusiform paravertebral abscesses or a gibbus [3,14,18,19] or by radiculomyelitis, myelitis, arachnoiditis (Figure 1), intradural or extraspinal tuberculomas (Figures 2,3,4), abscesses (Figure 5) or spinal syrigomyelic cavities. Tuberculous radiculomyelopathy characteristically appears with subacute paraparesis, radicular pain, paresthesia, bladder disorder and slowly progressive muscular weakness [3, 9, 14]. Muscle weakness is a late complication. In the neurological exam, there is sensitivity deficit, hypotonus and usually absence of deep reflexes. The plantar response may be extensor. Aabsence of deep reflexes provides a poor functional prognosis. Protein content in CSF of patients with paraplegia increases, becoming very high in some cases. This increase is related to partial or complete spinal blockage and especially with a gradual and progressive immunoallergic response to the presence of the tuberculoprotein and its antigens [3].

Cranial nerves are affected either secondary to entrapment in thick basilar exudates or because of increased intracranial pressure [9]. The loss of sight in TBM may be related to optochiasmatic arachnoiditis, third ventricular compression of optic chiasm in patients with severe hydrocephalus, optic nerve granulomas or ethambutol toxicity [9].

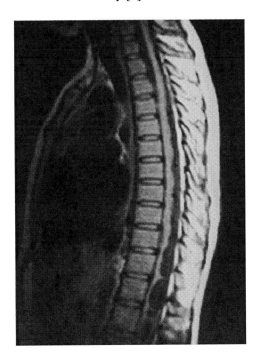

Figure 1. 42 years old patient. Sagital T1W spinal MRI shows myltiple leptomeningeal adherences and severe cord distortion.

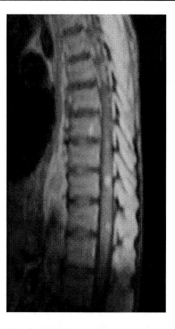

Figure 2. 17 years old patient. Sagital T1W spinal MRI with Gadolinium, shows multiple nodular enhansing spinal cord granulomas.

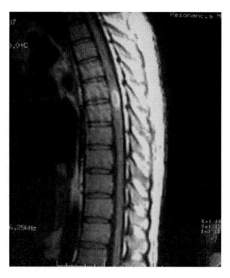

Figure 3. 56 years old patient. Sagital T1W spinal MRI with Gadolinium, shows a ring enhancing intramedulary granuloma.

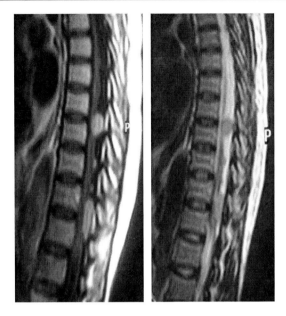

Figure 4. 35 years old patient. Sagital T1W with Gadolinium and T2W spinal MRI show intradural extramedulary granulomas and irregular leptomeningeal enhancement.

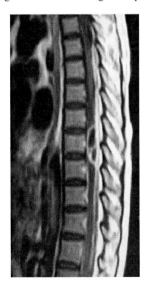

Figure 5. 28 years old patient. Sagital T1W spinal MRI with Gadolinium shows severe cord atrophy, meningeal enhancement and intradural extramedulary abscess.

Choroidal tubercles are infrequent funduscopic findings in patients with tuberculous meningitis. These lesions are considered pathognomonic for TBM. Choroidal tubercles are often associated with miliary tuberculosis [9]. In the examination of the fundus oculi, the choroidal tubercles are white, gray or yellow lesions with indistinct borders, surrounded by edema. Their size varies from 0.5 to 3 mm in diameter. Histologically choroidal tubercles represent caseated granulomas. Tubercle bacillus has been shown in choroidal tubercles [9].

The clinical features and CSF profiles of TBM are not modified by HIV infection. There are no significant differences between HIV-positive patients and HIV-negative patients, except for the presence of lymph node TB in 50% of HIV-positive patients, compared with 3% of HIV-negative patients. Some studies have reported a higher frequency of tuberculous intracerebral mass lesion in HIV-positive patients, mainly among intravenous drug users. Tuberculin skin tests are positive in about one third of patients, particularly in the early stages of HIV infection, while they develop an anergy with more advanced immunosuppresion [7].

PATHOLOGY

The pathological changes occurring in the cranium and spinal canal depend on various factors such as age, severity and duration of disease, patient's immunological condition or hypersensitivity, response to therapy and possibly the number and virulence of the bacillus, as well as the host's individual susceptibility to MT [3, 9,19,20]. Although the greatest impact of the disease takes place in the basal meninges and in the CSF, parenchymatous cerebral lesions, because of the direct extension of the inflammatory process or secondary to vascular changes, are found in most cases [3,19]. Diffuse pathological changes affect the arachnoid membrane and the subarachnoid space. Pathological characteristics are meningeal inflammation, fibrogelatinous basal exudates, vasculitis of the arteries traversing the exudates and obstruction of the flow of CSF resulting in hydrocephalus, which can appear early or late and be of variable degree [3, 9]. The inflammatory exudate predominating in the interpeduncular and pontine cisterns, can extend to the sylvian fissure and other cisternsleading to blockage of the foramina of Luschka and Magendie. Leptomeningeal exudate progressively surrounds and strangles the brain stem and its arteries [3, 9].

The optic chiasm and the roots of other cranial nerves arising from the ventral aspect of the brainstem are usually entrapped in thick exudates [21,22]. In addition, the exudate frequently covers the choroidal plexuses, the spinal canal, especially in the dorsal region and the ependyma of the ventricles, which has a granular aspect [3,9]. Exudates can be seen surrounding the lower part of the spinal cord and cauda equina resulting in tuberculous radiculomyelopathy [3,9]. Later the exudate can harden and calcify. In the meninges, choroidal plexuses, and ependyma, small nodes or tubercles more than 1 mm in diameter can be found [19,20]

Microscopically, the exudate is predominantly composed of lymphocytes and plasma cells with caseous necrotic foci. When the process becomes chronic, the exudate becomes a fibrous mass compromising the cranial nerves and the spinal cord, conditioning secondary neurological manifestations [3,19,20]. TBM can result in the formation of tuberculomas consisting of caseous necrotic material, epithelioid cell granuloma and mononuclear cell infiltration [9].

Obstruction to the flow of CSF occurs in the posterior fossa, as the thick exudate blocks openings of fourth ventricles, the sylvian aqueduct or the opening of the tentorium, developing hydrocephalus as a consequence. In addition to the inflammatory exudate, obstruction of the sylvian aqueduct is related to ependymitis or the presence of tuberculomas [3,19,20]. Hydrocephalus may develop late as a result of arachnoid adherences [3]. The brain tissue underlying the tuberculous exudate shows various degrees of edema, perivascular infiltration and a microglial reaction collectively termed as "border zone encephalitis." A microscopic pathological feature of tuberculous meningitis is the formation of epithelioid cell granulomas with Langhans giant cells, lymphocytic infiltrates and caseous necrosis. Exudates are prominently present around the sylvian fissure, basal cysterns, brainstem and cerebellum [9].

The distribution of tubercles along the pial vessels, the occasional location of tuberculous lesions in an arterial territory and the presence of dense and fibrinocellular gelatinous leptomeningeal exudate contribute to the development of pathological findings related to stroke in TM [3,23]. The leptomeningeal exudate initially located in the interpeduncular fossa is disseminated anteriorly and compromises the optic chiasm, anterior brain vessels and laterally the sylvian valley, surrounding the carotid artery, the middle cerebral artery and its penetrating branches [9].

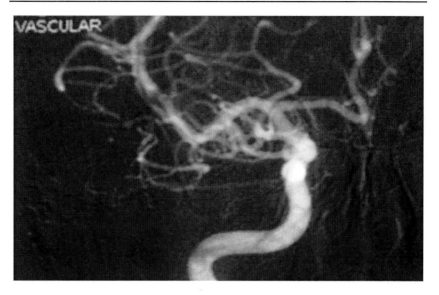

Figure 6. 27 years old patient. Cerebral angiography shows stenosis and intimal irregularity of the middle cerebral artery.

Stroke occurs especially in the advanced and severe stage of the disease in 15 to 57% of cases [18,19,23-25] and may be asymptomatic because it occurs more frequently in deep areas and not very manifest. Among children, infarcts of the basal ganglia and inner capsule have been associated with a poor prognosis [23-25]. Most strokes in TBM are multiple, bilateral and located in the basal ganglia, especially in the caudate, thalamus, anterior arm and knee of the inner capsule. These are attributed to compromise of the medial striatal perforating, thalamotuberal and thalamostriates arteries, which are immersed in the leptomeningeal exudate and can be compressed or displaced because of hydrocephalus. Cortical strokes can also occur because of the affectation of the proximal part of the middle (Figure 6), anterior and posterior cerebral arteries as well as the supraclinoid segments of the carotid arteries and the basilar artery. These findings have been documented in MRI, angiography and autopsy studies [3,9,23].

Changes in cerebral vessels are characterized by inflammation, spasm, constriction and eventually thrombosis of the vessels. Occlusion of cerebral arteries leads to infarction of the underlying tissue [9]. Arteritis is more common than infarct in autopsy studies. It has been suggested that cytokynes could play a role here, especially the tumoral necrosis factor, the endothelial vascular growth and the matrix of metaloproteinases in a damaged hematoencephalic barrier attracting leukocytes and liberating vasoactive autocoids. Without doubt, the prothrombic status may also contribute to the occlusion of the cerebral vessels in TBM. It has not been proven that the use of corticosteroids, antitubercular treatment and aspirin is able to reduce stroke frequency [23].

DIAGNOSIS

CSF examination is crucial in determining the diagnosis of TBM. CSF pressure is increased in about 50% of cases. Changes in CSF help to differentiate it from other meningitis. The macroscopic aspect of the fluid may be clear or xanthochromic and may show a film or small lumps [3, 9]. Characteristically, CSF shows lymphocytic pleocytosis, higher concentration of proteins and low concentration of glucose. In 9 to 15% of patients, the first CSF does not show pleocytosis [3,26]. Initial mononuclear pleocytosis may briefly change in direction to polymorphonuclear predominance when therapy starts, and this may be associated with clinical deterioration. This therapeutic paradox has been regarded as virtually pathognomonic for TBM [7]. In 81% of patients, moderate pleocytosis (between 5 and 500 cells/mm) can be found; below 100 cells/mm in 44% of cases. In 7% of patients there were between 500 and 1,500 cells/ml, and in 2% more than 1,500 cells/ml. In 72% of patients there was a predominance of lymphocytes [3], whereas 93% showed moderate elevation of proteins (between 30 and 500 mg/dl), 4% a substantial increase in proteins between 500 and 2,000 mg, and 2% a large increase of more than 2,000 mg/dl. In patients with a substantial increase in proteins, there is a high risk of affectation of the medulla. Glucose level declined to less than 45 mg/dl in 71% of cases, and in 10% it was less than 10 mg/dl [13]. The CSF changes reflect the individual reaction to the tuberculoprotein, which in some cases may not appear or is found to be diminished. In these cases, the white cell count or the level of proteins may be normal or slightly increased [3]. These small changes in CSF may be interpreted as excluding TM, which may be an error because it may be an authentic TBM or a serous form of TBM [3,18], which is a self-confined meningeal disease affecting children with active pulmonary tuberculosis and which is considered to be caused by a reaction to a primary or post-primary focus in the CNS [3]. Increased proteins in CSF are almost constant. Nevertheless, the gold standard for diagnosis is the demonstration of MT bacilli in CSF. Unfortunately smear for acid-fast bacillus is positive only in 5-30% of patients in the first sample, with increasing possibly in the following samples [3, 9,20,27]. Culture of MT from CSF is not always positive and it takes several weeks for a positive result. Conventional CSF culture in a Lowenstein-Jensen medium is positive in 45-90% of cases [3,9,20]. In HIV-associated TM, 69% positivity in smears and 87.9% positivity in bacterial culture have been demonstrated [9,28,29]. To increase the positivity of the smear examination, it is necessary to collect 10 cc of CSF and centrifuge it at high speeds. The smear must be examined for at least 30 minutes [3,26,30]. A combination of both microscopic examination and culture of several samples of CSF (sometimes as many as four are needed) provides the highest yield of positivity [3, 7].

Because of the lower percentage of identification of MT in the first CSF sample and its slow growth in the culture mediums, fast tests have been developed as early diagnostic help methods in TBM. The detection of MT DNA in CSF samples using polymerase chain reaction (PCR) is a widely used diagnostic method. A meta-analysis found a sensitivity of 56% for the commercial testing of PCR and a specificity of 98%. Sensitivity of PCR testing is higher in culture-positive patients [9,31,32]. A recent study observed that CSF filtrates contain a substantial amount of MT DNA [9], suggesting that the filtrates and not sediments are likely to reliably provide a PCR-based diagnosis [33]. The PCR test does not replace the conventional tests such as microscopic, culture and biopsy. Results of nucleic acid amplification test should be interpreted in conjunction with conventional test and clinical data [34]

When the results of smear, culture and PCR were compared in a study carried out in India, it was found that the sensitivity of CSF microscopy was only 3.3%, culture 26.7%, CT scan 60%, and PCR 66.7% [31-35]. These results, as well as others, show an increase in the percentage of positivity when diagnostic tests are combined, especially if they are conducted in various CSF samples [3, 9]. Greater positivity has been found when various diagnostic tests are associated with a higher degree of neurological deterioration of the patients, especially if, in these patients, the smear results are positive [3]. Similar results have been found with new methods such as Anti-Bacillus Calmette-Guérin antibody-secreting cell detection in CSF by an enzyme-linked immunospot assay, valuable because of its high degree of sensitivity [9,36,37].

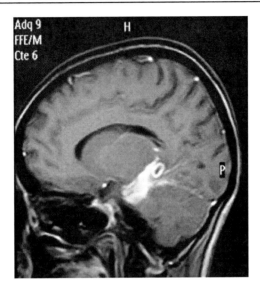

Figure 7. 17 years old patient. Axial and sagital T1W brain MRI with Gadolinium shows leptomeningeal enhancement around the mesencephalon and a supratentorial granuloma.

NEUROIMAGING

Computed Tomography (CT) and Magnetic Resonance Imaging (MRI) are valuable in diagnosis, evaluation of complications and prognosis of TBM. All patients with TBM must have imaging studies with and without contrast. Characteristic changes in CTimages include cysternal effacement, leptomeningeal enhancement, (Figure 7), cerebral infarcts(Figures 8 a,b), granulomas(Figure 9) and hydrocephalus (Figures 10 a,b c). In our series [13] of 310 patients, we found hydrocephalus in 35% of patients who had a complete recovery or mild or moderate deficit, in 64.3% of patients who had severe deficit, and in 73.7% of patients who died. Cysternal effacement was found in 19% of the patients who recovered without deficit or mild or moderate deficit, 42.9% that had severe deficit, and in 49.1% of those who died. Leptomeningeal enhancement showed 19.9% of patients who recovered without deficit or had mild deficit, 34.6% who had moderate deficit, 46.4% who had severe deficit, and 50.9% of patients who died. Infarcts were present jn 17.7% of patients without deficit or with slight or moderate deficit, 39.3% of patients who showed severe deficit, and in 42.1% of patients who died, with superficial location in 40% of cases and deep location in 60%. We found granulomas in 18% of cases. Prognosis is worse if the patient has hydrocephalus, cysternal effacement and deep infarcts.

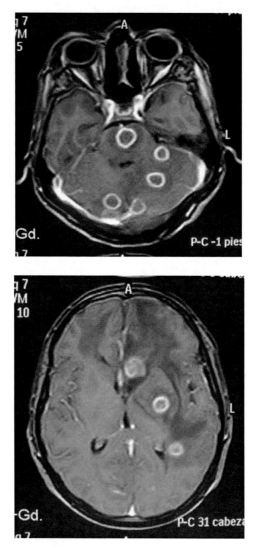

Figure 8A. 25 years old patient, December 2004. Axial T2W and T1W with Gadolinium brain MRI show multiple intraparenchymal granulomas, hypointense in T2 and ring enhancing in T1 images.

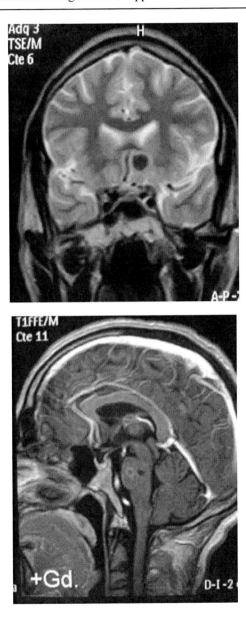

Figure 8B. 25 years old patient, August 2005. Coronal, axial and sagital T1W with Gadolinium, T2W, FLAIR and TW1 with Gadolinium show thalamic and pontine granulomas. The last one near a small infarct secondary to vasculitis.

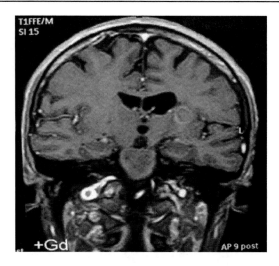

Figure 9. 34 years old patient. Coronal T2W and T1W with Gadolinium brain MRI show a hypointense in T2 and ring enhansing in T1W striatum granuloma.

THERAPY

The prognosis for TBM, which was almost invariably fatal in the early twentieth century, has improved substantially after the advent of streptomycin in the forties and isoniazid in the fifties [7]. The drugs for tuberculosis have been divided by general consensus into first-line drugs, which include isoniazid, rifampicin, ethambutol, pyrazinamide, and streptomycin, and second-line drugs which include4-aminosalicylic acid, ethionamide, cycloserine, and some aminoglycosides and quinolones [7]. Fluoroquinolones (levofloxacin, gatifluoxacin, and moxifluoxacin) are antimicrobial agents used in drug-resistant tuberculosis. Substitution of older fluoroquinolones, especially ciprofloxacin, into a regime meant for treating drug-resistant tuberculosis resulted in a higher rate of relapse [9]. The main therapeutic principle in TBM is that the antituberculous therapy must be administered as soon as the disease is suspected. Postponing start-up of treatment even for a few hours or days may increase morbi-mortality [3, 5]. When TBM is suspected, because antituberculous therapy is not particularly toxic in the short term, empirical treatment should be started as early as possible to reduce morbidity and mortality [3, 5, 7]. Antimicrobial therapy often must be administered empirically, much before bacteriological confirmation. Most first-line drugs, except ethambutol, penetrate the CSF satisfactorily. The concentration of isoniazid and pyrazinamide in CSF is below the minimum inhibitory concentration. These two drugs and streptomycin do not penetrate uninflamed meninges. Rifampicin is bactericidal, whereas streptomycin and ethambutol are tuberculostatic [7,9,37]. The concentration of rifampicin and streptomycin three hours after administration is over the inhibitory concentration but declined later. Corticosteroids had no effect on CSF penetration of antituberculous drugs [38].

There is no consensus about the optimal duration of TBM treatment. Widely accepted regimes include short 6 months and long 9 to 18 months duration treatment [3,5,7]. A 6-month therapeutic regime has proven to be effective with a morbidity and mortality ratio similar to that found in the longer course therapies [3,5]. Whenever drug resistance is unlikely, a regime with three drugs, rifampicin, isoniazid, and pyrazinamide (all daily), for two months and two drugs (isoniazid and rifampicin daily) for four additional months (10 months in children) seems a reasonable option in the adult [3, 5, 7]. The low toxicity of these drugs and their powerful sterilizing action has led them to be considered as the most important. Some authors recommend the initial use of a fourth drug for TBM, usually ethambutol [7], especially when there is pulmonary tuberculosis. The World Health Organization (WHO) recommends a category-based treatment for TBM [39]. For category-1 patients, the antituberculous treatment regime is divided into two phases: an initial intensive phase and a second phase. In the intensive phase, the antituberculous therapy regime includes a combination of four first-line drugs: isoniazid, rifampicin, streptomycin and pyrazinamide. The intensive phase continues for two months [9]. A regime without streptomycin is equally effective [5]. In the second phase, a two-drug regime, with isoniazid and rifampicin, is administered for at least four months [5, 9,13]. In patients with TBM, the second phase is usually extended to 7 or 12 months, especially for patients with delayed response as judged by mycobacterial cultures that remain positive or by inadequate resolution of symptoms and signs and in those cases where CSF continues with pleocytosis or proteins with amounts that are higher than normal [3,7, 9,13]. Some experts have recommended a twice-a-week drug regime [9]. Antituberculous therapy in HIV-positive patients remains the same as for HIV-negative patients [7,9,40,41].

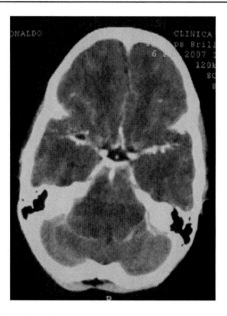

Figure 10A. 8 years old patient, February 2007. CT scan without and with contrast show diffuse brain hypodensity and basal meningeal enhancent with signs of vascular entrapment and vasculitis. Mild hyrocephalus.

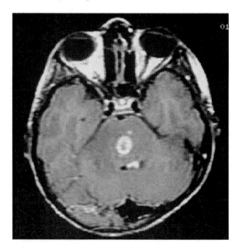

Figure 10 B. 8 years old patient, febrary 2007. Axial T1W brain MRI with Gadolinium, eigth months after treatment, shows pontine and intraventricuar granulomas.

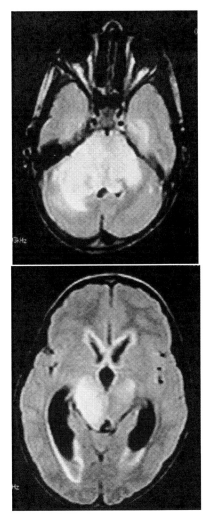

Figure 10C. 8 years old patient, March 2007. Axial T1W with Gadolinium and FLAIR brain MR images show multiple pontine and right middle cerebellar peduncle granulomas with severe edema, ependymitis and hydrocephalus with caseum in the occipital horns of the lateral ventricles.

Multidrug-resistant TBM should be considered if there is a history of contact with a patient of multidrug-resistant pulmonary tuberculosis, in patients that have previously received more than one incomplete or irregular treatment for pulmonary tuberculosis or TBM or a poor clinical response to antimicrobial therapy despite adequate treatment [42-44] When the patient that is being treated shows, after six months, pathological CSF, the treatment must be extended until CSF falls within normal limits [3, 4,13]. The regimes recommended for this type of patient must include at least five drugs. The treatment regime must include drugs that the patient has not received before and to which the patient's organism is susceptible. The regime must also include an injectable medication. In the five-drug regime, one of the antituberculous drugs must be fluoroquinolone [9]. The initial six-month phase must be followed by a continuation phase from 12 to 18 months. With the appearance of tuberculosis that is multidrug-resistant to at least isoniazid and rifampicin, any fluoroquinolone and at least one of the injectable drugs like amikasin, kanamycin and capreomycin [9] must be administered.

Immune reconstitution inflammatory syndrome (IRIS) is a potentially life-threatening condition which is seen in HIV-positive patients of tuberculosis [9]. This complication can be seen within three months after starting highly active antiretroviral therapy. IRIS is characterized by improvement in CD4 cell counts. Its differential diagnosis includes failure of the antituberculous treatment, drug reactions, paradoxical clinical deterioration, antituberculous and antiretroviral drugs interaction with loss of antiretroviral efficacy and alternative opportunistic conditions. IRIS may be severe enough to cause death [9,39,45,46].

The administration of antituberculous and antiretroviral drugs at the same time may produce significant interactions between the drugs, which could lead to a loss of effectiveness of the antiretroviral drugs [9]. In general, treatment with antituberculous drugs is reasonably well tolerated by patients. Hepatitis induced by antituberculous drugs does not reach unacceptable levels [5]. For successful treatment, it is a challenge to handle this complication. If a patient develops hepatitis induced by antituberculous drugs, treatment must be suspended temporarily. After liver function tests show that the patient has recovered, the therapeutic regime must start up again, with the gradual and progressive reintroduction of each one of the drugs until the complete dose is being administered. In TBM, it is advisable that at least two drugs that have no hepatotoxic effects (like ethambutol and streptomycin) be continued [3, 5, 9,47].

Therapy with corticosteroids continues to be controversial despite the recent Cochrane review, which recommends to use corticosteroids routinely in TBM, because they substantially reduce death and neurological disability after treatment. Nevertheless, our results do not show any benefits [3, 5,13].The Cochrane review [48] refers to a well-designed, randomized, double-blind, placebo-controlled trial conducted in Vietnam. In this study, the patients were randomly assigned to receive either dexamethasone or a placebo. Patients with grade II or grade III of British Medical Research Council (BMRC) TBM received intravenous dexamethasone for four weeks and then oral dexamethasone for four weeks. Patients with grade-I disease received two weeks intravenous dexamethasone and the four weeks of oral therapy. Nine months of follow-up treatment with dexamethasone was associated with a significantly improved survival. However, treatment with corticosteroids did not alter the combined outcome of death and severe disability. Grade-I patients showed a slightly significant benefit for the combined outcome [49]. Furthermore, the patients who received corticosteroids had slightly fewer adverse events as a result of the antituberculous drugs than those in the placebo group [9]. Some authors have shown that dexamethasone affects the prognosis of TBM, possibly because it reduces the incidence of hydrocephalus and cerebral infarct [50].The mechanism of action of the corticosteroids in TBM is not known. A recent study showed that dexamethasone decreased CSF matrix metalloproteinases-9 concentrations early in the course of the treatment. The authors suggest that this could be one of the mechanisms whereby the corticosteroids would improve the prognosis in TBM [51]. These results are not similar to those we have found in our series of 310 patients where steroids were used in patients with severe loss of consciousness, bilateral motor impairment, vasculitis, spinal tuberculosis and intracranial tuberculomas with intracranial hypertension and focal deficit [3, 5,13]. In our patients (Table 1), we do not use corticosteroids on grade-I patients or most grade-II patients. Nevertheless they had a better prognosis in terms of death and neurological disability. Corticosteroids were administered to 80 patients (25.8%). It was found, after completing the antituberculous treatment, that 49% of patients recovered completely, of which 43.4% were in grade I, 34.9% in grade II, and 21.7% in grade III. We found severe sequels in 17.9% of grade-I patients, in 32.1% of grade-II patients, and in 50.0% of grade-III patients. 5.3% of grade-I patients, 38.6% of grade-II patients, and 56.1% of grade-III of our patients died.The combined outcome of death and severe disability in our patients was 9.4 % of the cases that started the treatment in grade I, in 36.4 % of the patients that started in grade II and in 54.1 % of the patients who started treatment in grade III. In our study the use of corticoids was associated with a poor prognosis, may be because we used steroids in patients with severe tuberculosis, who have poor prognosis.

TUBERCULOMAS, TUBERCULOUS ABSCESSES, AND SPINAL-CORD INVOLVEMENT

Tuberculous granulomas (tuberculomas) are composed of a central zone of solid caseation necrosis that is surrounded by a capsule of collagenous tissue, epithelioid cells, multinucleated giant cells and mononuclear inflammatory cells. They contain a few bacilli in the necrotic center. Outside the capsule, there is parenchymal edema and astrocytic proliferation [7]. Tuberculomas can be found in the cerebrum, cerebellum, subarachnoid space, subdural space or epidural space [7]. In children, the tuberculomas tend to be infratentorial, whereas in adults they tend to be supratentorial. They can coexist with meningitis in 10 to 15% of cases and be multiple in more than one third of the patients [7,52,53].

Table 1. Funtional prognosis at discharge in 310 patients with TBM

BMRC	Number cases	Total	Mild or moderate	Severe sequelae	Death	Total
	Percent	recovery	sequelae			
BMRC	Count	66	23	5	3	97
Stage I	%	43.2	31.5	17.9	5.8	31.3
BMRC	Count	53	35	9	22	119
Stage II	%	34.9	47.9	32.1	38.6	38.3
BMRC	Count	33	15	14	32	94
Stage III	%	21.7	20.5	50	56.1	30.4
Total	Count	152	73	28	57	310
	%	49	23.5	9	18.4	100

BMRC = British Medical Research Council.
Stages = Stage I, Stage II, Stage III.

Clinical course is subacute or chronic, lasting weeks or months. Chest X-rays suggest pulmonary TB in 30 to 80% of patients. Mantoux test is positive in up to 85% of the patients. CSF findings are unremarkable or show slight abnormalities, and bacteriology is usually negative. The diagnosis is therefore made on the basis of neuroimaging findings, PPD results and response to antituberculous therapy [7,54,55]. In CT scans, tuberculomas may appear as solid enhancing rim enhancing or mixed lesions. On occasions, there is a central calcification surrounded by a hypodense area with a peripheral rim enhancement (target sign), a highly suggestive pattern, although not pathognomonic for TB [7,56]. On MRI images, tuberculomas appear as isointense to gray matter on T1-weighted images and many have a slightly hyperintense rim. Noncaseating lesions are bright on T2-weighted images. Caseating tuberculomas vary from isointense to hypointense on T2-weighted images and exhibit rim enhancement [7]. Tuberculomas may show a variable degree of perilesional edema, which is usually more prominent in the early stage [7,13]. Differential diagnosis includes neoplasias and other granulomatous processes such as sarcoidosis and parasitic diseases such as cysticercosis and toxoplasmosis [7].

With medical treatment, tuberculomas usually diminish in size and are completely resolved in three months. In some cases, the resolution extends over several months and sometimes years, leading to residual calcification. The medical treatment, which is similar to TBM, is initially recommended and surgery advised only if there is intolerable intracranial hypertension or failure of medical treatment. Mortality with chemotherapy regimes is inferior to 10% [7,9,13,57].

The development or growth of brain tuberculomas in the weeks following the start of antimicrobial treatment has been recognized as a paradoxical response [57-60]. This paradoxical reaction appears in 2% of cases with TBM [57]. The paradoxical response may be interpreted as a clinical deterioration occurring weeks after the start of therapy, sometimes associated with an increase in CSF pleocytosis, more commonly lymphocytic.Response may change transiently in the direction of polymorphonuclear predominance. This is interpreted as a hypersensitivity reaction to the massive release of mycobacterial proteins [7,57,59]. This response appears from three weeks up to various months after starting the antituberculous therapy [7,57]. Enlargement of existing cerebral tuberculomas along with an aggravation of anterior cerebral artery vasculitis, despite the appropriate treatment, has been described [61]. The paradoxical reaction also occurs during the antituberculous treatment in HIV-positive patients when antiretroviral therapy restores immune function [7]. Although there are no controlled studies, it has been suggested that therapy with corticosteroids improves prognosis [7,57].

When the caseous core of a tuberculoma liquefies, a tuberculous abscess results. The abscesses are usually larger and less frequent than tuberculomas. Frequently multiloculated, they often exert a greater impact on mass and edema. In contrast to the solid caseation and few organisms seen in tuberculomas, the abscess is formed by pus, where many bacilli can be found. The appearance recalls a typically pyogenic abscess. A TB abscess has a faster course and its clinical manifestations are more evident than in tuberculomas, with high fever, headache, focal neurological signs and impaired consciousness. The appropriate therapy includes antituberculous chemotherapy and surgical removal when necessary [7,57,62].

Spinal cord, roots and vertebral bodies can be affected by tuberculosis. Tuberculous myelitis and radiculomyelitis usually appear as an acute or subacute disease and, in a few cases, chronically. The CSF analysis reveals an increase in protein content with lymphocytic pleocytosis and, in one third of cases, low glucose levels. The mid-thoracic cord is the most commonly affected, followed by the lumbar and cervical regions. MRI shows uptake of the contrast surrounding the spinal cord and the roots and obliterating the subarachnoid space with focal or diffusely increased intramedullary signal on T2 weighted images and variable degrees of edema and mass effect [3, 7]. Spinal meningitis most frequently accompanies intracranial disease, although in certain cases it may occur alone [7]. Rarely tuberculomas occur in the spinal cord, either as intramedullary or dural lesions.Very infrequently intramedullary tuberculous abscesses have been reported. Tuberculous spondilitis affects the thoraco-lumbar region more frequently, with L1 being the most affected. Extended standard antimicrobial therapy is indicated in the spinal lesions. Systemic corticosteroids improve the prognosis of spinal cord lesions . Surgery must be considered on a case-by-case basis.

PROGNOSIS

In TBM, early diagnosis and treatment are important indicators for a better prognosis [3, 5,13]. Antituberculous treatment prevents death and disability in less than 50% of patients. Impairment of consciousness is significantly associated with mortality and lesser degree of impaired consciousness shows a significantly associated disability [3]. The association between impairment of consciousness and mortality suggest that severe intracranial damage with or without intracranial hypertension or hydrocephalus could be progressive or irreversible. The irreversibility of neurological impairment could be related to ischemia, edema, distortion of the adjacent structures or venous thrombosis. The findings of Ziehl or positive cultures for MT in CSF, accounting for a high concentration of bacilli, has been associated with disease severity and death. In imaging studies, cysternal effacement and exudate in cysterns and sylvian fissures have shown to be associated with disability and mortality [3,5,7,9,13].

Mortality is higher in patients younger than five years of age, older than 50 years of age, and those in whom illness has been present for longer than two months [3, 5, 9]. BMRC staging, which is a scale to assess the severity of TBM, has been related to the prognosis of disease and death. In grade-I patients of the BMRC, disease and death are low, whereas in grade-II patients they are moderate, and in grade-III patients, they are very high (Table 1). Other factors that have been associated with poor outcome include headache, convulsions, motor deficit and cerebral infarcts. High mortality (63.3%) has been reported in HIV patients [9]. Hemiparesis, paraparesis, quadriparesis, aphasia and loss of sight are common neurological impairments among surviving patients. In a study, complete neurological recovery was observed in 21.5% of the surviving patients. However in our series complete recovery was obtained in 43.4%of the patients [13,63].

REFERENCES

[1] Sinner, S. W. (2010). "Approach to the diagnosis and management of tuberculous meningitis."*Curr Infect Dis Rep*12 (4): 291-298.

[2] Marais, S., G. Thwaites, et al. (2010). "Tuberculous meningitis: a uniform case definition for use in clinical research." *Lancet Infect Dis*10 (11): 803-812.

[3] Alarcón F, Cevallos N, Narvaes (1994). "Meningitis Tuberculosa:Un Viejo y Nuevo problema", *Rev Ecuat Neurol.* 3:39-54.

[4] Moreira, J., F. Alarcon, et al. (2008). "Tuberculous meningitis: does lowering the treatment threshold result in many more treated patients?" *Trop Med Int Health*13 (1): 68-75.

[5] Alarcon F, Escalante L. (1990). "Tuberculous meningitis short course of chemothery. Arch Neurol. 47: 1313-1317.

[6] Thwaites, G. E. and J. F. Schoeman (2009). "Update on tuberculosis of the central nervous system: pathogenesis, diagnosis, and treatment." *Clin Chest Med*30 (4): 745-754, ix.

[7] Garcia-Monco, J. C. (1999). "Central nervous system tuberculosis."*NeurolClin*17 (4): 737-759.

[8] Garg, R. K. and M. K. Sinha (2011). "Tuberculous meningitis in patients infected with human immunodeficiency virus." *J Neurol*258 (1): 3-13.

[9] Garg, R. K. (2010). "Tuberculous meningitis."*ActaNeurolScand*122 (2): 75-90.

[10] Alarcon, F., G. Duenas, et al. (2000). "Movement disorders in 30 patients with tuberculous meningitis."*MovDisord*15 (3): 561-569.

[11] Alarcon, F., E. Tolosa, et al. (2001). "Focal limb dystonia in a patient with a cerebellar mass."*Arch Neurol*58 (7): 1125-1127.

[12] Alarcon, F., J. C. Maldonado, et al. (2011). "Movement disorders identified in patients with intracranial tuberculomas."*Neurologia*26 (6): 343-350.

[13] Alarcon F, Moreira J,Rivera J,Salinas R,Duenas G,Van den Ende J.Outcome of central nervous system tuberculosis: An alternative scoring system proposal. *Indian J Tuberculosis*.In press.

[14] Srikanth, S. G., A. B. Taly, et al. (2007). "Clinicoradiological features of tuberculous meningitis in patients over 50 years of age." *J NeurolNeurosurg Psychiatry*78 (5): 536-538.

[15] Dastur, D. K. and P. M. Udani (1966)."The pathology and pathogenesis of tuberculous encephalopathy."*ActaNeuropathol*6 (4): 311-326.

[16] Udani, P. M. and D. K. Dastur (1970). "Tuberculous encephalopathy with and without meningitis.Clinical features and pathological correlations."*J NeurolSci*10 (6): 541-561.

[17] Alarcon F, EspinosaF, Pesantes B,Banda H,Vinan I. (1988) Encefalopatia tuberculosa: presentacion de un caso y caracteristicas en TAC craneal. Arch de Neurobiol (Madrid) 51:213-215.

[18] Molavi, A. and J. L. LeFrock (1985). "Tuberculous meningitis."*Med Clin North Am*69 (2): 315-331.

[19] Tandon Pn. (1978) Tuberculous meningitis in Vinken PJ, Bruyn, Klawans HL,Eds. *Handbook of Clinical Neurology* Vol35, Amsterdam: North Holland 1978:195-265.

[20] Kocen RS. (1987) Tuberculosis of the Nervous System. in: Kennedy PGE,Johnson RT,Eds. *Infections of the Nervous System*, London;Butterworth: 23-42.

[21] Hanna, L. S., N. I. Girgis, et al. (1988). "Ocular complications in meningitis: "fifteen years study"." *MetabPediatrSystOphthalmol*11 (4): 160-162.

[22] Amitava, A. K., S. Alarm, et al. (2001). "Neuro-ophthalmic features in pediatric tubercular meningoencephalitis." *J PediatrOphthalmol Strabismus*38 (4): 229-234.

[23] Misra, U. K., J. Kalita, et al. (2011). "Stroke in tuberculous meningitis."*J NeurolSci*303 (1-2): 22-30.

[24] Chan, K. H., R. T. Cheung, et al. (2005). "Cerebral infarcts complicating tuberculous meningitis."*Cerebrovasc Dis*19 (6): 391-395.

[25] Leiguarda, R., M. Berthier, et al. (1988). "Ischemic infarction in 25 children with tuberculous meningitis."*Stroke*19 (2): 200-204.

[26] Udani, P. M. (1985). "Management of tuberculous meningitis."*Indian J Pediatr*52 (415): 171-174.

[27] Kennedy, D. H. and R. J. Fallon (1979). "Tuberculous meningitis."*JAMA*241 (3): 264-268.

[28] Torok, M. E., T. T. Chau, et al. (2008). "Clinical and microbiological features of HIV-associated tuberculous meningitis in Vietnamese adults."*PLoS One*3 (3): e1772.

[29] Thwaites, G. E., T. T. Chau, et al. (2004). "Improving the bacteriological diagnosis of tuberculous meningitis."*J ClinMicrobiol*42 (1): 378-379.

[30] Barnes, P. F., A. B. Bloch, et al. (1991). "Tuberculosis in patients with human immunodeficiency virus infection."*N Engl J Med*324 (23): 1644-1650.

[31] Desai, D., G. Nataraj, et al. (2006). "Utility of the polymerase chain reaction in the diagnosis of tuberculous meningitis."*Res Microbiol*157 (10): 967-970.

[32] Pai, M., L. L. Flores, et al. (2003). "Diagnostic accuracy of nucleic acid amplification tests for tuberculous meningitis: a systematic review and meta-analysis." *Lancet Infect Dis*3 (10): 633-643.

[33] Haldar, S., N. Sharma, et al. (2009). "Efficient diagnosis of tuberculous meningitis by detection of Mycobacterium tuberculosis DNA in cerebrospinal fluid filtrates using PCR." *J Med Microbiol*58 (Pt 5): 616-624.

[34] Desai, M. M. and R. B. Pal (2002). "Polymerase chain reaction for the rapid diagnosis of tuberculous meningitis."*Indian J Med Sci*56 (11): 546-552.

[35] Thwaites, G. E., M. Caws, et al. (2004). "Comparison of conventional bacteriology with nucleic acid amplification (amplified mycobacterium direct test) for diagnosis of tuberculous meningitis before and after inception of antituberculosis chemotherapy."*J ClinMicrobiol*42 (3): 996-1002.

[36] Thomas, M. M., T. S. Hinks, et al. (2008). "Rapid diagnosis of Mycobacterium tuberculosis meningitis by enumeration of cerebrospinal fluid antigen-specific T-cells."*Int J Tuberc Lung Dis*12 (6): 651-657.

[37] Moadebi, S., C. K. Harder, et al. (2007). "Fluoroquinolones for the treatment of pulmonary tuberculosis."*Drugs*67 (14): 2077-2099.

[38] Kaojarern, S., K. Supmonchai, et al. (1991). "Effect of steroids on cerebrospinal fluid penetration of antituberculous drugs in tuberculous meningitis."*ClinPharmacolTher*49 (1): 6-12.

[39] World Health Organization. (2002) *Treatment of tuberculosis: guidelines for national programmes,*3rd edn. Geneva,Switzerland: World Health Organization.

[40] Berenguer, J., S. Moreno, et al. (1992). "Tuberculous meningitis in patients infected with the human immunodeficiency virus."*N Engl J Med*326 (10): 668-672.

[41] Garg, R. K. and M. K. Sinha (2011). "Tuberculous meningitis in patients infected with human immunodeficiency virus." *J Neurol*258 (1): 3-13.

[42] Horn, D. L., D. Hewlett, Jr., et al. (1993). "RISE-resistant tuberculous meningitis in AIDS patient."*Lancet*341 (8838): 177-178.

[43] Patel, V. B., N. Padayatchi, et al. (2004). "Multidrug-resistant tuberculous meningitis in KwaZulu-Natal, South Africa."*Clin Infect Dis*38 (6): 851-856.

[44] Byrd, T. F. and L. E. Davis (2007). "Multidrug-resistant tuberculous meningitis."*CurrNeurolNeurosci Rep*7 (6): 470-475.

[45] Huttner, H. B., R. Kollmar, et al. (2004). "Fatal tuberculous meningitis caused by immune restoration disease." *J Neurol*251 (12): 1522-1523.

[46] McIlleron, H., G. Meintjes, et al. (2007). "Complications of antiretroviral therapy in patients with tuberculosis: drug interactions, toxicity, and immune reconstitution inflammatory syndrome." *J Infect Dis*196 Suppl 1: S63-75.

[47] Saukkonen, J. J., D. L. Cohn, et al. (2006). "An official ATS statement: hepatotoxicity of antituberculosis therapy." *Am J RespirCrit Care Med*174 (8): 935-952.

[48] Prasad K,Singh MB. (2008) *Corticosterois for managing tuberculous meningitis.* Cochrane Database Syst Rev;Art. No.: CD002244.DOI:10.1002/14651858. CD002244.pub 3.

[49] Thwaites, G. E., D. B. Nguyen, et al. (2004). "Dexamethasone for the treatment of tuberculous meningitis in adolescents and adults."*N Engl J Med*351 (17): 1741-1751.

[50] Thwaites, G. E., J. Macmullen-Price, et al. (2007). "Serial MRI to determine the effect of dexamethasone on the cerebral pathology of tuberculous meningitis: an observational study." *Lancet Neurol*6 (3): 230-236.

[51]   Green, J. A., C. T. Tran, et al. (2009). "Dexamethasone, cerebrospinal fluid matrix metalloproteinase concentrations and clinical outcomes in tuberculous meningitis."*PLoS One*4 (9): e7277.

[52]   Arseni, C. (1958). "Two hundred and one cases of intracranial tuberculoma treated surgically." *J NeurolNeurosurg Psychiatry* 21 (4): 308-311.

[53]   Jinkins, J. R. (1991). "Computed tomography of intracranial tuberculosis."*Neuroradiology* 33 (2): 126-135.

[54]   Loizou, L. A. and M. Anderson (1982). "Intracranial tuberculomas: correlation of computerized tomography with clinico-pathological findings." *Q J Med*51 (201): 104-114.

[55]   Mayers, M. M., D. M. Kaufman, et al. (1978). "Recent cases of intracranial tuberculomas." *Neurology*28 (3): 256-260.

[56]   Whiteman, M. L. (1997). "Neuroimaging of central nervous system tuberculosis in HIV-infected patients."*Neuroimaging Clin N Am*7 (2): 199-214.

[57]   Alarcòn F,Espinosa S,Dueñas G. (2001) Respuesta paradojica y desarrollo de tuberculomas intracraneales durante tratamiento antituberculoso: Reporte de seis casos. *Rev Ecuat Neurol.;*10: 43-49.

[58]   Nicolls, D. J., M. King, et al. (2005). "Intracranial tuberculomas developing while on therapy for pulmonary tuberculosis." *Lancet Infect Dis*5 (12): 795-801.

[59]   Garcia Monco JC, Ferreira E,Gomez-Beldarrain M. (2005) The therapeutic paradox in the diagnosis of tuberculous meningitis. *Neurology*; 65:191-192.

[60]   Afghani, B. and J. M. Lieberman (1994). "Paradoxical enlargement or development of intracranial tuberculomas during therapy: case report and review." *Clin Infect Dis*19 (6): 1092-1099.

[61]   Lee, S. I., J. H. Park, et al. (2008). "Paradoxical progression of intracranial tuberculomas and anterior cerebral artery infarction. "*Neurology*71 (1): 68.

[62]   Tyson, G., P. Newman, et al. (1978). "Tuberculous brain abscess."*SurgNeurol*10 (5): 323-325.

[63]   KalitaJ, MisraUK,RanjanP. (2007) Predictors of long –term neurological sequelae of tuberculous meningitis: a multivariate analysis.Eur J Neurol 2007;14:33-37 (Erratum in: Eur J Neurol;14:357.

In: Meningitis: Causes, Diagnosis and Treatment   ISBN 978-1-62100-833-0
Editors: G. Houllis et al. pp. 175-201   ©2012 Nova Science Publishers, Inc.

Chapter 4

MENINGITIS ASSOCIATED WITH AUTOIMMUNE DISEASES

Masakazu Nakamura[1] and Masaaki Niino[2,]*
[1]Department of Neurology, Hokkaido University Graduate School of
Medicine, Sapporo, Japan
[2]Department of Clinical Research, Hokkaido Medical Center, Sapporo,
Japan

ABSTRACT

Autoimmune diseases can be organ-specific or systemic, with the latter type affecting many different organs. As a neurological complication particularly of systemic autoimmune diseases such as systemic lupus erythematosus and Behçet disease, meningitis can occur at any stage of the disease and can be a main symptom as well as a prognostic factor. Mechanisms of meningitis associated with autoimmune diseases are still unclear, although disease-specific autoantibodies and cytokines are considered to play critical roles in the pathogenesis.

In meningitis associated with autoimmune disease, the main symptoms are fever, headache, nausea, and neck stiffness, which are similar to those presenting in infectious, malignant, or other forms of meningitis. The clinical course is also varied and can be acute, chronic, or recurrent, and thus is not that helpful in differential diagnosis. It is extremely difficult to prove that comorbid autoimmune disease is a direct

---
[*] Tel.: +81 11 6118111, Fax: +81 11 611 5820, E-mail: niino@hok-mc.hosp.go.jp

cause of meningitis, but the exclusion of other etiologies is essential for accurate diagnosis. Such diagnosis is made from a full set of physical and laboratory data and imaging findings. Furthermore, in patients with autoimmune diseases treated with immunosuppressive or immunomodulating agents, it is often difficult to differentiate meningitis associated with autoimmune disease from infectious or drug-induced meningitis.

Treatment options for meningitis related to autoimmune diseases are targeted to suppress activated autoimmunity, and immunosuppressive agents such as pulsed cyclophosphamide and steroids are often recommended for acute relapse or severe forms of the disease. Recently, new agents such as monoclonal antibodies have been tested in cases involving the central nervous system; however, their efficacy remains unclear.

In this chapter, we discuss autoimmune diseases with which meningitis can occur, and review the clinical features, diagnosis, and treatments for meningitis associated with autoimmune diseases.

INTRODUCTION

Meningitis can be observed during the course of autoimmune diseases. Diagnosis of meningitis is based on the signs of meningeal irritation, inflammatory findings in cerebrospinal fluid (CSF), and meningeal enhancement on brain magnetic resonance imaging (MRI), and this diagnostic procedure is the same as for meningitis of other etiologies. However, the typical symptoms of meningitis are often absent in autoimmune diseases,making meningitis associated with autoimmune diseasesoften difficult to diagnose. In some autoimmune diseases, meningitis is a critical complication of the central nervous system (CNS). In patients treated with corticosteroids and/or otherimmunosuppressants, the differential diagnosis of co-morbid meningitis in autoimmune diseases or infectionsis important for treatment, but it can be extremely difficult to diagnose. Carcinomatous meningitis can occur in patients treated long term with corticosteroids and other immunosuppressants. Moreover, nonsteroidal anti-inflammatory drugs (NSAIDs), which are often used for patients with autoimmune diseases, may also induce meningitis.

In patients with autoimmune diseases, meningitis can occur due to various causes, such as autoimmunity, infection, medication, or malignancy, with different prognoses. Here, we discuss autoimmune diseases in which meningitis can occur and review the clinical features, diagnosis, and treatment of meningitis associated with these diseases.

BEHÇET DISEASE

Behçet disease (BD) is an idiopathic vascular inflammatory multisystem disease characterized by recurrent oral and genital ulcers and uveitis [1, 2]. There is a geographical variation in its prevalence, with a higher rate in the region along the Silk Route from the Mediterranean basin to Japan and a very low rate in Europe and North America. There is a similar geographical variation in HLA-B51 sensitivity, which is strongly associated with this disease [3].

BD manifests neurological complications mainly in the CNS, which is termed neuro-Behçet disease (NBD) [4, 5]. Neurological complications commonly develop a few years after the onset of BD [6-8], although they can occur as the first symptom of BD [6, 9, 10]. Such complications are clinically important as they are the most serious causes of long-term mortality and morbidity in BD [11], even though the prevalence of NBD is low (around 5% in general, and about 10% in the area of highest prevalence of BD along the Silk Route [6-8, 12, 13]). CNS involvement shows two forms. The first is parenchymal type, which is characterized by any objective CNS abnormalities detected on neurological examination, neuroimaging, or CSF tests. These findings are based on small-vessel disease. Cases of parenchymal type BD mainly show brainstem or pyramidal tract syndrome, and many cases present neurological symptoms as acute attacks, while some present with a chronic progressive course [6, 7, 14]. The second is non-parenchymal (vascular) type, characterized by extra-axial large vessel disease (cerebral venous sinus thrombosis, intracranial aneurysm, or extracranial aneurysm/dissection). These cases have limited symptoms such as headache from intracranial hypertension [4, 5, 15].

Meningitis is usually observed as a comorbid finding with 70–80% of parenchymal type cases [6, 7, 14], whereas it occurs less frequently as the sole presentation (only 4 of 50 NBS cases in a UK report [7] and 1 of 200 cases in a Turkish study [6]). Fever and headache are common symptoms in the exacerbation of parenchymal neurological involvement. However, these symptoms are often observed as part of the comorbid systemic features, which include malaise, orogenital ulcers, skin lesions, and uveitis [7, 10, 12].

Headache due to direct neurological involvement is present in around 10% of patients, whereas primary headache (e.g. migraine and tension-type headache) accounts for 70% of headaches [16-20]. In addition, non-structural headache associated with systemic exacerbations of BD is frequently reported, and there is no evidence of direct CNS involvement in this type of headache [16, 18, 19].In the CSF, white blood cell counts are significantly raised with a neutrophil-dominant pattern in the early stage, changing into a lymphocyte-dominant pattern in the later stage of meningitis [5], and the protein level is also moderately increased, often above 1 g/dl [6-8, 14]. Raised white blood cell counts and protein levels in the CSF are thought to be poor prognostic factors [6, 7, 14]. Elevated interleukin-6 (IL-6) levels in the CSF are considered to be a feature of NBD, and are associated with disease activity and prognosis [21-24]. In addition, it has been suggested that CSF IL-6 levels higher than 20 pg/ml indicate a poor long-term prognosis [21].There are no specific treatments for meningitis in NBD, and treatments are the same as for other forms of NBD (Table 1). Parenchymal acute attacks in NBD are usually treated with corticosteroids, either high-dose intravenous methylprednisolone or oral prednisolone [4, 5]. These treatments are followed by a slow tapering of oral prednisolone over 2 to 3 months in order to avoid early relapse [25]. The efficacy of other immunosuppressive or immunomodulatory drugs, such as colchicine, azathioprine, cyclophosphamide, methotrexate, chlorambucil, mycophenolatemofetil, tacrolimus, and thalidomide, has been demonstrated for some systemic manifestations, but not fully for neurological involvement of BD [4, 5]. It has been reported that chlorambcil improves CSF pleocytosis with meningoencephalitis in BD [26], although its efficacy for NBD is still unclear. Cyclosporin A, commonly used for ocular involvement of BD, is not recommended for NBD due to neurotoxicity and the risk of inducing neurological complications [27-31]. For NBD with a chronic progressive course, weekly oral methotrexate was shown to slow the rate of deterioration in one study [23], but this finding has not been confirmed. Recently, the efficacy of monoclonal anti-tumor necrosis factor (TNF)-α antibody for NBD has been reported [32-37]. An expert panel recommended that the anti-TNFα antibody infliximab could be used for patients refractory to therapies with pulse cyclophosphamide and prednisolone, or those who relapse while on maintenance therapy with azathioprine or prednisolone [38].

Table1. Treatments for CNS manifestation of autoimmune diseases focusing on aseptic meningitis

autoimmune disease	meningitis related to autoimmune disease	1st-line therapy for acute attacks and maintenance	2nd-line therapy for refractory cases or to avoid adverse effects of corticosteroids	3rd-line therapy for severe or more refractory cases	Expected therapy (efficacy needs to be confirmed)
Behçet disease (BD)	neuro-Behçet disease (NBD) (parenchymal type involving aseptic meningitis)	corticosteroids	switch to or add immunosuppressants (cyclophosphamide, azathioprine, etc) except for cyclosporin A	monoclonal anti-TNFα antibody (infliximab)	
systemic lupus erythematosus (SLE)	neuropsychiatric SLE (NPSLE) involving aseptic meningitis	corticosteroids	combination with immunosuppressants (intravenous cyclophosphamide is recommended)	high-dose cyclophosphamide with autologous hematopoietic stem cell transplantation	mycophenolatemofetil monoclonal anti-CD20 antibody (rituximab)
rheumatoid arthritis (RA)	rheumatoid pachymeningitis (RPM)	corticosteroids	combination with immunosuppressants (cyclophosphamide or methotrexate)		
	rheumatoid leptomeningitis (RLM)	corticosteroids	switch to or add in immunosuppressants (cyclophosphamide, cyclosporin A, etc)	monoclonal anti-TNFα antibody (infliximab, etc)	
Sjögren's syndrome (SjS)	neurologic manifestation involving aseptic meningitis	corticosteroids	switch to or add in cyclophosphamide (intravenous administration is common)	other immunosuppressants (combination with corticosteroids or monotherapy)	monoclonal anti-CD20 antibody (rituximab or epratuzumab) monoclonal anti-TNFα antibody (infliximab or etanercept)
sarcoidosis	neurosarcoidosis (NS) involving aseptic meningitis	corticosteroids	combination with immunosuppressants	TNFα antagonist (pentoxifylline or thalidomide) monoclonal anti-TNFα antibody (infliximab)	

Most NBD patients have been shown to recover well from acute attacks, whereas after more than 10 years from onset of neurologic involvement, 20–50% of patients have at least mild neurological disabilities due to repeat relapses or conversion to a progressive disease course [4, 6-8, 14]. Optimal treatments for parenchymal neurological complications including meningitis are expected to be established to prevent neurological sequelae.

SYSTEMIC LUPUS ERYTHEMATOSUS

Systemic lupus erythematosus (SLE) is a chronic autoimmune disease characterized by multi-organ involvement, including the peripheral and central nervous systems. These neurological syndromes in SLE patients in which other causes have been excluded are termed neuropsychiatric syndromes of SLE (NPSLE), and classified by the American College of Rheumatism into 19 categories, one of which is aseptic meningitis [39]. NPSLE develops before or around the time of diagnosis of SLE [40]. NPSLE has been reported in 23.3–95.0% of patients with SLE, whereas the rate of aseptic meningitis is consistently very low (0–2%) [41-46]. These neurological manifestations are associated with a poor prognosis [40, 47, 48].

The pathogenesis of NPSLE is considered to be due to many factors, including microangiopathy, premature atherosclerosis, autoantibody production, and intrathecal production of pro-inflammatory cytokines [49, 50]. Accumulating evidence indicates that collapse of the integrity of the blood–brain barrier,mainly due to the up-regulated expression of adhesion molecules on vascular endothelial cells, which is attributed to pro-inflammatory cytokines and autoantibodies, is critical for development of NPSLE [51-53]. Anti-phospholipid antibodies were reported to be associated with thrombotic events, including stroke [54] and cognitive dysfunction [55-57] in SLE patients. Antibodies against ribosome P were reported to be associated with psychosis, depression, and NPSLE activities [58-60]. There have been some reports that anti-glutamate receptor antibodies might be associated with cognitive dysfunction and/or depression, but this is still controversial [61, 62].

Meningitis associated with SLE generally consists of aseptic meningitis as NPSLE (see above), infectious septic or aseptic meningitis, or drug-induced aseptic meningitis (DIAM; especially by NSAIDs). Many defects of the immune system in SLE, such as complement protein and receptor deficiency, impaired spleen function [63-65], and decreased T cell count and function [66, 67], increase the risk of infection. In addition, corticosteroids and immunosupressants commonly used for SLE lead to immune insufficiency [66-68]. Thus, infectious meningitis should always be kept in mind in the diagnosis of SLE patients.The infectious agents *Listeria monocytogenes* [69], *Mycobacterium tuberculosis* [70], and *Cryptococcusneoformans* [71] should be considered. It has been reported that SLE patients are predisposed to NSAID-related meningitis (DIAM) [72]. In particular, they tend to show some specificity for ibuprofen, and a specific cell–cell-mediated immunity to ibuprofen has been reported [73, 74]. DIAM is also important in the differential diagnosis of meningitis in SLE in those patients treated with NSAIDs.

Signs of meningeal irritation (fever, headache, nausea, vomiting, and neck stiffness) usually accompany these three types of meningitis, and the nature of these symptoms does not differ among the three types [75, 76]. Thus, it is important to have an understanding of chronic headaches without meningitis (such as migraine, tension-type headache, or intracranial hypertension) which are often observed in NPSLE (20–70%) [41-44, 46].

In the CSF of SLE cases with aseptic meningitis, mild pleocytosis predominantly of lymphocytes is usually observed, and mildly to moderately elevated protein is reported [45, 77-79]. Although there have been some reports of decreased CSF glucose levels in SLE, whether these findings are disease-specific has not yet been confirmed [77, 80]. Higher cell counts, higher protein level, and lower glucose level might suggest septic meningitis; however, these findings are not always crucial differential points [75, 76]. Culture, stain (gram, india ink, and acid-fast bacillus), latex agglutination test (for some bacteria), and PCR (containing virus) are essential to diagnose infectious meningitis. It is difficult to discriminate with CSF findings between NPSLE and DIAM following administration of NSAIDs as the cause of aseptic meningitis.

The optimal treatment for aseptic meningitis with SLE as NPSLE is not clear. Antibiotics and a stress dose of steroids are often provided as primary treatment while waiting for laboratory tests to confirm or rule out septic meningitis [75, 76]. It seems that full recovery could be expected in aseptic meningitis as NPSLE, whereas septic meningitis is likely to cause psychosis (cognitive dysfunction and depression) and some focal signs [75, 76]. For DIAM, it takes a few days to recover after drug withdrawal, and this course is helpful to diagnosis [72]. Steroids alone or in combination with immunosuppressive therapy are generally recommended for NPSLE [81, 82] (Table 1). Cyclophosphamide is often selected as monthly intravenous (500–1000 mg/m^2) doses for a 6-month induction period followed by quarterly maintenance doses for a period of 2 years for severe NPSLE [83]. Recently, it has been reported that high-dose cyclophosphamide (200 mg/m^2), with or without autologous hematopoietic stem cell transplantation, is effective for severe NPSLE with other organ involvement [84-88]. Mycophenolatemofetil [89] and rituximab [90, 91] have also demonstrated potentially beneficial effects for SLE.

RHEUMATOID ARTHRITIS

Rheumatoid arthritis (RA) is a systemic inflammatory disease in which the joints are the main targets but other organs such as skin, eyes, lungs, blood vessels, and the nervous system may be involved [92]. Pachymeningitis and leptomeningitis are rare CNS complications of RA. These two forms have been discriminated by pathological findings mainly at autopsy, although brain MRI findings or gadolinium enhancement of the dura mater or leptomeninx have recently been used in clinical practice. With regard to symptoms, cranial nerve palsy is characteristic of pachymeningitis, but rarely of leptomeningitis. Pathophysiologic mechanisms and optimal treatments have not yet been fully clarified for either type of meningitis.

i) Rheumatoid Pachymeningitis (RPM)

RPM usually occurs at either the very early or late stage of RA, although it can precede systemic involvement of RA in rare cases. The gender ratio of RPM is equal. Headache and cranial nerve palsy are the main symptoms, and optic nerve involvement is common [93, 94]. Cranial nerve palsy may be caused either by constriction of the nerves by a thickened dura mater or by direct invasion of the inflammatory cells [95]. RPM can also involve hydrocephalus [96], sinus thrombosis [96], transient ischemic attack [97], and intracranial hypotension [98]. Serum rheumatoid factor (RF) is positive in almost all cases [93, 94]. CSF sometimes shows slight pleocytosis, and protein levels are usually elevated [93, 96, 99, 100]. RF in the CSF is often used as a diagnostic marker [99, 101]. The pathology of the biopsied dura mater is most significant for diagnosis. In autopsy specimens, typical rheumatoid nodules are observed as central necrosis surrounded by elongated histiocytes and mononuclear inflammatory cells, whereas biopsy specimens usually show inflammatory cells and fibrosis, and rarely demonstrate rheumatoid nodules probably because of limited tissue sampling [93, 94, 102]. However, MRI is currently the most useful diagnostic tool for RPM. MRI can detect thickening of the dura mater with linear and/or nodular enhancement in idiopathic hypertrophic pachymeningitis [103, 104]. In images without contrast enhancement, the thickened dura is hyperintense on T1-weigted images and hypointense on T2-weighted images [105]. Lesions are likely to be observed in the tentorium involving the falxcerebri and in the tentorium cerebelli [93, 99, 100, 106]. Treatments have not yet been established for RPM. Several decades ago, patients died soon after the onset of RPM in spite of corticosteroid administration [102], which is one of the reasons why many patients were diagnosed by autopsy, although there were some reports of successful treatment by corticosteroids alone [94, 99]. Recently, a combination of corticosteroids and other immunosuppressants (cyclophosphamide [100] or methotrexate [94]) have been indicated as effective treatment options (Table 1). Various prognoses have been reported: almost complete remission and no relapse, some sequalae, and death [93, 94, 102].

ii) Rheumatoid Leptomeningitis

Rheumatoid leptomeningitis (RLM) can occur with or without arthritis activity and even as a first symptom of RA. It is noted that meningeal signs are often lacking, but focal signs (e.g. hemiparesis, sensory disturbance of extremities, and seizures) and mental state abnormalities (e.g. disturbed consciousness and delirium) can be present. Serum RF is commonly positive. In the CSF, protein levels are usually elevated, whereas pleocytosis is not usually observed [94, 97, 107-114]. IL-6 levels in the CSF might indicate leptomeningitis [113]. The level of TNF-α in the CSF is controversial; it may [110] or may not be elevated [113] in leptomeningitis. Brain MRI scans reveal leptomeningeal enhancement and high intensity of the subarachnoid spaces on fluid-attenuated inversion recovery (FLAIR) images and diffusion weighted images (DWIs). Leptomeningeal lesions are usually focal, and focal signs are often observed [94, 97, 107-114]. Recently, it was reported that DWIs showed patchy high intensity in pia mater lesions which demonstrated high intensity on FLAIR images [112]. Corticosteroids are the drugs most commonly used to treat leptomeningitis and are effective for many patients. The other immunosuppressants, cyclophosphamide and cyclosporine A, are also reported to be useful [94, 97, 107-114]. Taken together, it seems appropriate to select corticosteroids as a first step in treating rheumatoid meningitis, and change or add other immunosuppressants when corticosteroids are ineffective or have to be stopped because of adverse effects. Anti-TNFα antibodies are expected to cure RLM, whereas pachymeningitis and/or leptomeningitis can occur during the administration of infliximab [107] and adalizumab [115] (Table 1).

SJöGREN'S SYNDROME

Sjögren's syndrome (SjS) is an autoimmune disease characterized by mononuclear infiltration and destruction of the salivary glands leading to xerostomia and xerophthalmia with extraglandular manifestations. SjS is classified as either primary or secondary disease; primary SjS occurs by itself and secondary SjS occurs after the onset of another connective tissue disease.

In SjS, the nervous system can be widely involved with predominance of peripheral nervous system involvement (e.g. polyneuropathy) [116, 117]. The CNS may be involved in up to 20% of cases with SjS [118, 119], with symptoms including myelopathy, multiple sclerosis-like syndrome, aseptic meningitis, or meningoencephalitis [120-122]. Aseptic meningitis and meningoencephalitis have been reported to occur in 20% of patients with CNS complications of SjS [120].Aseptic meningitis and meningoencephalitis are generally described as acute forms of the disease [120]; subacute or chronic forms have also been reported [123, 124]. In the acute forms, patients show acute-onset signs of meningeal irritation (e.g. fever, nausea, headache, and neck stiffness), sometimes with focal signs and seizures [120]. By contrast, the subacute or chronic forms may lack any or show very few of these meningeal signs, and unexpected symptoms such as cranial nerve palsies and cognitive dysfunction are sometimes presented [123, 124].

Serum tests often reveal anti-nuclear antibodies, RF, anti-Ro/SS-A antibodies, and anti-La/SS-B antibodies. Anti-Ro/SS-A antibodies are considered to be associated with CNS vasculitis in SjS, which might reflect the underlying pathology of meningitis and meningoencephalitis in SjS [119, 121, 125]. The CSF commonly shows mild and moderate pleocytosis, consisting predominantly of polymorphonuclear leukocytes at onset, and then mononuclear cells. Elevated protein levels are also commonly observed. IntrathecalIgG synthesis is also present, and oligoclonal bands are often detected [120, 126]. IL-6 in the CSF might be an indicator of CNS complications of SjS [127]. Specific autoantibodies against recurrent aseptic meningitis in the serum and CSF, recognizing 56-kD and 44-kD nuclear antigens of the CNS neurons, meningeal cells, and cells of other systemic organs, have been reported recently [128]. Brain computed tomography (CT) and MRI may show diffuse leptomeningeal and subarachnoid enhancement, which are not disease-specific findings [120, 123].

Most cases of aseptic meningitis become less severe or completely resolve in response to corticosteroid administration [120, 123, 128] (Table 1).Cyclophosphamide may be recommended as second-line treatment when meningoencephalitis is refractory to corticosteroids. Other immunosuppressants such as azathioprine, cyclosporine, methotrexate, chlorambucil, and tacrolimus may also be effective as monotherapy or in combination with corticosteroids [127, 129-132]. Recently, rituximab has been reported to successfully treat CNS manifestation of SjS [133]. However, B-cell targeted monoclonal antibodies (rituximab and epratuzumab) have not been considered as established treatment options, in contrast to anti-TNFα antibodies (infliximab and *etanercept*) [134]. Plasmapheresis and intravenous immunoglobulin might be worth considering in refractory cases for acute relief of symptoms [134, 135].

SARCOIDOSIS

Sarcoidosis is a multisystem inflammatory granulomatous disease with the characteristic pathological finding of noncaseating granuloma. The enhanced helper T-cell response is considered to be an important inducer of the disease, although its etiology remains unclear. It usually develops between the ages of 20 and 40 years, and predominantly affects the lungs, anterior uvea, lymph nodes, and skin [136, 137]. The prevalence of sarcoidosis remarkably differs among races; for example, 3–10 per 100,000 population in Caucasians and 35–80 per 100,000 in African Americans in North America [138].

Sarcoidosis can involve both peripheral and central nervous system, and is known as neurosarcoidosis (NS). NS occurs in less than 10% of clinically diagnosed sarcoidosis [139-141]. However, post-mortem studies have revealed that only 50% of cases with NS are diagnosed antemortem, suggesting that subclinical neurological manifestations may be more common [142, 143]. The diagnostic criteria of NS require nervous system pathological findings, and include the Kveim-Siltzbachtest (with potential infection transfer and other disadvantages), chest X-ray, and serum angiotensin-converting enzyme (ACE), which are poorly sensitive for NS for defining probable or possible disease [144]. This might be one of the reasons for the low rate of antemortem diagnosis of NS. Some investigators have proposed changing these three criteria to high-definition chest CT, bronchoalveolar lavage with a CD4:CD8 ratio >3.5, and a CD4:CD8 ratio >5 in the CSF.However, more data are needed to confirm the reliability of these criteria [145].

NS manifestations are various, such as cranial neuropathy, myelopathy, seizures, and headaches, and meningitis is also a common complication. Meningeal signs are of major importance in NS; however, meningitis may not be noticed until CSF analysis is conducted, because CSF pleocytosis is observed in as many as 50–70% of NS patients [144, 146-149]. Meningeal enhancement on brain MRI might also be diagnostic evidence in the absence of signs of meningeal irritation. Meningitis as NS may be acute, subacute, or chronic [139-141], and its symptoms may occur in the early course of the disease along with other neurological complications of NS [141, 144], which makes it difficult to diagnose. In the CSF, mild to moderate pleocytosis (10–200 cells/mm^3) with lymphocyte predominance and elevated protein levels (about 2.6 g/l) are commonly observed. Glucose concentration in the CSF is often decreased. IntrathecalIgG production is reported in some patients. Oligoclonal bands are detected in 20–80% of NS patients [144, 146-149]. The CSF ACE level is used as an indicator of diagnosis and disease activity, as ACE is thought to be derived from sarcoid granulomas in CSF [150, 151]. However, the rate of CSF ACE activity in NS is wide and CSF ACE activity could also be observed in other conditions such as infection and malignancy [152]. Taken together, it is currently suggested that CSF ACE activity should be considered as a supplementary index in diagnosis and treatment decision-making. Intracranial NS generally involves the leptomeninges and brain parenchyma attached to the meninges, especially in the basal cisterns. Brain MRI usually shows a nodular or diffuse thickening of the affected meninges, and focal parenchymal lesions in white matter and hypothalamic regions [149, 153]. The latter lesions are hyperintense on T2-weighted images and isointense on T1-weighted images, resembling multiple sclerosis in which the lesions have a mainly periventricular distribution [154]. The concomitant meningeal thickening could be one of the differential diagnostic points [147, 155]. Specific treatments for NS have not been identified, but general treatments are available for sarcoidosis (Table 1). First-line therapy for NS is corticosteroid administration; however, adverse effects with high dosage over a long duration and relapses accompanied by tapering are often experienced [144, 153]. In order to avoid these problems, use of other immunosuppressants should be considered. Although there have been some reports of NS treated with methotrexate [156, 157], cyclosporine [158], azathioprine [147], mycophenolatemofetil [159], or cyclophosphamide [160], it is unclear which drugs are most efficacious currently. TNFα may have a pathogenic role in NS via formation of granulomas in sarcoidosis, and the TNFα antagonistspentoxifylline and thalidomide are expected to ameliorate the symptoms of NS [153, 161, 162]. A monoclonal antibody against TNFα, infliximab, has shown efficacy for refractory sarcoidosis involving NS [163-168].

OTHER AUTOIMMUNE DISEASES

Mixed connective tissue disease (MCTD) [169], Vogt-Koyanagi-Harada disease (KVH) [170], ANCA-associated vasculitis (AAV) [171], primary angiitis of the CNS [172], multiple sclerosis [173], and neuromyelitisoptica [174] are also known to exacerbate aseptic meningitis. In each disease, the clinical significance of detecting meningitis is different. In KVH, it is an important finding for diagnosis of the disease. Although meningitis is a rare complication of MCTD and AAV, the complication of meningitis might require more aggressive treatment in those diseases. Wegener's granulomatosis and microscopic polyangiitis in AAV are well known to include hypertrophic pachymeningitis. These two diseases are important in the differential diagnosis of "idiopathic" hypertrophic pachymeningitis [175-178].

CONCLUSION

Meningitis associated with autoimmune diseases is often difficult to diagnose because autoimmune diseases have various frequencies of occurrence, various clinical courses, and different examination findings as well as a lack of definite evidence to differentiate them from other etiologies such as infection and drugs. Disease-specific pathogenetic mechanisms of meningitis remain unclear, which has resulted in a lack of consensus regarding the optimal treatment and prognosis. Future studies are required to elucidate the pathogenesis of meningitis associated with autoimmune diseases in order to advance future treatment and improve the prognosis of the patients with autoimmune diseases.

REFERENCES

[1] Sakane T, Takeno M, Suzuki N, Inaba G. Behcet's disease. *N. Engl. J. Med.* 1999 Oct 21;341(17):1284-91.

[2] Verity DH, Wallace GR, Vaughan RW, Stanford MR. Behcet's disease: from Hippocrates to the third millennium. *Br. J. Ophthalmol.* 2003 Sep;87(9):1175-83.

[3] Verity DH, Marr JE, Ohno S, Wallace GR, Stanford MR. Behcet's disease, the Silk Road and HLA-B51: historical and geographical perspectives. *Tissue Antigens.* 1999 Sep;54(3):213-20.

[4] Siva A, Saip S. The spectrum of nervous system involvement in Behcet's syndrome and its differential diagnosis. *J. Neurol.* 2009 Apr;256(4):513-29.

[5] Al-Araji A, Kidd DP. Neuro-Behcet's disease: epidemiology, clinical characteristics, and management. *Lancet Neurol.* 2009 Feb;8(2):192-204.

[6] Akman-Demir G, Serdaroglu P, Tasci B. Clinical patterns of neurological involvement in Behcet's disease: evaluation of 200 patients. The Neuro-Behcet Study Group. *Brain.* 1999 Nov;122 (Pt 11):2171-82.

[7] Kidd D, Steuer A, Denman AM, Rudge P. Neurological complications in Behcet's syndrome. *Brain.* 1999 Nov;122 (Pt 11):2183-94.

[8] Siva A, Kantarci OH, Saip S, Altintas A, Hamuryudan V, Islak C, et al. Behcet's disease: diagnostic and prognostic aspects of neurological involvement. *J. Neurol.* 2001 Feb;248(2):95-103.

[9] Wechsler B, Dell'lsola B, Vidailhet M, Dormont D, Piette JC, Bletry O, et al. MRI in 31 patients with Behcet's disease and neurological involvement: prospective study with clinical correlation. *J. Neurol. Neurosurg. Psychiatry.* 1993 Jul;56(7):793-8.

[10] Joseph FG, Scolding NJ. Neuro-Behcet's disease in Caucasians: a study of 22 patients. *Eur. J. Neurol.* 2007 Feb;14(2):174-80.

[11] Kural-Seyahi E, Fresko I, Seyahi N, Ozyazgan Y, Mat C, Hamuryudan V, et al. The long-term mortality and morbidity of Behcet syndrome: a 2-decade outcome survey of 387 patients followed at a dedicated center. *Medicine* (Baltimore). 2003 Jan;82(1):60-76.

[12] Al-Araji A, Sharquie K, Al-Rawi Z. Prevalence and patterns of neurological involvement in Behcet's disease: a prospective study from Iraq. *J. Neurol. Neurosurg. Psychiatry.* 2003 May;74(5):608-13.

[13] Serdaroglu P, Yazici H, Ozdemir C, Yurdakul S, Bahar S, Aktin E. Neurologic involvement in Behcet's syndrome. A prospective study. *Arch. Neurol.* 1989 Mar;46(3):265-9.

[14] Al-Fahad SA, Al-Araji AH. Neuro-Behcet's disease in Iraq: a study of 40 patients. *J. Neurol. Sci.* 1999 Nov 30;170(2):105-11.

[15] Siva A, Altintas A, Saip S. Behcet's syndrome and the nervous system. *Curr. Opin. Neurol.* 2004 Jun;17(3):347-57.

[16] Borhani Haghighi A, Aflaki E, Ketabchi L. The prevalence and characteristics of different types of headache in patients with Behcet's disease, a case-control study. *Headache.* 2008 Mar;48(3):424-9.

[17] Kidd D. The prevalence of headache in Behcet's syndrome. *Rheumatology* (Oxford). 2006 May;45(5):621-3.

[18] Aykutlu E, Baykan B, Akman-Demir G, Topcular B, Ertas M. Headache in Behcet's disease. *Cephalalgia.* 2006 Feb;26(2):180-6.

[19] Saip S, Siva A, Altintas A, Kiyat A, Seyahi E, Hamuryudan V, et al. Headache in Behcet's syndrome. *Headache.* 2005 Jul-Aug;45(7):911-9.

[20] Monastero R, Mannino M, Lopez G, Camarda C, Cannizzaro C, Camarda LK, et al. Prevalence of headache in patients with Behcet's disease without overt neurological involvement. *Cephalalgia.* 2003 Mar;23(2):105-8.

[21] Akman-Demir G, Tuzun E, Icoz S, Yesilot N, Yentur SP, Kurtuncu M, et al. Interleukin-6 in neuro-Behcet's disease: association with disease subsets and long-term outcome. *Cytokine.* 2008 Dec;44(3):373-6.

[22] Hirohata S, Isshi K, Oguchi H, Ohse T, Haraoka H, Takeuchi A, et al. Cerebrospinal fluid interleukin-6 in progressive Neuro-Behcet's syndrome. *Clin. Immunol. Immunopathol.* 1997 Jan;82(1):12-7.

[23] Hirohata S, Suda H, Hashimoto T. Low-dose weekly methotrexate for progressive neuropsychiatric manifestations in Behcet's disease. *J. Neurol. Sci.* 1998 Aug 14;159(2):181-5.

[24] Wang CR, Chuang CY, Chen CY. Anticardiolipin antibodies and interleukin-6 in cerebrospinal fluid and blood of Chinese patients with neuro-Behcet's syndrome. *Clin. Exp. Rheumatol.* 1992 Nov-Dec;10(6):599-602.

[25] Siva A, Fresko II. Behcet's Disease. *Curr. Treat Options Neurol.* 2000 Sep;2(5):435-48.

[26] O'Duffy JD, Robertson DM, Goldstein NP. Chlorambucil in the treatment of uveitis and meningoencephalitis of Behcet's disease. *Am. J. Med.* 1984 Jan;76(1):75-84.

[27] Kotter I, Gunaydin I, Batra M, Vonthein R, Stubiger N, Fierlbeck G, et al. CNS involvement occurs more frequently in patients with Behcet's disease under cyclosporin A (CSA) than under other medications--results of a retrospective analysis of 117 cases. *Clin. Rheumatol.* 2006 Jul;25(4):482-6.

[28] Mitsui Y, Mitsui M, Urakami R, Kihara M, Takahashi M, Kusunoki S. Behcet disease presenting with neurological complications immediately after conversion from conventional cyclosporin A to microemulsion formulation. *Intern Med.* 2005 Feb;44(2):149-52.

[29] Kato Y, Numaga J, Kato S, Kaburaki T, Kawashima H, Fujino Y. Central nervous system symptoms in a population of Behcet's disease patients with refractory uveitis treated with cyclosporine A. *Clin. ExperimentOphthalmol.* 2001 Oct;29(5):335-6.

[30] Serkova NJ, Christians U, Benet LZ. Biochemical mechanisms of cyclosporine neurotoxicity. *Mol. Interv.* 2004 Apr;4(2):97-107.

[31] Kotake S, Higashi K, Yoshikawa K, Sasamoto Y, Okamoto T, Matsuda H. Central nervous system symptoms in patients with Behcet disease receiving cyclosporine therapy. *Ophthalmology.* 1999 Mar;106(3):586-9.

[32] Sarwar H, McGrath H, Jr., Espinoza LR. Successful treatment of long-standing neuro-Behcet's disease with infliximab. *J. Rheumatol.* 2005 Jan;32(1):181-3.

[33] Fujikawa K, Aratake K, Kawakami A, Aramaki T, Iwanaga N, Izumi Y, et al. Successful treatment of refractory neuro-Behcet's disease with infliximab: a case report to show its efficacy by magnetic resonance imaging, transcranial magnetic stimulation and cytokine profile. *Ann. Rheum. Dis.* 2007 Jan;66(1):136-7.

[34] Kikuchi H, Aramaki K, Hirohata S. Effect of infliximab in progressive neuro-Behcet's syndrome. *J. Neurol. Sci.* 2008 Sep 15;272(1-2):99-105.

[35] Licata G, Pinto A, Tuttolomondo A, Banco A, Ciccia F, Ferrante A, et al. Anti-tumour necrosis factor alpha monoclonal antibody therapy for recalcitrant cerebral vasculitis in a patient with Behcet's syndrome. *Ann. Rheum. Dis.* 2003 Mar;62(3):280-1.

[36] Ribi C, Sztajzel R, Delavelle J, Chizzolini C. Efficacy of TNF {alpha} blockade in cyclophosphamide resistant neuro-Behcet disease. *J. Neurol Neurosurg. Psychiatry.* 2005 Dec;76(12):1733-5.

[37] Pipitone N, Olivieri I, Padula A, D'Angelo S, Nigro A, Zuccoli G, et al. Infliximab for the treatment of Neuro-Behcet's disease: a case series and review of the literature. *Arthritis Rheum.* 2008 Feb 15;59(2):285-90.

[38] Sfikakis PP, Markomichelakis N, Alpsoy E, Assaad-Khalil S, Bodaghi B, Gul A, et al. Anti-TNF therapy in the management of Behcet's disease--review and basis for recommendations. *Rheumatology* (Oxford). 2007 May;46(5):736-41.

[39] The American College of Rheumatology nomenclature and case definitions for neuropsychiatric lupus syndromes. *Arthritis Rheum.* 1999 Apr;42(4):599-608.

[40] Hanly JG, Urowitz MB, Sanchez-Guerrero J, Bae SC, Gordon C, Wallace DJ, et al. Neuropsychiatric events at the time of diagnosis of systemic lupus erythematosus: an international inception cohort study. *Arthritis Rheum.* 2007 Jan;56(1):265-73.

[41] Ainiala H, Loukkola J, Peltola J, Korpela M, Hietaharju A. The prevalence of neuropsychiatric syndromes in systemic lupus erythematosus. *Neurology.* 2001 Aug 14;57(3):496-500.

[42] Sanna G, Bertolaccini ML, Cuadrado MJ, Laing H, Khamashta MA, Mathieu A, et al. Neuropsychiatric manifestations in systemic lupus erythematosus: prevalence and association with antiphospholipid antibodies. *J. Rheumatol.* 2003 May;30(5):985-92.

[43] Brey RL, Holliday SL, Saklad AR, Navarrete MG, Hermosillo-Romo D, Stallworth CL, et al. Neuropsychiatric syndromes in lupus: prevalence using standardized definitions. *Neurology.* 2002 Apr 23;58(8):1214-20.

[44] Afeltra A, Garzia P, Mitterhofer AP, Vadacca M, Galluzzo S, Del Porto F, et al. Neuropsychiatric lupus syndromes: relationship with antiphospholipid antibodies. *Neurology.* 2003 Jul 8;61(1):108-10.

[45] Kasitanon N, Louthrenoo W, Piyasirisilp S, Sukitawu W, Wichainun R. Neuropsychiatric manifestations in Thai patients with systemic lupus erythematosus. *Asian Pac. J. Allergy Immunol.* 2002 Sep;20(3):179-85.

[46] Sibbitt WL, Jr., Brandt JR, Johnson CR, Maldonado ME, Patel SR, Ford CC, et al. The incidence and prevalence of neuropsychiatric syndromes in pediatric onset systemic lupus erythematosus. *J. Rheumatol.* 2002 Jul;29(7):1536-42.

[47] Harel L, Sandborg C, Lee T, von Scheven E. Neuropsychiatric manifestations in pediatric systemic lupus erythematosus and association with antiphospholipid antibodies. *J. Rheumatol.* 2006 Sep;33(9):1873-7.

[48] Bernatsky S, Clarke A, Gladman DD, Urowitz M, Fortin PR, Barr SG, et al. Mortality related to cerebrovascular disease in systemic lupus erythematosus. *Lupus.* 2006;15(12):835-9.

[49] Hanly JG. Neuropsychiatric lupus. *Curr. Rheumatol. Rep.* 2001 Jun;3(3):205-12.

[50] Jennekens FG, Kater L. The central nervous system in systemic lupus erythematosus. Part 2. Pathogenetic mechanisms of clinical syndromes: a literature investigation. *Rheumatology* (Oxford). 2002 Jun;41(6):619-30.

[51] Ainiala H, Hietaharju A, Dastidar P, Loukkola J, Lehtimaki T, Peltola J, et al. Increased serum matrix metalloproteinase 9 levels in systemic lupus erythematosus patients with neuropsychiatric manifestations and brain magnetic resonance imaging abnormalities. *Arthritis Rheum.* 2004 Mar;50(3):858-65.

[52] Zaccagni H, Fried J, Cornell J, Padilla P, Brey RL. Soluble adhesion molecule levels, neuropsychiatric lupus and lupus-related damage. *FrontBiosci.* 2004 May 1;9:1654-9.

[53] Abbott NJ, Mendonca LL, Dolman DE. The blood-brain barrier in systemic lupus erythematosus. *Lupus.* 2003;12(12):908-15.

[54] Cervera R, Khamashta MA, Font J, Sebastiani GD, Gil A, Lavilla P, et al. Morbidity and mortality in systemic lupus erythematosus during a 10-year period: a comparison of early and late manifestations in a cohort of 1,000 patients. *Medicine* (Baltimore). 2003 Sep;82(5):299-308.

[55] McLaurin EY, Holliday SL, Williams P, Brey RL. Predictors of cognitive dysfunction in patients with systemic lupus erythematosus. *Neurology.* 2005 Jan 25;64(2):297-303.

[56] Hanly JG, Hong C, Smith S, Fisk JD. A prospective analysis of cognitive function and anticardiolipin antibodies in systemic lupus erythematosus. *Arthritis Rheum.* 1999 Apr;42(4):728-34.

[57] Menon S, Jameson-Shortall E, Newman SP, Hall-Craggs MR, Chinn R, Isenberg DA. A longitudinal study of anticardiolipin antibody levels and cognitive functioning in systemic lupus erythematosus. *Arthritis Rheum.* 1999 Apr;42(4):735-41.

[58] Yoshio T, Masuyama J, Ikeda M, Tamai K, Hachiya T, Emori T, et al. Quantification of antiribosomal P0 protein antibodies by ELISA with recombinant P0 fusion protein and their association with central nervous system disease in systemic lupus erythematosus. *J. Rheumatol.* 1995 Sep;22(9):1681-7.

[59] Schneebaum AB, Singleton JD, West SG, Blodgett JK, Allen LG, Cheronis JC, et al. Association of psychiatric manifestations with antibodies to ribosomal P proteins in systemic lupus erythematosus. *Am.J. Med.* 1991 Jan;90(1):54-62.

[60] Reichlin M. Ribosomal P antibodies and CNS lupus. *Lupus.* 2003;12(12):916-8.

[61] Lapteva L, Nowak M, Yarboro CH, Takada K, Roebuck-Spencer T, Weickert T, et al. Anti-N-methyl-D-aspartate receptor antibodies, cognitive dysfunction, and depression in systemic lupus erythematosus. *Arthritis Rheum.* 2006 Aug;54(8):2505-14.

[62] Omdal R, Brokstad K, Waterloo K, Koldingsnes W, Jonsson R, Mellgren SI. Neuropsychiatric disturbances in SLE are associated with antibodies against NMDA receptors. *Eur. J. Neurol.* 2005 May;12(5):392-8.

[63] Cunha BA. Infections in nonleukopenic compromised hosts (diabetes mellitus, SLE, steroids, and asplenia) in critical care. *Crit. Care Clin.* 1998 Apr;14(2):263-82.

[64] Mitchell SR, Nguyen PQ, Katz P. Increased risk of neisserial infections in systemic lupus erythematosus. *Semin. Arthritis Rheum.* 1990 Dec;20(3):174-84.

[65] Wilson JG, Ratnoff WD, Schur PH, Fearon DT. Decreased expression of the C3b/C4b receptor (CR1) and the C3d receptor (CR2) on B lymphocytes and of CR1 on neutrophils of patients with systemic lupus erythematosus. *Arthritis Rheum.* 1986 Jun;29(6):739-47.

[66] Noel V, Lortholary O, Casassus P, Cohen P, Genereau T, Andre MH, et al. Risk factors and prognostic influence of infection in a single cohort of 87 adults with systemic lupus erythematosus. *Ann. Rheum. Dis.* 2001 Dec;60(12):1141-4.

[67] Bermas BL, Petri M, Goldman D, Mittleman B, Miller MW, Stocks NI, et al. T helper cell dysfunction in systemic lupus erythematosus (SLE): relation to disease activity. *J. Clin. Immunol.* 1994 May;14(3):169-77.

[68] Pryor BD, Bologna SG, Kahl LE. Risk factors for serious infection during treatment with cyclophosphamide and high-dose corticosteroids for systemic lupus erythematosus. *Arthritis Rheum.* 1996 Sep;39(9):1475-82.

[69] Kraus A, Cabral AR, Sifuentes-Osornio J, Alarcon-Segovia D. Listeriosis in patients with connective tissue diseases. *J. Rheumatol.* 1994 Apr;21(4):635-8.

[70] Victorio-Navarra ST, Dy EE, Arroyo CG, Torralba TP. Tuberculosis among Filipino patients with systemic lupus erythematosus. *Semin. Arthritis Rheum.* 1996 Dec;26(3):628-34.

[71] Hung JJ, Ou LS, Lee WI, Huang JL. Central nervous system infections in patients with systemic lupus erythematosus. *J. Rheumatol.* 2005 Jan;32(1):40-3.

[72] Moris G, Garcia-Monco JC. The challenge of drug-induced aseptic meningitis. *Arch. Intern. Med.* 1999 Jun 14;159(11):1185-94.

[73] Berliner S, Weinberger A, Shoenfeld Y, Sandbank U, Hazaz B, Joshua H, et al. Ibuprofen may induce meningitis in (NZB X NZW)F1 mice. *Arthritis Rheum.* 1985 Jan;28(1):104-7.

[74] Shoenfeld Y, Livni E, Shaklai M, Pinkhas J. Sensitization to ibuprofen in systemic lupus erythematosus. *JAMA.* 1980 Aug 8;244(6):547-8.

[75] Kim JM, Kim KJ, Yoon HS, Kwok SK, Ju JH, Park KS, et al. Meningitis in Korean patients with systemic lupus erythematosus: analysis of demographics, clinical features and outcomes; experience from affiliated hospitals of the Catholic University of Korea. *Lupus.* 2011;20(5):531-6.

[76] Baizabal-Carvallo JF, Delgadillo-Marquez G, Estanol B, Garcia-Ramos G. Clinical characteristics and outcomes of the meningitides in systemic lupus erythematosus. *Eur. Neurol.* 2009;61(3):143-8.

[77] Gibson T, Myers AR. Nervous system involvement in systemic lupus erythematosus. *Ann. Rheum. Dis.* 1975 Oct;35(5):398-406.

[78] Canoso JJ, Cohen AS. Aspectic meningitis in systemic lupus erythematosus. Report of three cases. *Arthritis Rheum.* 1975 Jul-Aug;18(4):369-74.

[79] Johnson RT, Richardson EP. The neurological manifestations of systemic lupus erythematosus. *Medicine* (Baltimore). 1968 Jul;47(4):337-69.

[80] Andrianakos AA, Duffy J, Suzuki M, Sharp JT. Transverse myelopathy in systemic lupus erythematosus. Report of three cases and review of the literature. *Ann. Intern. Med.* 1975 Nov;83(5):616-24.

[81] Bertsias GK, Ioannidis JP, Aringer M, Bollen E, Bombardieri S, Bruce IN, et al. EULAR recommendations for the management of systemic lupus erythematosus with neuropsychiatric manifestations: report of a task force of the EULAR standing committee for clinical affairs. *Ann. Rheum. Dis.* 2010 Dec;69(12):2074-82.

[82] Bertsias GK, Boumpas DT. Pathogenesis, diagnosis and management of neuropsychiatric SLE manifestations. *Nat. Rev. Rheumatol.* 2010 Jun;6(6):358-67.

[83] Klippel JH. Indications for, and use of, cytotoxic agents in SLE. *Baillieres Clin. Rheumatol.* 1998 Aug;12(3):511-27.

[84] Jayne D, Passweg J, Marmont A, Farge D, Zhao X, Arnold R, et al. Autologous stem cell transplantation for systemic lupus erythematosus. *Lupus.* 2004;13(3):168-76.

[85] Traynor AE, Barr WG, Rosa RM, Rodriguez J, Oyama Y, Baker S, et al. Hematopoietic stem cell transplantation for severe and refractory lupus. Analysis after five years and fifteen patients. *Arthritis Rheum.* 2002 Nov;46(11):2917-23.

[86] Traynor AE, Schroeder J, Rosa RM, Cheng D, Stefka J, Mujais S, et al. Treatment of severe systemic lupus erythematosus with high-dose chemotherapy and haemopoietic stem-cell transplantation: a phase I study. *Lancet.* 2000 Aug 26;356(9231):701-7.

[87] Petri M, Brodsky R. High-dose cyclophosphamide and stem cell transplantation for refractory systemic lupus erythematosus. *JAMA.* 2006 Feb 1;295(5):559-60.

[88] Burt RK, Traynor A, Statkute L, Barr WG, Rosa R, Schroeder J, et al. Nonmyeloablative hematopoietic stem cell transplantation for systemic lupus erythematosus. *JAMA.* 2006 Feb 1;295(5):527-35.

[89] Ginzler EM, Dooley MA, Aranow C, Kim MY, Buyon J, Merrill JT, et al. Mycophenolate mofetil or intravenous cyclophosphamide for lupus nephritis. *N. Engl. J. Med.* 2005 Nov 24;353(21):2219-28.

[90] Leandro MJ, Edwards JC, Cambridge G, Ehrenstein MR, Isenberg DA. An open study of B lymphocyte depletion in systemic lupus erythematosus. *Arthritis Rheum.* 2002 Oct;46(10):2673-7.

[91] Looney RJ, Anolik JH, Campbell D, Felgar RE, Young F, Arend LJ, et al. B cell depletion as a novel treatment for systemic lupus erythematosus: a phase I/II dose-escalation trial of rituximab. *ArthritisRheum.* 2004 Aug;50(8):2580-9.

[92] Sofat N, Malik O, Higgens CS. Neurological involvement in patients with rheumatic disease. *QJM.* 2006 Feb;99(2):69-79.

[93] Otsuka M, Fujiwara T, Kuwata Y, Yamada S, Ueki A. [A case of rheumatoid pachymeningitis]. *Rinsho Shinkeigaku.* 1997 Sep;37(9):834-40.

[94] Starosta MA, Brandwein SR. Clinical manifestations and treatment of rheumatoid pachymeningitis. *Neurology.* 2007 Mar 27;68(13):1079-80.

[95] Agildere AM, Tutar NU, Yucel E, Coskun M, Benli S, Aydin P. Pachymeningitis and optic neuritis in rheumatoid arthritis: MRI findings. *Br. J. Radiol.* 1999 Apr;72(856):404-7.

[96] Cellerini M, Gabbrielli S, Maddali Bongi S, Cammelli D. MRI of cerebral rheumatoid pachymeningitis: report of two cases with follow-up. *Neuroradiology.* 2001 Feb;43(2):147-50.

[97] Chowdhry V, Kumar N, Lachance DH, Salomao DR, Luthra HS. An unusual presentation of rheumatoid meningitis. *J. Neuroimaging.* 2005 Jul;15(3):286-8.

[98] Kurne A, Karabudak R, Karadag O, Yalcin-Cakmakli G, Karli-Oguz K, Yavuz K, et al. An unusual central nervous system involvement in rheumatoid arthritis: combination of pachymeningitis and cerebral vasculitis. *Rheumatol. Int.* 2009 Sep;29(11):1349-53.

[99] Ii Y, Kuzuhara S. Rheumatoid cranial pachymeningitis successfully treated with long-term corticosteroid. *Rheumatol. Int.* 2009 Mar;29(5):583-5.

[100] Yucel AE, Kart H, Aydin P, Agildere AM, Benli S, Altinors N, et al. Pachymeningitis and optic neuritis in rheumatoid arthritis: successful treatment with cyclophosphamide. *Clin. Rheumatol.* 2001;20(2):136-9.

[101] Markenson JA, McDougal JS, Tsairis P, Lockshin MD, Christian CL. Rheumatoid meningitis: a localized immune process. *Ann. Intern. Med.* 1979 May;90(5):786-9.

[102] Bathon JM, Moreland LW, DiBartolomeo AG. Inflammatory central nervous system involvement in rheumatoid arthritis. *Semin. ArthritisRheum.* 1989 May;18(4):258-66.

[103] Hatano N, Behari S, Nagatani T, Kimura M, Ooka K, Saito K, et al. Idiopathic hypertrophic cranial pachymeningitis: clinicoradiological spectrum and therapeutic options. *Neurosurgery.* 1999 Dec;45(6):1336-42; discussion 42-4.

[104] Kupersmith MJ, Martin V, Heller G, Shah A, Mitnick HJ. Idiopathic hypertrophic pachymeningitis. *Neurology.* 2004 Mar 9;62(5):686-94.

[105] Martin N, Masson C, Henin D, Mompoint D, Marsault C, Nahum H. Hypertrophic cranial pachymeningitis: assessment with CT and MR imaging. *AJNR Am. J. Neuroradiol.* 1989 May-Jun;10(3):477-84.

[106] Shintani S, Shiigai T, Tsuruoka S. Hypertrophic cranial pachymeningitis causing progressive unilateral blindness: MR findings. *Clin. Neurol.Neurosurg.* 1993 Mar;95(1):65-70.

[107] Chou RC, Henson JW, Tian D, Hedley-Whyte ET, Reginato AM. Successful treatment of rheumatoid meningitis with cyclophosphamide but not infliximab. *Ann. Rheum. Dis.* 2006 Aug;65(8):1114-6.

[108] Claassen J, Dwyer E, Maybaum S, Elkind MS. Rheumatoid leptomeningitis after heart transplantation. *Neurology.* 2006 Mar 28;66(6):948-9.

[109] Jones SE, Belsley NA, McLoud TC, Mullins ME. Rheumatoid meningitis: radiologic and pathologic correlation. *AJR Am. J.Roentgenol.* 2006 Apr;186(4):1181-3.

[110] Kato T, Hoshi K, Sekijima Y, Matsuda M, Hashimoto T, Otani M, et al. Rheumatoid meningitis: an autopsy report and review of the literature. *Clin. Rheumatol.* 2003 Dec;22(6):475-80.

[111] Matsushima M, Yaguchi H, Niino M, Akimoto-Tsuji S, Yabe I, Onishi K, et al. MRI and pathological findings of rheumatoid meningitis. *J. Clin. Neurosci.* 2010 Jan;17(1):129-32.

[112] Matsuura D, Ohshita T, Nagano Y, Ohtsuki T, Kohriyama T, Matsumoto M. [Case of rheumatoid meningitis: findings on diffusion-weighted image versus FLAIR image]. *Rinsho Shinkeigaku.* 2008 Mar;48(3):191-5.

[113] Shimada K, Matsui T, Kawakami M, Hayakawa H, Futami H, Michishita K, et al. Diffuse chronic leptomeningitis with seropositive rheumatoid arthritis: report of a case successfully treated as rheumatoid leptomeningitis. *Mod. Rheumatol.* 2009;19(5):556-62.

[114] Yaguchi M, Yaguchi H. Unilateral supratentorial lesion due to rheumatoid meningitis on MRI. *Intern. Med.* 2008;47(21):1947-8.

[115] Ahmed M, Luggen M, Herman JH, Weiss KL, Decourten-Myers G, Quinlan JG, et al. Hypertrophic pachymeningitis in rheumatoid arthritis after adalimumab administration. *J. Rheumatol.* 2006 Nov;33(11):2344-6.

[116] Mauch E, Volk C, Kratzsch G, Krapf H, Kornhuber HH, Laufen H, et al. Neurological and neuropsychiatric dysfunction in primary Sjogren's syndrome. *Acta Neurol. Scand.* 1994 Jan;89(1):31-5.

[117] Govoni M, Bajocchi G, Rizzo N, Tola MR, Caniatti L, Tugnoli V, et al. Neurological involvement in primary Sjogren's syndrome: clinical and instrumental evaluation in a cohort of Italian patients. *Clin. Rheumatol.* 1999;18(4):299-303.

[118] Alexander EL, Provost TT, Stevens MB, Alexander GE. Neurologic complications of primary Sjogren's syndrome. *Medicine* (Baltimore). 1982 Jul;61(4):247-57.

[119] Binder A, Snaith ML, Isenberg D. Sjogren's syndrome: a study of its neurological complications. *Br. J. Rheumatol.* 1988 Aug;27(4):275-80.

[120] Alexander EL, Alexander GE. Aseptic meningoencephalitis in primary Sjogren's syndrome. *Neurology.* 1983 May;33(5):593-8.

[121] Alexander GE, Provost TT, Stevens MB, Alexander EL. Sjogren syndrome: central nervous system manifestations. *Neurology.* 1981 Nov;31(11):1391-6.

[122] De Backer H, Dehaene I. Central nervous system disease in primary Sjogren's syndrome. *Acta Neurol. Belg.* 1995;95(3):142-6.

[123] Rossi R, Valeria Saddi M. Subacute aseptic meningitis as neurological manifestation of primary Sjogren's syndrome. *Clin. Neurol. Neurosurg.* 2006 Oct;108(7):688-91.

[124] Caselli RJ, Scheithauer BW, O'Duffy JD, Peterson GC, Westmoreland BF, Davenport PA. Chronic inflammatory meningoencephalitis should not be mistaken for Alzheimer's disease. *Mayo Clin. Proc.* 1993 Sep;68(9):846-53.

[125] Alexander EL, Hirsch TJ, Arnett FC, Provost TT, Stevens MB. Ro(SSA) and La(SSB) antibodies in the clinical spectrum of Sjogren's syndrome. *J.Rheumatol.* 1982 Mar-Apr;9(2):239-46.

[126] Delalande S, de Seze J, Fauchais AL, Hachulla E, Stojkovic T, Ferriby D, et al. Neurologic manifestations in primary Sjogren syndrome: a study of 82 patients. *Medicine* (Baltimore). 2004 Sep;83(5):280-91.

[127] Hoshina T, Yamaguchi Y, Ohga S, Kira R, Ishimura M, Takada H, et al. Sjogren's syndrome-associated meningoencephalomyelitis: cerebrospinal fluid cytokine levels and therapeutic utility of tacrolimus. *J. Neurol. Sci.* 2008 Apr 15;267(1-2):182-6.

[128] Ishida K, Uchihara T, Mizusawa H. Recurrent aseptic meningitis: a new CSF complication of Sjogren's syndrome. *J. Neurol.* 2007 Jun;254(6):806-7.

[129] Vincent TL, Richardson MP, Mackworth-Young CG, Hawke SH, Venables PJ. Sjogren's syndrome-associated myelopathy: response to immunosuppressive treatment. *Am. J. Med.* 2003 Feb 1;114(2):145-8.

[130] Hawley RJ, Hendricks WT. Treatment of Sjogren syndrome myelopathy with azathioprine and steroids. *Arch. Neurol.* 2002 May;59(5):875; author reply 6.

[131] Williams CS, Butler E, Roman GC. Treatment of myelopathy in Sjogren syndrome with a combination of prednisone and cyclophosphamide. *Arch. Neurol.* 2001 May;58(5):815-9.

[132] Rogers SJ, Williams CS, Roman GC. Myelopathy in Sjogren's syndrome: role of nonsteroidal immunosuppressants. *Drugs.* 2004;64(2):123-32.

[133] Yamout B, El-Hajj T, Barada W, Uthman I. Successful treatment of refractory neuroSjogren with Rituximab. *Lupus.* 2007;16(7):521-3.

[134] Ozgocmen S, Gur A. Treatment of central nervous system involvement associated with primary Sjogren's syndrome. *Curr. Pharm. Des.* 2008;14(13):1270-3.

[135] Gerraty RP, McKelvie PA, Byrne E. Aseptic meningoencephalitis in primary Sjogren's syndrome. Response to plasmapheresis and absence of CNS vasculitis at autopsy. *Acta Neurol. Scand.* 1993 Oct;88(4):309-11.

[136] Moller DR, Chen ES. What causes sarcoidosis? *Curr. Opin. Pulm. Med.* 2002 Sep;8(5):429-34.

[137] Iannuzzi MC, Rybicki BA, Teirstein AS. Sarcoidosis. *N. Engl. J. Med.* 2007 Nov 22;357(21):2153-65.

[138] Rybicki BA, Iannuzzi MC. Epidemiology of sarcoidosis: recent advances and future prospects. *Semin. Respir. Crit. Care Med.* 2007 Feb;28(1):22-35.

[139] Oksanen V. Neurosarcoidosis: clinical presentations and course in 50 patients. *Acta Neurol. Scand.* 1986 Mar;73(3):283-90.

[140] Chen RC, McLeod JG. Neurological complications of sarcoidosis. *Clin.Exp. Neurol.* 1989;26:99-112.

[141] Stern BJ, Krumholz A, Johns C, Scott P, Nissim J. Sarcoidosis and its neurological manifestations. *Arch. Neurol.* 1985 Sep;42(9):909-17.

[142] James DG, Sharma OP. Neurosarcoidosis. *Proc. R. Soc. Med.* 1967 Nov 1;60(11 Part 1):1169-70.

[143] Iwai K, Tachibana T, Takemura T, Matsui Y, Kitaichi M, Kawabata Y. Pathological studies on sarcoidosis autopsy. I. Epidemiological features of 320 cases in Japan. *Acta Pathol. Jpn.* 1993 Jul-Aug;43(7-8):372-6.

[144] Zajicek JP, Scolding NJ, Foster O, Rovaris M, Evanson J, Moseley IF, et al. Central nervous system sarcoidosis--diagnosis and management. *QJM.* 1999 Feb;92(2):103-17.

[145] Marangoni S, Argentiero V, Tavolato B. Neurosarcoidosis. Clinical description of 7 cases with a proposal for a new diagnostic strategy. *J. Neurol.* 2006 Apr;253(4):488-95.

[146] Pawate S, Moses H, Sriram S. Presentations and outcomes of neurosarcoidosis: a study of 54 cases. *QJM.* 2009 Jul;102(7):449-60.

[147] Joseph FG, Scolding NJ. Neurosarcoidosis: a study of 30 new cases. *J. Neurol. Neurosurg. Psychiatry.* 2009 Mar;80(3):297-304.

[148] Sharma OP. Neurosarcoidosis: a personal perspective based on the study of 37 patients. *Chest.* 1997 Jul;112(1):220-8.

[149] Nowak DA, Widenka DC. Neurosarcoidosis: a review of its intracranial manifestation. *J. Neurol.* 2001 May;248(5):363-72.

[150] Oksanen V, Fyhrquist F, Somer H, Gronhagen-Riska C. Angiotensin converting enzyme in cerebrospinal fluid: a new assay. *Neurology*. 1985 Aug;35(8):1220-3.

[151] Tahmoush AJ, Amir MS, Connor WW, Farry JK, Didato S, Ulhoa-Cintra A, et al. CSF-ACE activity in probable CNS neurosarcoidosis. *Sarcoidosis Vasc. Diffuse Lung Dis*. 2002 Oct;19(3):191-7.

[152] Dale JC, O'Brien JF. Determination of angiotensin-converting enzyme levels in cerebrospinal fluid is not a useful test for the diagnosis of neurosarcoidosis. *Mayo Clin. Proc*. 1999 May;74(5):535.

[153] Joseph FG, Scolding NJ. Sarcoidosis of the nervous system. *Pract.Neurol*. 2007 Aug;7(4):234-44.

[154] Miller DH, Kendall BE, Barter S, Johnson G, MacManus DG, Logsdail SJ, et al. Magnetic resonance imaging in central nervous system sarcoidosis. *Neurology*. 1988 Mar;38(3):378-83.

[155] Khaw KT, Manji H, Britton J, Schon F. Neurosarcoidosis--demonstration of meningeal disease by gadolinium enhanced magnetic resonance imaging. *J. Neurol. Neurosurg. Psychiatry*. 1991 Jun;54(6):499-502.

[156] Lower EE, Baughman RP. The use of low dose methotrexate in refractory sarcoidosis. *Am. J. Med. Sci*. 1990 Mar;299(3):153-7.

[157] Soriano FG, Caramelli P, Nitrini R, Rocha AS. Neurosarcoidosis: therapeutic success with methotrexate. *Postgrad. Med. J*. 1990 Feb;66(772):142-3.

[158] Stern BJ, Schonfeld SA, Sewell C, Krumholz A, Scott P, Belendiuk G. The treatment of neurosarcoidosis with cyclosporine. *Arch Neurol*. 1992 Oct;49(10):1065-72.

[159] Androdias G, Maillet D, Marignier R, Pinede L, Confavreux C, Broussolle C, et al. Mycophenolate mofetil may be effective in CNS sarcoidosis but not in sarcoid myopathy. *Neurology*. 2011 Mar 29;76(13):1168-72.

[160] Bullmann C, Faust M, Hoffmann A, Heppner C, Jockenhovel F, Muller-Wieland D, et al. Five cases with central diabetes insipidus and hypogonadism as first presentation of neurosarcoidosis. *Eur. J.Endocrinol*. 2000 Apr;142(4):365-72.

[161] Baughman RP, Strohofer SA, Buchsbaum J, Lower EE. Release of tumor necrosis factor by alveolar macrophages of patients with sarcoidosis. *J. Lab. Clin. Med*. 1990 Jan;115(1):36-42.

[162] Zheng L, Teschler H, Guzman J, Hubner K, Striz I, Costabel U. Alveolar macrophage TNF-alpha release and BAL cell phenotypes in sarcoidosis. *Am. J. Respir. Crit. Care Med.* 1995 Sep;152(3):1061-6.

[163] Doty JD, Mazur JE, Judson MA. Treatment of sarcoidosis with infliximab. *Chest.* 2005 Mar;127(3):1064-71.

[164] Sollberger M, Fluri F, Baumann T, Sonnet S, Tamm M, Steck AJ, et al. Successful treatment of steroid-refractory neurosarcoidosis with infliximab. *J. Neurol.* 2004 Jun;251(6):760-1.

[165] Carter JD, Valeriano J, Vasey FB, Bognar B. Refractory neurosarcoidosis: a dramatic response to infliximab. *Am. J. Med.* 2004 Aug 15;117(4):277-9.

[166] Morcos Z. Refractory neurosarcoidosis responding to infliximab. *Neurology.* 2003 Apr 8;60(7):1220-1; author reply -1.

[167] Santos E, Shaunak S, Renowden S, Scolding NJ. Treatment of refractory neurosarcoidosis with Infliximab. *J. Neurol. Neurosurg. Psychiatry.* 2010 Mar;81(3):241-6.

[168] Pettersen JA, Zochodne DW, Bell RB, Martin L, Hill MD. Refractory neurosarcoidosis responding to infliximab. *Neurology.* 2002 Nov 26;59(10):1660-1.

[169] Fujita Y, Fujii T, Nakashima R, Tanaka M, Mimori T. Aseptic meningitis in mixed connective tissue disease: cytokine and anti-U1RNP antibodies in cerebrospinal fluids from two different cases. *Mod. Rheumatol.* 2008;18(2):184-8.

[170] Ginsberg L, Kidd D. Chronic and recurrent meningitis. *Pract. Neurol.* 2008 Dec;8(6):348-61.

[171] Zhang W, Zhou G, Shi Q, Zhang X, Zeng XF, Zhang FC. Clinical analysis of nervous system involvement in ANCA-associated systemic vasculitides. *Clin. Exp. Rheumatol.* 2009 Jan-Feb;27(1 Suppl 52):S65-9.

[172] Birnbaum J, Hellmann DB. Primary angiitis of the central nervous system. *Arch. Neurol.* 2009 Jun;66(6):704-9.

[173] Pohl D, Rostasy K, Reiber H, Hanefeld F. CSF characteristics in early-onset multiple sclerosis. *Neurology.* 2004 Nov 23;63(10):1966-7.

[174] Wingerchuk DM, Lennon VA, Pittock SJ, Lucchinetti CF, Weinshenker BG. Revised diagnostic criteria for neuromyelitis optica. *Neurology.* 2006 May 23;66(10):1485-9.

[175] Nagashima T, Maguchi S, Terayama Y, Horimoto M, Nemoto M, Nunomura M, et al. P-ANCA-positive Wegener's granulomatosis presenting with hypertrophic pachymeningitis and multiple cranial

neuropathies: case report and review of literature. *Neuropathology.* 2000 Mar;20(1):23-30.

[176] Furukawa Y, Matsumoto Y, Yamada M. Hypertrophic pachymeningitis as an initial and cardinal manifestation of microscopic polyangiitis. *Neurology.* 2004 Nov 9;63(9):1722-4.

[177] Kono H, Inokuma S, Nakayama H, Yamazaki J. Pachymeningitis in microscopic polyangiitis (MPA): a case report and a review of central nervous system involvement in MPA. *Clin. Exp. Rheumatol.* 2000 May-Jun;18(3):397-400.

[178] Takahashi K, Kobayashi S, Okada K, Yamaguchi S. Pachymeningitis with a perinuclear antineutrophil cytoplasmic antibody: response to pulse steroid. *Neurology.* 1998 Apr;50(4):1190-1.

In: Meningitis: Causes, Diagnosis and Treatment   ISBN 978-1-62100-833-0
Editors: G. Houllis et al. pp. 203-223   ©2012 Nova Science Publishers, Inc.

Chapter 5

MENINGITIS: DIAGNOSTIC TECHNIQUES AND TREATMENT

Sandip K. Dash[1], Minakshi Sharma[2] and Ashok Kumar[1]

[1]Institute of Genomics and Integrative Biology (CSIR),
Mall Road, Delhi, India
[2]Department of Zoology, M. D. University, Rohtak, Haryana, India

ABSTRACT

Meningitis is a bacterial, viral and fungal infection causing inflammation of the protective membrane covering the brain and spinal cord (meninges). Viral and other forms of meningitis are mild and get cured automatically within one or two week. Whereas, bacterial meningitis is life threatening disease if not being diagnosed or treated in time. Meningitis is contagious infection and can spread from one person to another by coughing, sneezing and through close contact.The diagnosis of the disease is carried out from CSF and blood of patients mostly by culture, latex agglutination, biochemical tests, PCR, MALDI, microarray and nucleic acid sensors. The treatment, prevention and therapy of especially bacterial meningitis are discussed in this chapter.

INTRODUCTION

Meningitis is a serious life threatening disease that causes inflammation of the meninges in the brain and spinal cord of the patients. Survey of literature suggests that Hippocrates was first person to realize the existence of meningitis. The bacterial infection underlying meningitis was first reported in 1887 by Austrian bacteriologist Anton Weichselbaum, who termed the word meningococcus [1]. The first recorded major outbreak of the meningitis occurred in Geneva in 1805 followed by Europe and United States. The epidemic form of meningitis appeared in Africa during 1840. Later on, spread worldwide in 20th century starting with a major epidemic swapping in Nigeria and Ghana during 1905-08. During late of 20th century the disease was developed into epidemics in Africa and pandemics in Asia. The endemic form of meningitis has an incident of 1-5 per one lakh population annually while epidemics cases have an effecting rate of 500 per one lakh [2]. Herrick (1919) described meningitis as "no other infection so quickly slays", this holds true still [2]. Lassen (1951) pointed that meningitis under endemic conditions is mostly a disease of infants and young children while under epidemic conditions it can be widely distributed in all age-groups [3].

Patients with meningitis do not always display typical clinical signs or characteristic laboratory parameters at the time of admission. Symptoms of the disease vary with severity and age group of the patients. Meningitis causes swelling of brain tissue and increase of pressure inside the skull resulting in lethargy, seizures, loss of consciousness and sometimes leads to coma or death. The inflammation of the meninges may lead to abnormalities of the cranial nerves resulting in visual abnormalities and hearing loss after an episode of meningitis. In infants the primary symptoms include excessive crying, excessive sleepiness, difficulty with feeding and bulging of the soft spot on the top of the head. Main symptom in adults include fever, headache, stiff neck, irritability, nausea, vomiting and may be purple or red rashes on the body. Meningitis is associated with additional problems like sepsis, very low blood pressure, increased heart beat, disseminated intravascular coagulation and occasionally gangrene of limbs. Severe meningococcal infections may result in hemorrhaging of the adrenal glands leading to Waterhouse-Friderichsen syndrome, which is often lethal.

1. CAUSES

Meningitis can be caused by viruses, fungi or bacteria. Different forms of parasites can also lead to meningitis. Some time meningitis results as a secondary sequel of a disease different from bacterial meningitis or as a consequence of drugs taken against a disease. The various causes of meningitis are illustrated below.

1.1. Viral and Fungal Meningitis

Viruses that can cause meningitis include enteroviruses, herpes simplex virus type 2 and varicella zoster virus. Fungal meningitis is rare and seen mostly in people with immune deficiency such as AIDS. Fungal meningitis is mostly caused by *Cryptococcus neoformans*. Viral and fungal meningitis are mild and get cured automatically within a week or two.

1.2. Bacterial Meningitis

Bacterial meningitis or sepsis is most dangerous form of meningitis which may be lethal. The types of bacteria cause bacterial meningitis may vary with age group of the patients. Neonatal bacterial meningitis is mainly due to transmission of *Streptococcus agalactiae* and *Escherichia coli* K1 from the maternal genital tract to newborn infant [4]. Children and adults are mostly affected by *Haemophilus influenzae, Streptococcus pneumoniae* and *Neisseria meningitidis* [5]. Exceptional cases of bacterial meningitis may include *Bacteroides fragilis, Achromobacter xylosoxidans, Gordona aurantiaca, Lactobacillus sp., Corynebacterium aquaticum, Streptococcus mitis, Staphylococcus aureus, Pasteurella multocida, H. influenzae* type f and *Psychrobacter immobilis. N. menigitidis* is the most etiological agent for bacterial meningitis [6].

The cause of meningitis in a patient when fail to illustrate clearly, the condition is called as aseptic meningitis. This is usually due to viral or bacterial infection that has partially treated with antibiotic or by infection in a space adjacent to the meninges (sinusitis). Aseptic meningitis may also result from infection with spirochetes, a type of bacteria that includes *Treponema pallidum* (cause syphilis) and *Borrelia burgdorferi* (cause Lyme disease).

1.3. Non Pathogenic Meningitis

Meningitis caused by organisms other than bacteria, viruses and fungi can be termed as non-pathogenic meningitis. Meningitis due to infection by amoeba such as *Naegleria fowleri* is known as amoebic meningitis. Amoebic meningitis mainly spreads from freshwater sources. Some of the parasites like *Angiostrongylus cantonensis* and *Gnathostoma spinigerum* cause parasitic meningitis. This type of meningitis is characterized by increased number of eosinophils in the CSF of the patient. Tuberculosis, syphilis, cryptococcosis and coccidioidomycosis are rare causes of parasitic meningitis. Meningitis may occur as the result of several non-infectious causes: spread of cancer to the meninges (malignant meningitis) and certain drugs or antibiotics. It may also be caused by several inflammatory conditions such as sarcoidosis (neurosarcoidosis), connective tissue disorders (systemic lupus erythematosus) and certain forms of vasculitis (inflammation of blood vessel). Epidermoid cysts and dermoid cysts may cause meningitis by releasing irritant matter into the subarachnoid space.

2. DIAGNOSIS

Viral and other forms of meningitis are mild and get cured automatically within a week or two whereas bacterial meningitis is highly dreadful and lethal. The disease spreads very rapidly and delayed diagnosis may lead to death. Therefore, etiological diagnosis of the bacterial meningitis is important for detection of specific bacteria. The primary suspicion of bacterial meningitis is based on specific symptoms shown by the patients. Symptoms of meningococcal disease closely resemble with influenza and migraine headache. Therefore, further confirmation of the disease is required by different methods described below.

2.1. Traditional Methods

All traditional methods used for diagnosis of bacterial meningitis are old, time consuming and show minimum specificity and sensitivity particularly, in those patients with prior antibiotic treatment. Therefore, these methods were slowly replaced by advanced methods. Traditional methods of diagnosis mainly involve culture of bacteria and then detection of those either through antigen antibody reaction or through pathogen specific substance produced in the culture media. Culture based detection through lumbar puncture or spinal tap is a conventional method of diagnosis. In this method small amount of cerebrospinal fluid (CSF) is drawn from meninges of suspected patient. The collected CSF is centrifuged for sedimentation and supernatant is divided into three tubes for chemical, microbiological and cytological tests. While, the sediment is cultured in either 5% sheep blood agar or chocolate agar with an enrichment broth like thioglycolate, Columbia, brucella or peptone for 48 - 72h. The bacterial culture can be tested for E-test (antimicrobial susceptibility for *N. meningitidis*) [7].Typical laboratory parameters of patients suffering from bacterial meningitis include elevated count of leukocytes, protein and lactate in CSF or blood. The other traditional methods are as follows:

Counterimmunoelectrophoresis (CIE) involves application of an electric current across immunodiffusion agar facilitating diffusion of specific bacterial antigenic protein and corresponding antibody towards each other. Immunoprecipitation of antigen and antibody takes around 30-60 min [8]. Although CIE is highly specific but is less sensitive [9]. Therefore, this method was gradually replaced by latex agglutination test.

Latex agglutination (LA) test involves latex polystyrene beads adsorbed with broad range of monoclonal antibodies to react with specific bacterial surface protein present in the CSF of patients. Agglutination of specific antigen and antibody forms clumps. Test kits such as Directigen, Bactigen and Wellcogen are available in the market based on the principle of LA. The LA test is not suitable for detection of *N. meningitidis* in urine of the patients [10].

Coagglutination assay (COAG) contains bacterial suspensions of *S. aureus*. The outer membrane protein of these bacteria bind to Fc region of IgG while, the free Fab region of the antibody bind with specific bacterial protein from CSF. This multi antigen-antibody agglutination can be detected. Detection efficacy of COAG is 50-100ng/ml of bacterial protein present in the CSF of patient [11]. A kit was developed on the basis of coagglutination assay known as Phadebact CSF test kit.

2.2. Microscopy

CSF or blood of the patient is centrifuged at 25°C for pellet formation. Thereafter, the pellet is dried and differentially stained to visualize under microscope. Pathogenic condition of the sample is determined by counting number of bacteria and other components like leukocytes and proteins.

Microscopy can detect bacterial count within the range of 10^1-10^9 CFU/ml. The various staining methods under microscopy are described below:

Gram staining is an initial method to differentiate Gram-negative bacteria from Gram-positive bacteria on the basis of cell wall structure. Membrane of Gram-positive bacteria is surrounded by thick peptidoglycan layer (20-50 nm) which stain violet with Gram stain. Gram-negative bacteria contain a thin wall of petidoglycan (2-3 nm) and a second outer membrane of lipopolysaccharide. Therefore, cell wall of Gram-negative bacteria does not stain by Gram stain and retains pink color of the counter stain. The evaluated detection efficacy and sensitivity of this method is about 75% and 10^3CFU/ml respectively [12].

Acridine staining involves use of acridine orange to produce fluorescent image under fluorescent microscope. Bacteria appear bright red and leukocytes appear pale green under high magnification of fluorescent microscope. Acridine staining is advantageous over Gram stain for its 10 fold higher detection efficacies [13].

Wayson staining method (fuchsine, methylene blue, ethanol and phenol) is simple, quick and sensitive in comparison to Gram staining. In a Wayson stained slide under microscope bacteria appear dark blue, protein appears light blue and leukocytes appear light blue or purple [14]. A Wayson stained slide cannot be further Gram stained.

Quellung method uses specific antiserum against the outer capsular polysaccharide of bacteria. It can be used to confirm the presence of organisms with morphology typical to *S. pneumoniae, N. meningitidis* or *H. influenzae* type b [4]. The antiserum agglutinates with corresponding surface antigen to produce swollen and clear capsule under oil immersion microscope. However, results of microscopy, chemical and hematological examinations of CSF may be inconclusive or totally misleading especially in case of mild bacterial meningitis. This may result in delay of pre-mediated prophylaxis or treatment.

2.3. Rapid Detection Methods

Both COAG and LA tests include series of enzyme reactions which may lead to uncertainty in results. Sensitivity of these techniques ranges from 60-90% [15]. CIE, COAG and LA are most efficient in detecting *H. influenzae* antigens. CIE is least efficient for detection of *Streptococcus* group B antigens while COAG and LA test are least efficient for detection of *N. meningitidis* antigens [4]. In order to overcome short comings of both traditional and microscopy methods of diagnosis, some of the following rapid and advanced methods were developed for diagnosis.

Enzyme immonoassay (EIA) involves immobilized enzymes bound to Fc site of different monoclonal antibodies, free Fab site of these antibodies bind to specific bacterial protein present in the CSF or blood of patients. Addition of particular substrate to the enzyme is changed into detectable colored product [7]. The test can detect bacterial antigen concentrations 0.1-5.0 ng/ml. EIA can detect *H. influenzae* type b, *S. pneumoniae* and *N. meningitidis* antigens in CSF [4]. The sensitivity and specificity of this test is 84-100% and 89-100%, respectively. EIA takes several hours for completion and also need multiple controls. Therefore, EIA is better suited for testing specimens in a batch mode than for testing of individual CSF sample. Bang (2000) reported that bacterial membrane lipopolysaccharide (LPS) can coagulate blood of the *Limulus polyphemus* within 1h of exposure [16]. It was later found that the factor responsible for this is *Limulus amoebocyte* lysate (LAL). Under optimal conditions (36-38°C, pH 6.0-7.5), if LAL is exposed to very small amount of LPS from bacteria, can induce clotting [17]. The LAL assay is a highly sensitive and specific assay for the detection of endotoxin in CSF. LAL assay can detect approximately 10^3 CFU/ml of Gram-negative bacteria. Ross *et al* (1975) developed a bedside adaptation of the "gel endpoint" method for diagnosis of meningitis [18]. Dwelle *et al* (1987) simplified the assay to a microslide gelation test with sensitivity of 97.3% and false negative of 99.9% [19]. LAL assays have a sensitivity of 93% and a specificity of 99.4%. Bacteria that have been detected in CSF by LAL tests include *H. influenzae* type b, *N. meningitidis, E. coli, Pseudomonas sp., Serratia marcescens, Klebsiella pneumonia* and other Gram-negative *Bacilli* [4]. However, not all reports gave the LAL test approval for diagnosis of meningitis. Sarif and McCracken (1975) reported a sensitivity of 71% and false-positive rate of 14% for diagnosis of neonatal meningitis in CSF [20]. Their research elicited that LAL test is not sensitive enough for diagnosis of bacterial meningitis in neonates.

Gas-liquid chromatography (GLC) was first used in clinical microbiology for identification of anaerobic bacteria. Presence of microbial metabolites like amines, carbohydrates and short-chain fatty acids in the host body can be evaluated by GLC for detection of the type and number of bacteria present. Application of GLC for detection of microorganisms in CSF is still in pre-developmental stage. Brice *et al* (1979) used GLC technique to establish chromatography patterns for five bacterial agents responsible for meningitis: *S. pneumoniae, H. influenzae, N. meningitidis, S. aureus* and *E. coli* [21]. His group concluded that GLC may be a useful assay for rapid laboratory diagnosis of bacterial meningitis. As this method requires expensive equipments and highly demanding techniques hence it is not preferred for diagnosis of bacterial meningitis.

2.4. Polymerase Chain Reaction (PCR)

Since 1995, PCR was started to be used as a gold-standard method for diagnosis of bacterial meningitis. Mohamed *et al* (2003) used direct PCR method for detection of bacterial meningitis from CSF of patients during an outbreak of meningitis in Sudan [22]. During earlier period of PCR based detection, patient's blood and CSF were used for diagnosis but Staquet *et al* (2007) used skin biopsy for RT-PCR [23]. PCR is a rapid method for amplification of DNA and detection of small quantities of DNA. Generally PCR is used for diagnosis of meningitis at low bacterial count.

Kotileinen *et al* (1998) developed a broad range PCR method for detection of *N. meningitidis* [24]. They initially screened CSF samples from patients using primers MS37 and MS38 by counting G and C content (Gram-positive bacteria have low G and C nucleotide count as compared to Gram-negative bacteria). Clinical CSF samples, after heating at 94°C for 10 min, PCR was carried out using universal primers of 16S RNA. In order to reduce the time consumed by agarose gel electrophoresis, Seward and Towner (2000) used multiplex PCR and immunoassay (IA) for detection of *N. meningitidis* [25].

Real-time PCR is highly sensitive detection technique since it is fluorescence based [26]. Diggle *et al* (2003) developed dual-labeled end-point fluorescence PCR (DEF-PCR) with a reporter dye carboxyfluorescein at 5´-end and a quencher dye carboxy-tetramethylrhodamine at 3´-end for detection of meningococcal meningitis [27]. The probe gets hybridized to specific DNA sequence during PCR product formation but is subsequently digested by 5´-exonuclease activity of *Taq* DNA polymerase during primer extension. The´ released reporter dye causes increase in fluorescence emission. The PCR product formed during RT-PCR is analyzed via altered decrease and increase in fluorescence emissions using a fluorimeter.

2.5. Matrix-Assisted LASER Desorption/Ionization (MALDI)

PCR tests often have number of limitations and challenges such as susceptibility to inhibitory substances, laborious and time consuming for the culture of bacteria and isolation of nucleic acid. To overcome this problem, Gudlavalleti *et al* (2009) applied proteomic approach for detection of *Neisseria sp.* using AP-MALDI MS (atmospheric-MALDI mass spectrometry) [28]. MALDI-MS is being used from past as a powerful technique for rapid identification of microorganisms but AP-MALDI has been developed very recently which provides both decoupled ion production and specificity therefore, it is more preferably used over MALDI-MS. In this method 10^3-10^4 heat-inactivated bacterial cells were placed on C^{18} coated MALDI target plate at 50°C from which bacterial proteins were selectively extracted with 50% NH_4OH. Extracted proteins were digested *in situ* on the probe via addition of trypsin (immobilized on beads) followed by acetonitrile. Sample spots were allowed to dry and subsequently washed with water. Generated peptides were subjected to AP-MALDI MS analysis after addition of matrix (10 mg of α-cyano-4-hydroxycinnamic acid in 1ml of 70% acetonitrile containing 0.1% tri-fluoroacetic acid). Jesse *et al* (2010) used isoelectric focusing for expression and quantification of several proteins from the pathogen [29]. Proteins with significant higher spot were stained with colloidal coomassie dye and identified by MALDI TOF-MS. These highly expressed proteins were used as biomarkers.

2.6. Microarray

Microarray is an advance and promising technique for diagnosis of any disease. Tong *et al* (2005) first time used 16S microarray for detection of neonatal bacterial meningitis using patient's blood [30]. Ben *et al* (2008) used isolated genomic DNA from CSF samples of patients for microarray [31]. His group designed three specific probes (one for each of positive, negative and control) for all of the twenty types of bacteria responsible for causing bacterial meningitis. The heated CSF samples were used in PCR for amplification of specific regions of 16S RNA sequence and the amplicons were hybridized with DNA probes.

DNA microarray can either be constructed by direct synthesis of oligonucleotide on the solid surface (like affymetrix microarray) or by immobilization of earlier synthesized oligonucleotides on the specific substrate

[32]. Surface of the slides can be coated with polylysine or aminopropyle to increase the efficacy of oligonucleotide binding. Carboxyl-amine, thiol-disulfide, amine-aldehyde, aldehyde-oxyamine, biotin-streptavidin, gold-thiol, zirconylated-surface-phosphate and epoxide-amine are some of the commonly used covalent linkage for DNA array. Mahajan *et al* (2009) used thio-ether linkage fabrication technique for detection of human bacterial meningitis in Indian patients [33]. In this method thiol-modified DNA probe were immobilized on silanized glass slide and hybridized with fluorescent tetrachlorofluorescein (TET) labeled DNA sample (Figure 1).

After hybridization, the slide was scanned under LASER scanner to quantify fluorescence intensity of the spot. Sethi e*t al* (2010) used SU-8(glycidyl ether of bisphenol A) coated glass slides for efficient immobilization of aminoalkyl-, thiophosphoryl- and phosphorylated oligonucleotides [34]. The immobilized probes were hybridized with complementary DNA from *N. meningitidis* for detection of meningococcal disease. Jarvinen *et al* (2009) used PCR-microarray based detection method for detection of *N. meningitidis* from CSF samples [35]. In this method, they produced ssDNA amplicon in three phases of PCR. These amplicons were directly hybridized with ssDNA probe.

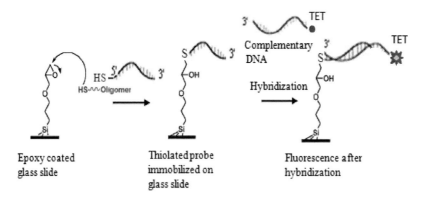

Figure 1. Immobilization of thiolated oligonucleotides onto epoxy coated glass slide and hybridization with TET labeled complementary DNA from bacteria.

2.7. Nucleic Acid Sensors

Nucleic acid sensor is rapidly taking over traditional methods of diagnosis due to simplicity, economical value, error free and small size [36]. In biosensor based detection, interfacial to the sensing electrode and current obtained thereof in the steady state is being employed for sensing various analytes. When difference in current is not significant at low target concentration, electrochemical impedance spectroscopy (EIS) technique is more favorable than other techniques [37]. Thiolated DNA can be well ordered onto a gold surface via use of spacer molecules between DNA and thiol moiety. Chemical bonding of the thiol group with gold can induce immobilization of probes on gold surface (Figure 2). Constructing probe layer with well-defined surface chemistry and preventing non-specific binding can improve efficacy of DNA biosensor. Change in resistance or capacitance of the interface are induced by hybridization of complementary DNA with the probe. An electrochemical DNA biosensor for detection of bacterial meningitis caused by *N. meningitidis* was developed by Patel *et al* (2009) using thiol-labeled probe. Immobilized probe onto gold surface was charecterised by using atomic force microscopy (AFM), Fourier transform infrared spectroscopy (FT-IR) [38]. Patel *et al* (2010) developed a *ctrA* gene based electrochemical DNA sensor for detection of meningococcal disease with a sensitivity range 7-42 ng/μl [39].

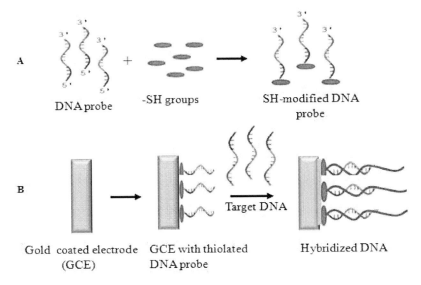

Figure 2. Diagrammatic representation (A) Preparation of thiol-labeled DNA probe from thiol molecule and probe (B)Hybridization of complementary target DNA with immobilized probe.

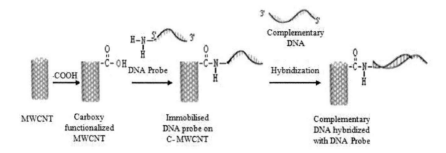

Figure 3. Schematic representation for immobilization of DNA probe on COOH-MWCNT and hybridization with complementary DNA from *N. meningitidis.*

Carbon nanotubes (CNTs) are one of the important nanomaterials for nucleic acid sensors. The single-walled carbon nanotubes (SWCNTs) or multi-walled carbon nanotubes (MWCNTs) can be functionalized on surface by attaching carbonyl or other reacting groups. DNA oligomer (probe) are then immobilized on it (Figure 3) followed by hybridization with complementary DNA from pathogen. The hybridization can be detected through electrochemical response using cyclic voltammeter (CV), differential pulse voltammeter (DPV) or by electrochemical impedance spectroscopy (EIS).

Metal nanoparticles deposited on an electrode are used to enhance impedance by allowing immobilization of DNA probe [40]. Gold nanoparticles deposited on the electrode are employed as a platform for immobilization of thiolated DNA probe followed by hybridization with complementary DNA. The difference in R_{ct} values of EIS study before and after hybridization shows a linear relation with the concentration of the target DNA. Bonnani *et al* (2008) utilized streptavidin-coated gold nanoparticles to improve R_{ct} signal [41]. Biotinylated oligomers were immobilized on a strepatvidin coated glass electrode through streptavidin-biotin linkage. The immobilized DNA probe was hybridized with complementary DNA oligomers.

3. TREATMENT

Now days, the preliminary treatment of meningococcal disease includes hospitalization, intensive care and intravenous administration of antibiotics. Despite of these all, mortality due to meningitis still remains high [42].

3.1. Host Immune Defense

The bacteria responsible for causing meningitis, after invasion into host bloodstream may produce menigococcemia (at mild endotoxin production) or sepsis (at severe case). Although, meningococcemia is associated with a short febrile flu-like episode but sepsis may lead to maculopapular or petechial rashes in the body and nodular or ecchymotic lesions. The host produces cytokines like TNF and IL1 in response to endotoxins produced by the pathogen (known as endotoxin responsiveness). Moreover, bactericidal antibodies and other serum components along with terminal complement factor of complement system in the body reveals an important host defense mechanism. Several investigators have recently observed that patients with deficiencies in the terminal components of the complement cascade (C5, C6, C7 and C8) have a predisposition for bacteremic infections with about 6000 folds higher propensity.

3.2. Prevention

Capsular polysaccharides of meningococci shield them from host complement reaction. Therefore, immune system of the body requires a protective level of anticapsular polysaccharides to initiate bacteriolysis. Serogroups A, B and C meningococci account for about 90% cases of meningitis with the remainder being caused by serogroup W135 and Y. Epidemic form of the disease is mainly contributed by serogroup A [43]. Effective vaccines against serogroup of *N. meningitidis* A, C, Y and W135 have already been developed but not for serogroup B which is responsible for most meningococcal disease in the United States and Europe [44, 45]. Progress towards a vaccine against serogroup B is proving quite difficult due to the protective capsule which is made of homopolymer of (2-8)-linked sialic acid. The capsule of serogroup B is relatively poor immunogen to human as it shares epitopes which are expressed on normal human neural cell adhesion molecule, N-CAM1 [46]. Indeed, generating immune responses against the serogroup B capsule might prove fatal. The *N. meningitidis* serogroup C conjugate (MCC) vaccine lunched in Europe and North America just recently consists of a conjugated form of α-2,9-linked polysialic capsule of serogroup C and a carrier protein.

Two injections of group A polysaccharide, starting at age of three months elicit a booster response of antibodies and at age group six year need reinjection of these vaccines for long-lived protective antibody response [47, 48]. Antibody level elicited by these vaccines remains same irrespective of the age (18-24 month of age) and place [49]. Therefore, group A polysaccharide has been licensed by many countries and certified by WHO [43]. Group C polysaccharide does not elicit protective antibodies in children aged less than two years and reinjection in this age group results in diminished antibody level against this antigen and group C polysaccharide is not allowed in children of age below than two years.

The introduction of haemophilus vaccines in the late 20th century led to remarkable fall in corresponding meningitis [49]. Since, newborn infants can produce antibodies to proteins such as tetanus toxoid but not for polysaccharide antigens. At present, the quadrivalent vaccines (made from polysaccharides) are tried to be conjugated with a carbohydrate to produce conjugate vaccines. This conjugate vaccine results in antibody response against both the protein and the carbohydrate. Pilot studies have shown that conjugant vaccines evoke high titers of anticapsular antibody against bacteremic infections like sepsis, meningitis and arthritis. Such a vaccine may not only be consistently immunogenic in all ages but would be directed against two bacterial structures one-two punch.

3.3. Therapy

At the beginning acute bacterial meningitis must be differentiated from "aseptic meningitis", a condition of frequent occurrence for which no specific therapy is available. In the pre-antibiotic era, the treatment for meningitis was done through spinal drainage (introduced by Quincke in 1895), serotherapy and skilled nursing. Although, spinal drainage got success in few cases but suffered from failure in lot of cases and slowly replaced by serum therapy. Nevertheless, in 1936 Sturdee pointed out that serotherapy is useful if applied at early stage of the disease. Later, serotherapy was also gradually replaced by penicillin therapy. In 1906 penicillin was first reported to be effective in meningitis [50]. As some of the meningococci are penicillin resistant, a broad spectrum of third generation cephalosporin is recommended as first line antimicrobial treatment [51]. Either cefotaxime 200 mg/kg/day in three or four divided doses, or ceftriaxone 80 mg/kg/day in a single daily dose are suitable [52]. For meningitis and septicemia in infants 1-3 month old, additional ampicillin 200 mg/kg/day is recommended [53], to ensure activity against *Escherichia coli*, *Listeria monocytogenes* and *Salmonella sp.* [54, 55].

Parenteral benzylpenicillin given by the general practitioner significantly reduced the mortality due to meningitis [53]. Intravenous route is more preferable for this but intramuscular or intraosseous route are also acceptable.

Rifampicin 20 mg/kg once daily for four days [56] eliminated meningitis with a sensitivity of 90% in United States. These drugs were discarded since the resistance of pathogens to this drug is increasing during the past several years [57, 58]. Rifampicin should also be avoided in persons wearing soft contact lenses to avoid staining of the lens. Because of high toxic potentialities, sulfonamides and chloramphenicol must be used cautiously and should be avoided during the late stage of pregnancy. In 2002, evidence emerged that treatment with steroids can improve the prognosis of bacterial meningitis. Dexamethasone is one of the highly studied steroid and easily available therefore, used as preferable therapeutic agent [59]. But this drug proves effective if given at early stage of the disease. However, this is associated with a number of adverse effects. The meningitis caused by *H. influenzae* requires ampicillin and chloramphenicol as most preferable and effective drugs [52]. Ampicillin is associated with lot of serious sensitivity reactions and development of staphylococcal enteritis. On the other hand, chloramphenicol has the possibility of inducing aplastic anemia with a mortality rate of 50%. Aplastic anemia appears about some weeks or months after stopping drug intake.Therefore, it should be used cautiously. Benzylpenicillin is the most preferred drug against meningococcal meningitis [60]. In case of sulphonamide resistant group-meningococcal infection ampicillin and chloramphenicols can be used as an alternative. Benzylpenicillin can also be effectively used to treat pneumococcal meningitis with ampicillin as an alternative but no chloramphenicol [49]. *Staphylococcus aureus* is the organism that causes staphylococcal meningitis mostly in new born babies. Cloxacillin and methicillin are still being used as appropriate drugs against staphylococcal meningitis.

CONCLUSION

Although, the scintillating advance in science has thumped over most of the dreadful diseases of mankind but meningitis is still proving an overwhelming threat for human life. The failure for accurate diagnosis and complete treatment of the disease has raised endemic form of the disease to epidemic form. Rapid and accurate diagnosis is essential both for effective public health management and time bound antibiotic mediated prophylaxis.

However, the diagnosis is hindered due to a number of technical short comings, which proves to be the most challenging problem for the researchers worldwide. The inefficacy for eradication of any disease is equally shared by ignorance of the people and bankruptcy at pre-stage treatment. Recent advances in the field of diagnosis of bacterial meningitis such as DNA biosensor and nanosensors can save life of several people especially during outbreak of the disease.

REFERENCES

[1]   Weichselbaum, A. (1987) http://www.ehow.com/facts 5485019 history-meningitis.html.
[2]   Herrick, W. W., Dannenberg, A. M. (1919) Observations on the cerebrospinal fluid of acute disease. *JAMA,* 73, pp.1321-1328.
[3]   Lassen, H. C. A., Neukirch, F. (1951) On Streptomycin therapy in tuberculous meningitis and in miliary tuberculosis. *J. Int. Med.,* 141, pp.110-124.
[4]   Gray, L. D., Fedorko, D. P. (1992) Laboratory diagnosis of bacterial meningitis. *Clin. Microbiol. Rev.,* 5, pp.130-145.
[5]   Peltola, H. (2000) Worldwide *Haemophilus influenzae* type b disease at the beginning of the 21st century: global analysis of the disease burden 25 years after the use of the polysaccharide vaccine and a decade after the advent of conjugates. *Clin. Microbiol. Rev.,* 13, pp.302-317.
[6]   Hart, C. A., Rogers, T. R. F. (1993) Meningococcal disease. *J. Med. Microbiol.,* 39, pp.3-25.
[7]   Hughes, J. H., Biedenbach, D. J., Jones, R. N. (1993) E-test as susceptibility test and epidemiologic tool for evaluation of *N.meningitidis* isolates. *J. Clin. Microbiol.,*31(12), pp.3255-3259.
[8]   Beuvery, E. C., van Rossum, F., Lauwers, S., Coignau, H. (1979) Comparison of counterimmunoelectrophoresis and ELISA for diagnosis of bacterial meningitis. *Lancet,* 1, pp.208-208.
[9]   Granoff, D. M., Murphy, T. V., Ingram, D. L., Cates, K. L. (1986) Use of rapidly generated results in patient management. *Diagn. Microbiol. Infect. Dis.,* 4, pp.157-166.
[10]   Ingram, D. L., Suggs, D. M., Pearson, P. W. (1982) Detection of group B Streptococcal disease with the Wellcogen Strep B latex agglutination test. *J. Clin. Microbiol.,* 16, pp.656-658.

[11] Fung, J. C., Tilton, R. C. (1985) Detection of bacterial antigens by counterimmuno-electrophoresis, coagglutination and latex agglutination. *Am. Soc. Microbiol.*, 4, pp.883-890.

[12] Greenlee, J. E. (1990) Approach to diagnosis of meningitis. Cerebrospinal fluid evaluation. *Infect. Dis. Clin. N. Am.*, 4, pp.583-597.

[13] Lauer, B. A., Reller, L. B., Mirrett, S. (1981) Comparison of acridine orange and Gram stains for detection of microorganisms in cerebro spinal fluid and other clinical specimens. *J. Clin. Microbiol.*, 14, pp.201-205.

[14] Sheridon, E. A., Ramsay, A. R., Short, J. M., Stepniwska, V.,Simpson, A. J. H. (2007) Evaluation of the Wayson stain for the rapid diagnosis of melioidosis. *J. Clin. Microbiol.*, 45, pp.1669-1670.

[15] Carpenter, R. R., Petersdorf, R. G. (1962) The clinical spectrum of bacterial meningitis. *Am. J. Med.*, 33, pp.262-274.

[16] Bang, F. (2000) A bacterial disease of *Limulus polyphemus. Bull. Johns Hopkins Hosp.*, 98(5), pp.325-351.

[17] Nachum, R. (1990) Detection of Gram negative bacterial meningitis by clinical application of *Limulus amoebocyte* lysate test. *N. Eng. J. Med.*, 289, pp.931-973.

[18] Ross, S. R., Rodriguez, W., Controni, G., Korengold, G., Watson, S., Khan, W. (1975) Limulus lysate test for Gram-negative bacterial meningitis bedside application. *JAMA*, 233, pp.1366-1369.

[19] Dwelle, T. L., Dunkle, L. M., Blair, L. (1987) Correlation of cerebrospinal fluid endotoxin like activity with clinical and laboratory variables in Gram-negative bacterial meningitis in children. *J. Clin. Microbiol.*, 25, pp.856-858.

[20] Sarif, L. D., McCracken, G. H., Schiffer, M. S., Glode, M. P., Robbins, J., Orskov, I., Orskov, F. (1975) Epidemiology of *Escherichia coli* KI in healthy and diseased newborns. *Lancet*, 1, pp.1099-1104.

[21] Brice, J. L., Tornabene, T. G., Laforce, F. M. (1979) Diagnosis of bacterial meningitis by gas-liquid chromatography. Chemotyping studies of *Streptococcus pneumoniae, Haemophilus influenzae, Neisseria meninngitidis, Staphylococcus aureus* and *E. coli. Infect. Dis.*,140, pp.443-452.

[22] Mohamed, I., Paula, M., Anders, B., Magnus, U., Nageeb, S., Per, O. (2003) PCR of cerebrospinal fluid for diagnosis of bacterial meningitis during meningococcal epidemics: an example from Sudan. *Scand. J. Infect. Dis.*, 35, pp.719-723.

[23] Staquet, P., Lemee, L., Verdier, E., Bonmarchand, G., Laudenbach, V., Michel, C., Lemeland, J., Marret, S., Blanc, T. (2007) Detection of *Neisseria meningitidis* DNA from skin lesion biopsy using real-time PCR: usefulness in the etiological diagnosis of purpura fulminans. *Intensive Care Med.*, 33, pp.1168-1172.

[24] Kotilainen, P., Jalava, J., Meurman, O., Lehtonen, O., Rintala, E., Seppa, O., Eerola, E., Nikkari, S. (1998) Diagnosis of meningococcal meningitis by broad-range bacterial PCR with cerebrospinal fluid. *J. Clin. Microbiol.*, 36, pp.2205-2209.

[25] Seward, R. J., Towner, K. J. (2000) Evaluation of a PCR-immunoassay technique for detection of *Neisseria meningitidis* in cerebrospinal fluid and peripheral blood. *J. Med. Microbiol.*, 49, pp.451-456.

[26] Livak, K. J., Flood, S. J., Mamro, J., Giusti, W., Deetz, K. (1995) Oligonucleotide with fluorescent dye at opposite ends provide a quenched probe system useful for detecting PCR product and nucleic acid hybridization. *PCR Method Appl.*, 4, pp.357-362.

[27] Diggle, M. A., Smith, K., Girvan, E. K., Clarke, S. C. (2003) Evaluation of a fluorescence-based PCR method for identification of serogroup A meningococci. *J. Clin. Microbiol.*, 41, pp.1766-1768.

[28] Gudlavalleti, S. K., Sundaram, A. K., Razumovski, J. D. (2009) Application of atmospheric pressure matrix-assisted laser desorption/ionization mass spectrometry for rapid identification of *Neisseria* species. *J. Biomol. Tech.*, 19, pp.200-204.

[29] Jesse, S., Steinacker, P., Lehnert, S., Sdzuj, M., Cepek, L., Tumani, H., Jahn, O., Schmidt, H., Otto, M. (2010) A proteomic approach for the diagnosis of bacterial meningitis. *PLoS One*, 6, pp.1-9.

[30] Tong, M., Shang, S., Wu, Y., Zhao, Z. (2005) Value of 16S RNA microarray detection in early diagnosis of neonatal septicemia. *World J. Pediatric.*, 2, pp.121-126.

[31] Ben, R., Kung, S., Chang, F., Lu, J., Feng, N., Hsieh, Y. (2008) Rapid diagnosis of bacterial meningitis using a microarray. *J. Formos Med. Assoc.*, 107, pp.448-453.

[32] Fenselau, C., Sethi, D., Seth, S., Kumar, A., Gupta, K. C. (2009) Construction of oligonucleotide microarray. *J. Formos Med. Assoc.*, 107, pp.448- 453.

[33] Mahajan, S., Sethi, D., Seth, S., Kumar, A., Kumar, P., Gupta, K. C. (2009) Construction of oligonucleotide microarrays (biochips) via thioether linkage for the detection of bacterial meningitis. *Bioconjugate Chem.*, 20, pp.1703-1710.

[34]   Sethi, D., Kumar, A., Gandhi, R. P., Kumar, P., Gupta, K. C. (2010) New protocol for oligonucleotide microarray fabrication using SU-8-coated glass microslides. *Bioconjugate Chem.*, 211, pp.703-708.

[35]   Jarvinen, A., Laakso, S., Piiparinen, P., Aittakorpi, A., Lindfors, M., Huopaniemi, L., Piiparinen, H., Mäki, M. (2009) Rapid identification of bacterial pathogens using a PCR and microarray-based assay. *BMC Microbiol.*, 9, pp.1-16.

[36]   Zhang, K., Zhang, M. H., Zhang, L. Y. (2008) Fabrication of a sensitive impedance biosensor of DNA hybridization based on gold nanoparticle modified gold electrode. *Electro. Anal.*, 20, pp.2127-2133.

[37]   Park, J., Park, S. (2009) DNA hybridization sensors based on electrochemical impedance spectroscopy as a detection tool. *Sensors,* 9, pp.9513-9532.

[38]   Patel, M. K., Solanki, P. R., Seth, S., Gupta, S., Khare, S., Malhotra, B. D., Kumar, A. (2009) ctrA gene based electrochemical DNA sensor for detection of meningitis. *Electrochem. Commun.*, 11, pp.969-973.

[39]   Patel, M. K., Solanki, P. R., Khare, S., Gupta, S., Malhotra, B. D., Kumar, A. (2010) Electrochemical DNA sensor for *Neisseria meningitidis* detection. *Biosens. Bioelectron.*, 25, pp.2586-2591.

[40]   Xu, Y., Cai, H., He, P. G., Fang, Y. Z. (2004) Probing DNA hybridization by impedance measurement based on cds oligonucleotide conjugates. *Electro. Anal.,* 16, pp.150-155.

[41]   Bonanni, A., Esplandiu, M. J., del Valle, M. (2008) Signal amplification for impedimetric genosensing using gold-streptavidin nanoparticles. *Electrochim. Acta,* 53, pp.4022-4029.

[42]   Kreger, B. E., Craven, D. E., Carling, P. C., McCabe, W. R. (1980) Gram-negative bacteremia. III. Reassessment of etiology, epidemiology and ecology in 612 patients. *Am. J. Med.*, 68, pp.332-343.

[43]   World Health Organization (1976) Requirements for meningococcal polysaccharide vaccine. *WHO*, 23, pp.50-75.

[44]   Al'Aldeen, A. A., Cartwright, K. A. (1996) *Neisseria meningitidis*: vaccines and vaccine candidates. *J. Infect. Dis.*, 33, pp.153-157.

[45]   Artenstein, M. S., Gold, R., Zimmerly, J. G., Wyle, F. A., Schneider, H., Harkins, C. (1970) Prevention of meningococcal disease by group C polysaccharide vaccine. *N. Engl. J. Med.,* 282, pp.417–420.

[46]   Finne, J., Leinonen, M., Makela, P. H. (1983) Antigenic similarities between brain components and bacteria causing meningitis: implications for vaccine development and pathogenesis. *Lancet*, 2, pp.355-357.

[47]   Käyhty, H., Karanko, V., Peltola, H., Sarna, S., Mäkelä, P. H. (1980) Serum antibodies to capsular polysaccharide vaccine of group A *Neisseria meningitidis* followed for three years in infants and children. *J. Infect. Dis.*, 142, pp.861-868.

[48]   Zangwill, K. M., Stout, R. W., Carlone, G. M., Pais, L., Harekeh, H., Mitchell, S. (1994) Duration of antibody response after meningococcal polysaccharide vaccination in U.S. Air Force personnel. *J. Infect. Dis.*, 169, pp.847-852.

[49]   Lieberman, J. M., Chiu, S. S., Wong, V. K., Partidge, S., Chang, S. J., Gheeslin, L. L. (1996) Safety and immunogenicity of a serogroup A/C *Neisseria meningitidis* oligosaccharide-protein conjugate vaccine in young children. A randomized controlled trial. *JAMA,* 275, pp.1499-1503.

[50]   WHO (2003) Detecting meningococcal meningitis epidemics in highly-endemic African countries. *Weekly Epidem. Rec.,* 78, pp.294-256.

[51]   Nadel, S., Habibi, P., Levin, M. (1995) Management of meningococcal septicemia. *Care of the Critically Ill*, 11, pp.33-38.

[52]   Peltola, H., Anttila, M., Renkonen, O. V. (1989) Randomised comparison of chloramphenicol, ampicillin, cefotaxime and ceftriaxone for childhood bacterial meningitis. *Lancet*, 333, pp.1281-1287.

[53]   Dowd, J. M., Blink, D., Miller, C. H., Frand, P. F., Pierce, W. E. (1966) Antibiotic prophylaxis of carriers of sulfadiazine-resistant meningococci. *J. Infect. Dis.*, 116, pp.473-480.

[54]   Gotschlich, E. C., Austrian, R., Cvjetanovic, B., Robbins, J. B. (1978) Prospects for the prevention of bacterial meningitis with polysaccharide vaccines. *Bull. WHO*, 56, pp.509–518.

[55]   Klein, N., Heyderman, R., Levin, M. (1992) Antibiotic choices for meningitis beyond the neonatal period. *Arch. Dis. Child.*, 67, pp.157-161.

[56]   Granoff, D. M., Daum, R. S. (1980) Spread of *Haemophilus influenzae* type b: recent epidemiological and therapeutic considerations. *J. Pediatr.*, 97, pp.854-860.

[57]   Feldman, H. A. (1967) Sulfonamide-resistant meningococci. *Ann. Rev. Med.*, 18, pp.495-506.

[58]   van de Beek, D., de Gans, J., McIntyre, P., Prasad, K. (2008) Corticosteroids for acute bacterial meningitis. *Cochrane Database of Systematic Reviews*, 4, pp.1-52.

[59]   de Gans, J., van de Beek, D. (2002) Dexamethasone in adults with bacterial meningitis. *New Eng. J. Med.*, 347, pp.1549-1556.

[60]   Cartwright, K., Reilly, S., White, D., Stuart, J. (1992) Early treatment with parenteral penicillin in meningococcal disease. *BMJ*, 305, pp.143-152.

In: Meningitis: Causes, Diagnosis and Treatment   ISBN 978-1-62100-833-0
Editors: G. Houllis et al. pp. 225-240   ©2012 Nova Science Publishers, Inc.

Chapter 6

BACTERIAL MENINGITIS: NOVEL DISSEMINATION AND INVASION ROUTES

*Aristotelis S. Filippidis[1], Ioannis D. Siasios[1], Eftychia Z. Kapsalaki[2] and Kostas N. Fountas[1]**

Departments of Neurosurgery[1] and Diagnostic Radiology[2],
University Hospital of Larissa, School of Medicine,
University of Thessaly, Larissa, Greece

INTRODUCTION

Bacterial meningitis is an infection of arachnoid membrane, subarachnoid space, and cerebrospinal fluid caused by bacteria. It is an infectious disease ranked among the top ten infectious causes of death [1]. A small number of pathogens such as Escherichia coli, group B Streptococcus (a.k.a. Streprococcus agalactiae), S. pneumoniae, Haemophilus influenzae type b (Hib), Neisseria meningitidis, and Listeria monocytogenes can cause meningitis in neonates, children, and adults with pathogenetic mechanisms elusive to scientists several years ago. The major pathogens of bacterial meningitis are Streptococcus pneumoniae and Neisseria meningitidis, accounting for 80% of the cases observed in community-acquired, bacterial

* Correspondence: Kostas N. Fountas M.D., Ph.D. Biopolis, Larisa, 40011, Greece. Tel: +30-2413 502738. Fax: +30-2413 501014. E-mail: fountas@med.uth.gr and knfountasmd@excite.com.

meningitis in adults [2]. Nowadays, pneumococci are the most important cause of bacterial meningitis in children and adults worldwide. Haemophilus influenzae has disappeared in developed countries due to the wide employment of programs of successful vaccination. The incidence of the disease ranges from 1.1 to 2 per 100,000 population in USA [3-5] and Western Europe [6]. However, in Africa the incidence rises to 12 cases per 100,000 population per year [7]. The risk of disease is highest in individuals younger than 5 years and older than 60 years. In the adult subgroup (patients older than 16 years of age) the annual incidence of bacterial meningitis is 4 to 6 cases per 100,000 people [2]. Predisposing factors such as a previous splenectomy, malnutrition, or sickle cell disease have been identified [1, 8-10]. Bacterial meningitis can also be identified as a complication in 0.8 to 1.5% of patients undergoing craniotomy, and in 4 to 17% of patients with internal ventricular catheters. The incidence of meningitis after moderate or severe head trauma is up to 1.4% [11]. Leakage of cerebrospinal fluid (CSF) is the major risk factor for the development of meningitis, although most that occur after trauma remain undetected.

Besides classical meningitis, meningococci frequently cause systemic disease including fulminant gram-negative sepsis, and disseminated intravascular coagulopathy. The World Health Organization estimates that least 500,000 new symptomatic infections per year occur worldwide, leading to at least 50,000 deaths [12].

Bacterial meningitis remains a significant cause of morbidity and mortality throughout the world, despite the progress of antimicrobial therapy, especially in developing countries because of lack of preventive medical services, such as vaccination programs. Mortality rates are up to 34% [2, 13-15], while more than 50% of the survivors suffer from long-term neurological sequelae [3, 15-17]. The evolution of the disease can frequently result into a medical emergency with devastating consequences whenever inappropriate treatment is administered. However, mortality and morbidity vary by age and geographical location of the patient as well as the underlying pathogen. Patients at risk for high mortality and morbidity include newborns, those living in low-socioeconomical status, and those infected with Gram-negative bacilli and Streptococcus pneumoniae. Severity of illness on presentation (e.g. low Glasgow Coma Scale score), infection with resistant organisms, and incomplete knowledge of the pathogenesis of meningitis are additional factors contributing to increase mortality and morbidity. Age at infection is a crucial epidemiological factor. Different bacteria are the causative organisms of bacterial meningitis at different ages. Group B haemolytic Streptococcus, gram negative rods, Streptococcus pneumoniae, and Listeria monocytogenes are the main causes of neonatal and early childhood bacterial meningitis, and their presence is attributed to the acquisition through an infected maternal genital canal [18]. Streptococcus pneumoniae, Neisseria meningitis and Haemophilus influenzae type b appear usually responsible for meningitis occurring among patients with ages ranging between 6 months to 6 years [19, 20]. Epidemiology changes again between 6 years and 60 years, when Neisseria meningitis and Streptococcus pneumoniae predominate. In addition to this unacceptable mortality, there is a high rate of neurologic sequelae in children and adults who survive after episodes of bacterial meningitis.

High morbidity imposes the need to study the pathogenesis and pathophysiology of bacterial meningitis in an attempt to improve the response to conventional antimicrobial therapy. Many researchers have tried to analyze the pathogenesis of bacterial meningitis in an effort to develop new treatment approaches. Bacterial meningitis is an infectious disease that requires multidisciplinary and specialized medical treatment. Better understanding of the infection route, concerning the cascade of events that spread the disease from the primary infection site of the nasopharynx or the middle ear, would aid in the development of more effective treatment strategies [1, 9].

PATHOGENETIC MECHANISMS OF BACTERIAL MENINGITIS

In order to identify any novel invasion and dissemination routes we have to provide first the established theories concerning the pathogenesis of bacterial meningitis. The theories are tailored to each pathogen in focus. Common ground is the evolution of a chain of events in a susceptible individual [1, 9, 10, 18].

Colonization of nasopharynx or middle ear by the involved bacteria (Streptococcus pneumoniae, Neisseria meningitis or Haemophilus influenzae type b) is the first step. Many of the major meningeal pathogens possess surface characteristics that enhance mucosal colonization. Appropriate virulence factors such as fimbriae, a polysaccharide capsule, LPS, hemocin, or pili, found on many bacteria, often mediate their adhesion to host cells or invasion. Fimbriae are considered significant virulence factors for the adherence of H. influenzae to upper respiratory tract epithelial cells. Lack of fimbrial expression impairs the ability of H. influenzae type b to colonize the nasopharynx. Natural antibodies such as IgA, found predominantly in mucosal secretions, may inhibit the adherence of microorganisms to mucosal surfaces, while their pathogenetic role is elusive. The presence of high concentrations of circulating IgA antibodies to N. meningitidis may paradoxically permit the development or exacerbate the progression of invasive disease by blocking the beneficial effects of IgG and IgM antibodies. IgA1 proteases produced by many pathogenic Neisseria, Haemophilus, and Streptococcus species may facilitate the adherence of bacterial strains to mucosal surfaces. This can be achieved through local destruction of IgA.

The second step involves the invasion of the nasopharyngeal mucosal epithelium and the entry of the pathogens to the submucosal layer. This step requires specific virulence factors that the pathogenic bacteria should bear. For example, hemocin, the bacteriocin produced by H. influenzae, is strongly associated with type b encapsulated strains, and may play a role in host nasopharyngeal colonization or in facilitating systemic invasion.

A critical step engulfed by current models in the evolution of the bacterial meningitis, is the entrance of pathogens to the bloodstream and to the systemic circulation. It is speculated that the rich vascular network of the nasal submucosal layer or the lung circulation are the sites of entry to the bloodstream. Bacterial survival in a hostile environment is crucial for the development of meningitis. The role of bacterial capsule is the most important virulence factor in this regard. It inhibits neutrophil phagocytosis and provides resistance to classic complement-mediated bactericidal activity. These bacterial defense mechanisms favor bloodstream survival and facilitate intravascular replication. The most common meningeal pathogens (H. influenzae, N. meningitidis, S. pneumoniae, E. coli, and Streptococcus agalactiae) are all encapsulated, providing thus an evolutionary mechanism for circumventing the host defense mechanisms. Capsular types are associated disproportionately with the development of bacterial meningitis, providing evidence about certain tropism [1, 9, 10].

Neonatal meningitis is an example. About 84% of cases of neonatal meningitis due to E. coli are caused by strains bearing the K1 antigen, which is antigenically related to the capsular material of serogroup B meningococci and type III group B streptococci. In the absence of K1-specific host antibody, these organisms are profoundly resistant to phagocytosis. A critical and effective number of the pathogenic bacterial population is needed in the bloodstream to have positive blood cultures. This is not always true since positive blood cultures are not the rule of thumb whenever a diagnosis for bacterial meningitis is possible [18, 21-23].

The next critical step is the entry of the pathogen into the CSF. The pathogen should survive and overcome two barriers, the blood-brain barrier (BBB), and the blood-CSF barrier (choroid plexus) in order to gain access to the meninges [1, 9, 10, 24-26]. Current theories accept that the site of entry to the CSF is the choroid plexus or the brain endothelium although this is not clear [1]. Early studies with an experimental rat model suggested that the route of invasion from the bloodstream to the CSF was through the dural venous sinus system. Further studies of infant rats and primates demonstrated that bacteria may enter the CSF via the choroid plexus. Its exceptionally high rate of blood flow, may permit the delivery of more bacterial organisms to this site than to any other anatomic locations. Sampling of CSF compartments early during bacterial meningitis has demonstrated higher bacterial concentrations in the lateral ventricles than in the cisterna magna, lumbar subarachnoid space, or supracortical subarachnoid space. As time progresses an equilibrium state is reached in these other CSF locations, however the existent data suggest that the initial bacterial entry into CSF in the lateral ventricles, is through the choroid plexi. A virulence factor armamentarium is important in these steps too. This is also true for the cellular site preference of the bacteria. Extracellular bacteria possess and utilize different dissemination and invasion mechanisms comparing to intracellular bacteria [1, 10, 22, 27].

Mechanisms used by microbial pathogens to enter the CNS are usually divided according to the cellular route involved, and whether the organisms breach endothelial cells of blood-brain barrier or specialized epithelial cells of blood-CSF barriers. These routes of entry are commonly referred to as 1) intercellular, i.e., passing between cells, 2) transcellular, i.e., passing through cells, 3) leukocyte-monocyte facilitated, i.e., a Trojan horselike mechanism, suggesting that bacteria may gain access to the CSF along with the migrating monocytes, or 4) nonhematogenous [1, 8-10, 22, 27].

The most common routes of entry for extracellular bacteria are the intercellular and transcellular routes. For most of the organisms considered here, the cellular and molecular mechanisms that enable neuroinvasion are largely unknown or are just now being discovered. Finally, the pathogen should survive within the subarachnoid space (SaS) in order to be able to infect the meninges, and initiate a cascade of events, which eventually lead to neuronal damage. The bacterial survival in the subarachnoid space can be attributed to the low CSF complement and antibody levels, and the suboptimal opsonic activity of the CSF leucocytes [1, 10, 22, 27]. Bacterial meningitis results in increased permeability of the blood-brain barrier (BBB) and this can be achieved through the orchestration and combined action of a variety of cytokines and virulence factors. The major sites of the BBB are the arachnoid membrane, choroid plexus epithelium, and cerebral microvascular endothelium. Following bacterial invasion of the subarachnoid space, a secondary bacteremia may result from the local CNS suppurative process, allowing the meningeal pathogen to continuously enter and leave the CSF compartment under quite dynamic circumstances [1, 8-10, 22, 27].

IDENTIFYING THE POTENTIAL FOR ALTERNATIVE ROUTES OF INVASION AND DISSEMINATION

Blood cultures remain a diagnostic tool aiding the diagnosis of bacterial meningitis, however meningitis can be present with negative blood cultures and positive CSF cultures. The entry of the pathogen into the bloodstream and the systemic circulation is thought to be a crucial event in the chain of evolution of bacterial meningitis. This step follows the nasal submucosal invasion and then leads to meningeal invasion. A frequent example of meningitis with negative blood cultures is seen in neonatal meningitis. Often there is absence of bacteraemia, while CSF culture is the test of choice that leads to the establishment of the correct diagnosis in this subgroup of patients. Garges et al. [28] studied 92 neonates with bacterial meningitis. In this subgroup only 57 neonates (62%) had positive blood cultures in proven neonatal meningitis cases. Another study by Rosenstein et al. [22] reported that Neisseria meningitidis can be isolated from the bloodstream in about three quarters of the infected patients. Rosenstein et al. report that meningococcemia can be identified in only 5-20% of patients [22]. Current pathophysiologic theories engulf the bloodstream dissemination of the pathogenic bacteria as a cornerstone of the evolution of the disease. Thus, we would expect an increased incidence of septicaemia or meningococcemia in meningitis patients, which is not always true. However, literature reveals that the presence of the pathogenic bacteria in the blood, in levels adequate for culture identification is not a required phenomenon, or it is probably a delayed sign in specific cases.

The ability of pathogenic bacteria to appear in the bloodstream simultaneously with the meningeal inflammation is based on virulence factors that are genetically coded, as experiments conducted by Marra and Bringham have shown [29]. They used a novel mouse model of S. pneumoniae meningitis. They discovered that this pathogen could infect the brain of mice following respiratory tract infection in the absence of bacteraemia. Targeted mutations in a specific gene create the *galU* mutant S. pneumoniae strain. Experiments designed with this strain and intrabullar injections of gerbils showed a constant defect in its dissemination in the bloodstream while it could always infect the meninges. These observations could suggest that possibly the pneumonococcal invasion of the central nervous system could be independent of bacteraemia and it is probably a mistake to correlate them [9, 29]. According to Tunkel and Scheld [10], sustained bacteraemia is not the only factor responsible for meningeal invasion and thus meningitis.

Recently, Sjölinder et al. described a mouse model of bacterial meningitis in which they used an intranasal inoculation of Neisseria meningitidis [30]. In their model, bacteremia was absent in about 20% of proven, lethal meningitis. This subgroup had already extensive meningeal damage detected in the microscopic level, with dismal prognosis. Additionally, they managed to identify a threshold level for bacteraemia, which was necessary to lead to the evolution of meningococcal sepsis.

Virulence in bacterial strains and tropism are key factors. Viridans streptococci, which produce constant and prominent bacteraemia during infective endocarditis, rarely lead to bacterial meningitis. There is a relation between the magnitude of bacteraemia and the development of meningitis when the causative organisms are E. coli, S. pneumoniae or H. influenzae type b [9]. This observation leads to the possible existence of a threshold level of bacteraemia, appropriate for meningeal invasion, and this has been proven in animal models too [9, 30].

Literature observations described previously indicate that meningeal infection and inflammation can precede the appearance of a positive blood culture that is associated with meningeal inflammation [18, 21-23, 30]. It seems that a threshold level for bacteremia exists. This could imply that there is a shortcut for the pathogenic bacteria to reach and infect the meninges before they appear in the bloodstream. Another possible explanation could be that blood cultures have a lower sensitivity to detect bacterial colonies than CSF diagnostic tests, which is not true in the modern era. We propose that the presence in the bloodstream and systemic circulation of the underlying pathogen could represent the wide dissemination of the organism after meningeal invasion, so negative blood cultures could refer to a window period time frame. The window time frame corresponds to the period that bacteria infected the meninges via an anatomic shortcut but they were not widely disseminated in the blood stream to be detected with blood cultures.

This piece of evidence triggers us to think that new routes of infection could possibly exist. These new routes could bypass systemic circulation or occur in a parallel way with systemic dissemination. This alternative route for the pathogen to enter the subarachnoid space may represent a faster route, like an anatomical shortcut.

The varied percentages of bacteraemia reported in the literature and the limitations of the theory of bloodstream dissemination preceding meningeal inflammation are not the only points of argument for the existence of an alternative infection route. It is much more difficult for bacteria to survive by following a bloodstream dissemination hypothesis, because they have more enemies to fight.

The entrance to the bloodstream requires the survival of the pathogens in the blood. Current theories [1, 9, 10, 18] utilize the existence of proven virulence factors in the causative bacteria like a polysaccharide capsule, or the implementation of a defense mechanism deficiency of the host (i.e. deficiency of the complement system) [1, 9, 10]. Crossing from blood to CSF is the next critical step. The pathogens have to cross two quite strong barriers, the BBB and the blood-CSF barrier. Tight junctions, low level of pinocytosis in the BBB, and specific carrier and transport systems secure the brain from external invasions [1, 9, 10, 24, 25]. The choroid plexus bears fenestrated capillaries and venules but there is an external barrier covering, which is continuous with the ependyma of the ventricles, and thus acts as an active transport epithelium with occluding tight junctions [26]. The utilization of distinct virulence features is required to overcome these barriers. These are the pathogen's phase variation and paracellular or intracellurar BBB crossing, intracellular macrophage survival, transcytosis and receptor expression for adhesion, crossing and immune system deception [1, 8-10, 22, 27]. The existence of barriers could possibly lead to a prolonged exposure of the involved pathogen to host's defense mechanisms. This could be a tactical advantage for the host defense mechanisms. However, the cascade of events in bacterial meningitis is quite fast and disastrous. Peralta et al. reported that patients with meningitis belong to the subgroup with early positive blood cultures indicating a strong virulence due to short time to positivity in blood cultures of patients with S. pneumoniae [31]. The existence of alternative routes that could bypass blood-brain and blood-CSF barriers could provide a more safe and adequate passage for meningitis pathogens, without any delays in the infectious process correlating with a fulminant clinical picture.

NASAL LYMPHATICS AND OLFACTORY NERVES AS ALTERNATIVE INVASION AND DISSEMINATION ROUTES

In 2008, Filippidis and Fountas proposed that one of these alternative routes could be a non-hematogenous route, the nasal lymphatic network, which communicates with the cortical subarachnoid space via the perineural spaces of the olfactory nerves. This suggestion was based on rising and strong evidence about the presence of lymphatics in the brain [32].

Cerebrospinal fluid production via the choroid plexus and its absorption via the arachnoid villi to the cerebral venous sinuses had remained in the traditional CSF physiology textbooks as a widely accepted doctrine. However, the last fifteen years, there were a few reports describing the presence of a functional and anatomical connection between the extracranial lymphatics (especially nasal submucosal and cervical lymphatics) and the subarachnoid space via the perineural spaces and the cribriform plate [33-39]. Zakharov et al. [40] proposed that this communication is the main mechanism of CSF absorption in sheep when intracranial pressure is within normal range, while the elevation of pressure activates an additional route of absorption via the arachnoid villi that act as pressure valves. The function of this mechanism is better expressed in neonatal lamb population [39]. In humans, a microscopic autopsy study related to drainage routes and subarachnoid hemorrhage was the first to provide similar evidence [41]. Later on, more studies proved the existence of this communication [36, 42]. The exact role of this communication in humans in CSF turnover, needs to be established under various intracranial pressure scenarios although it seems to play a significant role in CSF absorption [36, 42].

Inflammation can spread via hematogenous, lymphatic, and adjacent tissue routes. Nasopharyngeal mucosal adhesion and colonization is a critical step for bacterial pathogens involved in the dissemination of meningitis [9]. They should possess the ability to colonize and invade the nasal mucosa and thus reach the nasal submucosal layer. This layer shows a dense vascular network that leads to systemic circulation and a dense network of lymphatics, that communicates directly with the subarachnoid space [42, 43]. Then, the involved pathogen has two options. One option is to invade the blood vessels and enter the bloodstream and the systemic circulation, starting a long and uncertain journey through host defenses and barriers to the subarachnoid space.

We proposed that the other option is a non-hematogenous route. It could be an invasion of the nasal submucosal lymphatics that leads directly to the subarachnoid space via an olfactory nerve perineural route and penetration of the cribriform plate [32].

This hypothesis led to experimental approaches and further research [30]. In 2010, Sjölinder et al. [30] used a humanized Neisseria meningitis mouse model with intranasal challenge. In their experimental population, 20% of the mice had negative blood cultures while in the same time this subgroup suffered from lethal meningitis. A search for a non-hematogenous route identified via immunohistochemistry, the olfactory nerve-nasal musocal lymphatic system route, which is a functional and anatomical connection between the respiratory epithelium and CNS [30]. Their observations confirmed the hypothesis proposed by Filippidis and Fountas for the existence of a non-hematogenous route for bacterial meningitis [30,32]. Evidence for the existence of this route was also present in the world of parasites and specific amoebas like Naegleria fowleri. Amoebic meningoencephalitis due to Naegleria fowleri in susceptible individuals seems to follow an intranasal route of invasion and dissemination to the CNS [44].

Nasal lymphatics or olfactory nerves offer a direct, faster shortcut to subarachnoid space. Nasal lymphatics communicate with the perineural spaces of the olfactory nerves, which are bathed in CSF of the frontal cranial subarachnoid space [36, 42]. The frequent observation of meningeal infection with negative blood cultures could be attributed to the passage of the pathogens via this alternative route.

The presence of positive blood cultures could be a later event that demonstrates systemic, wide dissemination, or an event that occurs in parallel with the nasal lymphatic infiltration. In case that the nasal submucosal communication with the subarachnoid space is proven to be more functional in neonates, as it has been demonstrated in neonatal lambs [39], it may well explain the presence of high rate of negative blood cultures in cases of human neonatal meningitis [18].

The circumventing of the bloodstream does not mean that host defense mechanisms are absent. Crucial obstacles such as numerous encounters with lymphocytes and antibodies exist. Lymphocytes possess the ability to defend the host from viruses and tumor cells, while they play a secondary role to bacterial destruction via the implementation of antibodies [45]. Bacterial pathogens of meningitis need to be encountered by neutrophiles and macrophages in order to be killed [1, 9, 10, 18]. Thus, a lymphatic infection route or an olfactory nerve infection might provide a potential advantage of survival against the bloodstream route [30, 32, 44]. Individuals with host defense mechanisms deficiencies, such as a malfunctioning complement system or anatomical or functional asplenia, are these patients that nasopharyngeal bacterial colonization progresses eventually to meningitis [1, 9, 10].

Moreover, systemic lymphatics are characterized by the presence of unidirectional valves in their course. These valves serve as a one-way promoter of the transport processes while they prevent the backflow of harmful pathogens [46, 47]. The meticulous observation of the morphology and function of the existent valves along the nasal submucosal lymphatics that promote the outflow of CSF from the subarachnoid space could hinder the transport of pathogens under the proposed hypothesis. However, Kim et al. [47] showed that the lymphatics of the human nasal mucosa possess no distinct valve-like structures and thus bidirectional flow is possible. The absence of this unidirectional flow barrier would not hinder the pathogens from entering the subarachnoid space and thus infecting the meninges.

CONCLUSIONS

High morbidity and mortality are still a dreadful characterictic of bacterial meningitis in the modern era. The underlying pathophysiological mechanisms implicated in the development of meningitis are complex and elusive. According to the current theories, the chain of events that lead from nasopharyngeal colonization to meningeal inflammation require the invasion and the bypassing of quite delicate central nervous system barriers like the BBB and the blood-CSF barrier and the survival of the involved pathogen against all host's defense mechanisms. However, high rates of fulminant meningitis can be present with negative blood cultures.

The invasion of the subarachnoid space directly through the nasal lymphatics or olfactory nerves, is an uprising proposal which could possibly offer reasonable explanations to observations that cannot be interpreted by the current theories. This proposal was recently confirmed experimentally in animals creating a whole new field of research in the pathogenesis of bacterial meningitis. Experimental studies and clinical research are necessary for further validating the proposed theory, and for clarifying its role in explaining the underlying pathophysiology in cases of bacterial meningitis. The detection of the involved pathogen along the proposed nasal lymphatic route, through the olfactory perineural spaces or in the olfactory nerves of humans before evidence of bloodstream dissemination could further strengthen the proposed theory. Our proposed hypothesis may not apply to the sum of meningitis pathogens, therefore identification of those pathogens that are capable of invading and propagating via the nasal lymphatic-olfactory nerve route seems to be of paramount importance. It could probably provide evidence for this subgroup of meningitis with a fulminant picture and negative blood cultures. More efficient treatment strategies could be evolved, targeting directly the nasal lymphatic-olfactory nerve route could result in decreased morbidity and more favorable overall outcome.

REFERENCES

[1]   Koedel U, Scheld W, Pfister H. Pathogenesis and pathophysiology of pneumococcal meningitis. *The Lancet Infectious Diseases.* 2002 Dec 1;2(12):721-36.

[2]   van de Beek D, de Gans J, Tunkel AR, Wijdicks EF. Community-acquired bacterial meningitis in adults. *N. Engl. J. Med.* 2006 Jan 5;354(1):44-53.

[3]   Schuchat A, Robinson K, Wenger JD, Harrison LH, Farley M, Reingold AL, et al. Bacterial meningitis in the United States in 1995. Active Surveillance Team. *The New England journal of medicine.* [Research Support, Non-U.S. Gov't Research Support, U.S. Gov't, P.H.S.]. 1997 Oct 2;337(14):970-6.

[4]   Wenger JD, Hightower AW, Facklam RR, Gaventa S, Broome CV. Bacterial meningitis in the United States, 1986: report of a multistate surveillance study. The Bacterial Meningitis Study Group. *The Journal of infectious diseases.* 1990 Dec;162(6):1316-23.

[5]   Thigpen MC, Whitney CG, Messonnier NE, Zell ER, Lynfield R, Hadler JL, et al. Bacterial meningitis in the United States, 1998-2007. *The New England journal of medicine.* [Research Support, U.S. Gov't, P.H.S.]. 2011 May 26;364(21):2016-25.

[6]   S, Trollfors B, Claesson BA, Alestig K, Gothefors L, Hugosson S, et al. Incidence and prognosis of meningitis due to Haemophilus influenzae, Streptococcus pneumoniae and Neisseria meningitidis in Sweden. *Scand. J. Infect. Dis.* [Research Support, Non-U.S. Gov't]. 1996;28(3):247-52.

[7]   O'Dempsey TJ, McArdle TF, Lloyd-Evans N, Baldeh I, Lawrence BE, Secka O, et al. Pneumococcal disease among children in a rural area of

west Africa. *The Pediatric infectious disease journal*. [Research Support, U.S. Gov't, Non-P.H.S.]. 1996 May;15(5):431-7.

[8]   Kastenbauer S. Pneumococcal meningitis in adults: Spectrum of complications and prognostic factors in a series of 87 cases. *Brain*. 2003 May 1;126(5):1015-25.

[9]   Kim K. Neurological diseases: Pathogenesis of bacterial meningitis: from bacteraemia to neuronal injury. *Nat. Rev. Neurosci*. 2003 May 1;4(5):376-85.

[10]   Tunkel AR, Scheld WM. Pathogenesis and pathophysiology of bacterial meningitis. *Annu. Rev. Med*. 1993 Jan 1;44:103-20.

[11]   Baltas I, Tsoulfa S, Sakellariou P, Vogas V, Fylaktakis M, Kondodimou A. Posttraumatic meningitis: bacteriology, hydrocephalus, and outcome. *Neurosurgery*. 1994 Sep;35(3):422-6; discussion 6-7.

[12]   Stephens DS, Greenwood B, Brandtzaeg P. Epidemic meningitis, meningococcaemia, and Neisseria meningitidis. *Lancet*. [Review]. 2007 Jun 30;369(9580):2196-210.

[13]   van de Beek D, de Gans J, Spanjaard L, Weisfelt M, Reitsma JB, Vermeulen M. Clinical features and prognostic factors in adults with bacterial meningitis. *N. Engl. J. Med*. 2004 Oct 28;351(18):1849-59.

[14]   van de Beek D, de Gans J, Tunkel AR, Wijdicks EFM. Community-acquired bacterial meningitis in adults. *The New England journal of medicine*. 2006 Feb 04;354(1):44-53.

[15]   van de Beek D, Schmand B, de Gans J, Weisfelt M, Vaessen H, Dankert J, et al. Cognitive impairment in adults with good recovery after bacterial meningitis. *The Journal of infectious diseases*. 2002 Oct 1;186(7):1047-52.

[16]   Bohr V, Paulson OB, Rasmussen N. Pneumococcal meningitis. Late neurologic sequelae and features of prognostic impact. *Arch Neurol*. [Research Support, Non-U.S. Gov't]. 1984 Oct;41(10):1045-9.

[17]   de Gans J, van de Beek D. Dexamethasone in adults with bacterial meningitis. *The New England journal of medicine*. [Clinical Trial Multicenter Study Randomized Controlled Trial Research Support, Non-U.S. Gov't]. 2002 Nov 14;347(20):1549-56.

[18]   Garges H. Neonatal Meningitis: What Is the Correlation Among Cerebrospinal Fluid Cultures, Blood Cultures, and Cerebrospinal Fluid Parameters? *Pediatrics*. 2006 Apr 1;117(4):1094-100.

[19]   Ashwal S, Tomasi L, Schneider S, Perkin R, Thompson J. Bacterial meningitis in children: pathophysiology and treatment. *Neurology*. 1992 Apr 1;42(4):739-48.

[20] Hart C. Meningococcal disease and its management in children. *BMJ.* 2006 Sep 30;333(7570):685-90.

[21] Bell LM, Alpert G, Campos JM, Plotkin SA. Routine quantitative blood cultures in children with Haemophilus influenzae or Streptococcus pneumoniae bacteremia. *PEDIATRICS.* 1985 Dec 1;76(6):901-4.

[22] Rosenstein NE, Perkins BA, Stephens DS, Popovic T, Hughes JM. Meningococcal disease. *N. Engl. J. Med.* 2001 May 3;344(18):1378-88.

[23] Sullivan TD, LaScolea LJ, Jr., Neter E. Relationship between the magnitude of bacteremia in children and the clinical disease. *Pediatrics.* 1982 Jun;69(6):699-702.

[24] Saunders NR, Habgood MD, Dziegielewska KM. Barrier mechanisms in the brain, I. Adult brain. *Clin. Exp. Pharmacol. Physiol.* 1999 Jan 1;26(1):11-9.

[25] Saunders NR, Habgood MD, Dziegielewska KM. Barrier mechanisms in the brain, II. Immature brain. *Clin. Exp. Pharmacol. Physiol.* 1999 Feb 1;26(2):85-91.

[26] Segal MB. The choroid plexuses and the barriers between the blood and the cerebrospinal fluid. *Cell Mol. Neurobiol.* 2000 Apr 1;20(2):183-96.

[27] Drevets DA, Leenen PJ, Greenfield RA. Invasion of the central nervous system by intracellular bacteria. *Clin. Microbiol. Rev.* 2004 Apr 1;17(2):323-47.

[28] Garges HP. Neonatal Meningitis: What is the correlation among cerebrospinal fluid cultures, blood cultures, and cerebrospinal fluid parameters? *Pediatrics.* 2006 May 01;117(4):1094-100.

[29] Marra A, Brigham D. Streptococcus pneumoniae causes experimental meningitis following intranasal and otitis media infections via a nonhematogenous route. *Infect. Immun.* 2001 Dec 1;69(12):7318-25.

[30] Sjölinder H, Jonsson A-B. Olfactory nerve--a novel invasion route of Neisseria meningitidis to reach the meninges. *PLoS One.* 2010;5(11):e14034.

[31] Peralta G, Rodríguez-Lera MJ, Garrido JC, Ansorena L, Roiz MP. Time to positivity in blood cultures of adults with Streptococcus pneumoniae bacteremia. *BMC Infect. Dis.* 2006 Jan 1;6:79.

[32] Filippidis A, Fountas KN. Nasal lymphatics as a novel invasion and dissemination route of bacterial meningitis. *Medical hypotheses.* 2009 Jul;72(6):694-7.

[33] Boulton M, Armstrong D, Flessner M, Hay J, Szalai JP, Johnston M. Raised intracranial pressure increases CSF drainage through arachnoid

villi and extracranial lymphatics. *Am. J. Physiol.* 1998 Sep 1;275(3 Pt 2):R889-96.

[34] .Boulton M, Flessner M, Armstrong D, Mohamed R, Hay J, Johnston M. Contribution of extracranial lymphatics and arachnoid villi to the clearance of a CSF tracer in the rat. *Am. J. Physiol.* 1999 Mar 1;276(3 Pt 2):R818-23.

[35] Brinker T, Lüdemann W, Berens von Rautenfeld D, Samii M. Dynamic properties of lymphatic pathways for the absorption of cerebrospinal fluid. *Acta Neuropathol.* 1997 Nov 1;94(5):493-8.

[36] Caversaccio M, Peschel O, Arnold W. The drainage of cerebrospinal fluid into the lymphatic system of the neck in humans. *ORL J. Otorhinolaryngol. Relat. Spec.* 1996 Jan 1;58(3):164-6.

[37] Johnston M, Zakharov A, Koh L, Armstrong D. Subarachnoid injection of Microfil reveals connections between cerebrospinal fluid and nasal lymphatics in the non-human primate. *Neuropathol. Appl. Neurobiol.* 2005 Dec 1;31(6):632-40.

[38] Lüdemann W, Berens von Rautenfeld D, Samii M, Brinker T. Ultrastructure of the cerebrospinal fluid outflow along the optic nerve into the lymphatic system. Child's Nervous System : *OfficialJournal of the International Society for Pediatric Neurosurgery.* 2005 Feb 1;21(2):96-103.

[39] Papaiconomou C, Bozanovic-Sosic R, Zakharov A, Johnston M. Does neonatal cerebrospinal fluid absorption occur via arachnoid projections or extracranial lymphatics? *Am. J. Physiol. Regul. Integr. Comp. Physiol.* 2002 Oct 1;283(4):R869-76.

[40] Zakharov A, Papaiconomou C, Djenic J, Midha R, Johnston M. Lymphatic cerebrospinal fluid absorption pathways in neonatal sheep revealed by subarachnoid injection of Microfil. *Neuropathol. Appl. Neurobiol.* 2003 Dec 1;29(6):563-73.

[41] Löwhagen P, Johansson BB, Nordborg C. The nasal route of cerebrospinal fluid drainage in man. A light-microscope study. *Neuropathology and applied neurobiology.* 1994 Dec;20(6):543-50.

[42] Johnston M, Zakharov A, Papaiconomou C, Salmasi G, Armstrong D. Evidence of connections between cerebrospinal fluid and nasal lymphatic vessels in humans, non-human primates and other mammalian species. *Cerebrospinal Fluid Research.* 2004 Dec 10;1(1):2.

[43] Caversaccio M, Peschel O, Arnold W. The drainage of cerebrospinal fluid into the lymphatic system of the neck in humans. ORL; *Journal for*

Oto-Rhino-Laryngology and its Related Specialties. 1995 Dec 31;58(3):164-6.

[44] Jarolim KL, McCosh JK, Howard MJ, John DT. A light microscopy study of the migration of Naegleria fowleri from the nasal submucosa to the central nervous system during the early stage of primary amebic meningoencephalitis in mice. *J. Parasitol.* [Research Support, Non-U.S. Gov't]. 2000 Feb;86(1):50-5.

[45] Liu CC, Young LH, Young JD. Lymphocyte-mediated cytolysis and disease. *N. Engl. J. Med.* 1996 Nov 28;335(22):1651-9.

[46] Ikomi E, Zweifach BW, Schmid-Schonbein GW. Fluid pressures in the rabbit popliteal afferent lymphatics during passive tissue motion. *Lymphology.* 1997 Mar 1;30(1):13-23.

[47] Kim T, Lee S, Moon J, Lee H, Lee S, Jung H. Distributional characteristics of lymphatic vessels in normal human nasal mucosa and sinus mucosa. *Cell Tissue Res.* 2007 Feb 7;327(3):493-8.

In: Meningitis: Causes, Diagnosis and Treatment   ISBN 978-1-62100-833-0
Editors: G. Houllis et al. pp. 241-254   ©2012 Nova Science Publishers, Inc.

Chapter 7

CONTEMPORARY MANAGEMENT OF NOSOCOMIAL BACTERIAL MENINGITIS IN NEUROSURGICAL PRACTICE

Moncef Berhouma[*]

Department of Neurosurgery B
Pierre Wertheimer Hospital – Hospices Civils de Lyon
59 Boulevard Pinel 69394 Lyon Cedex 03 – France
University Claude Bernard Lyon 1 - France

ABSTRACT

Nosocomial meningitis are rare but potentially serious and life-threatening complications of both cranial and spinal surgeries as well as head injuries. In a postoperative neurosurgical context, an important issue consists in differentiating accurately bacterial meningitis from aseptic meningitis. This latter is mainly related to the release of blood products in the cerebrospinal fluid (CSF) and the use of dural substitutes or haemostatic substances. Clinical presentation and CSF characteristics are identical between both entities while aseptic meningitis' outcome is usually benign under corticosteroids. Prompt and aggressive antibiotic treatment is mandatory in the first hours of postoperative meningitis after accurate CSF and blood samplings and adequate cultures. Only the

[*] Corresponding author: Moncef BERHOUMA MD, MSc, Consultant Neurosurgeon, Associate Professor of Neurosurgery, Mail: berhouma.moncef@yahoo.fr, Phone: (0033) 06 77 96 03 44, Web page: www.wix.com/berhoumamoncef/home

absence of bacterial culture growth in the CSF at the 72nd hour justifies
the interruption of antibiotherapy in the postoperative course. This review
details the epidemiology and the risk factors of postoperative meningitis,
pathophysiology of central nervous system infection, pathogenesis of
chemical or aseptic meningitis, paraclinical exams and treatment
modalities according to meningitis type. Short term and long term
complications including hydrocephalus, ventriculitis and/or vasculitis,
may occur depending upon precocity of treatment, accuracy of antibiotic
choice and bacteriological diagnosis.

Keywords: Bacterial meningitis, postoperative meningitis, aseptic chemical
meningitis, meningismus, cranial surgery, spinal surgery, hydrocephalus,
external ventricular drainage, head injury, CSF leakage

INTRODUCTION

Nosocomial bacterial meningitis (NBM) is a serious and potentially lethal
complication of neurosurgical procedures including both cranial and spinal
surgeries. In the specific neurosurgical post-operative context, the diagnosis of
bacterial meningitis may be difficult because of the absence of specific
symptoms but also clinical and biological modifications secondary to the
neurosurgical procedure itself. In head injuries, bacterial meningitis can occur
in the immediate post-injury course or at distance, and is secondary to skull
base defect or calvarial penetrating trauma.

In practical, the onset of fever, meningismus and more than 100
leucocytes per ml in the cerebrospinal fluid (CSF) during the post-operative
course must lead to immediate intravenous empirical bi-antibiotherapy for 72
hours until CSF and blood cultures confirm or infirm definitely the diagnosis.

Table 1. Bacteriological profile of NBM

BACTERIOLOGICAL PROFILE OF NOSOCOMIAL POSTOPERATIVE MENINGITIS	
Gram positive cocci (45-75%)	Gram negative bacilli (30-35%)
Staphylococcus epidermidis Staphylococcus aureus Streptococcus pneumoniae Enterococcus faecalis	Escherichia coli Klebsiella pneumoniae Serratia marcescens Pseudomonas aeruginosa Enterobacter cloacae

PATHOGENESIS AND BACTERIOLOGICAL PROFILE

The central nervous system is protected by the blood-brain barrier and by the meningeal layers as well as the skull. Any interruption of these barriers provides an entry access to germs, as observed in neurosurgical procedures (cranial and spinal surgeries, internal or external CSF diversions, spinal anesthesia) as well as closed or open head injuries. (Table 1 should be inserted here)

Cranial Surgery

The incidence of nosocomial bacterial meningitis after craniotomy (excluding CSF diversion procedures) varies between 0.3 and 1.5 %. The related-mortality may reach up to 50% of infected patients. Interval between the neurosurgical procedure and meningitis onset varies from hours to months. Grossly, one third of NBM occurs during the first post-operative week, a second third during the second week, and a last third after the third week. Exceptionally, NBM may occur several years after surgery. In neurosurgical procedures, the main risk of developing NBM is directly related to CSF leak. Therefore, NBM prevention includes a rigorous watertight layer-by-layer closure technique.

The neurosurgical risk factors for NBM are listed in Table 2. In the neurosurgical postoperative context, NBM should be differentiated according to their onset period: Precocious meningitis (1 to 8 postoperative days) are specifically related to direct peroperative inoculation and staphylococcus is the most frequent germ while delayed meningitis (several weeks after surgery) are usually related to CSF leak (wound, ear, nose, scalp occipital pressure sores).

CSF Diversion Procedures

These procedures include internal ventricular catheters, external ventricular drainage, external and internal lumbar drainage, and lumbar punctures. For CSF internal shunts, the risk of NBM ranges from 4 to 17%. Colonization of the catheter and the shunt mechanism itself during the surgery is the major causal factor. A special care should be taken preoperatively for the skin preparation of the patient and the clearing of any septic focus elsewhere. Double gloving during the surgical implantation have been proven to lessen infection rates. In these internal shunts, infections may appear months or years after surgery.

Table 2. Risk factors of nosocomial bacterial meningitis following neurosurgical procedures

NEUROSURGICAL RISK FACTORS FOR NOSOCOMIAL BACTERIAL MENINGITIS
Post-operative CSF leak (wound, otorrhea, rhinorrhea, around the drain)
Skin infection on the site of scalp incision
Approach through nasal fossa, facial aeric sinuses, mastoid cells (skull base approaches)
Duration of surgery (more than 4 hours)
Revision surgery
Emergency surgery (particularly in trauma context)

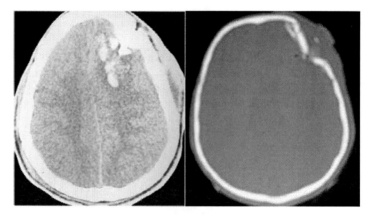

Figure 1. Open head injury by aggression with CSF leak from the wound. The patient developed meningitis within the first 24 hours. Wound neurosurgical debridement is mandatory immediately at admission to minimize the risk of meningitis.

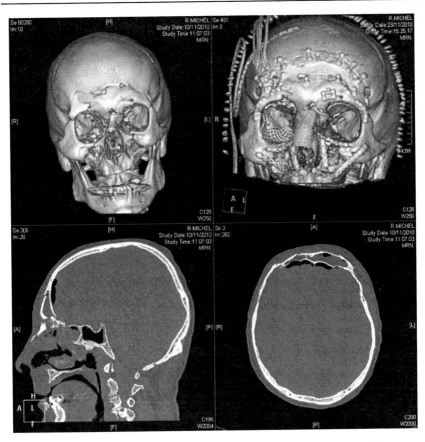

Figure 2. Closed head injury by frontal impact by a horse. Complex craniofacial fractures and anterior skull base defect involving frontal sinus leading to CSF rhinorrhea. Reparation includes closure of skull base defects and facial reconstruction (up and right panel).

External CSF diversions are frequently used in intensive care units dealing with head injuries and cerebral hemorrhages, for CSF diversion alone and/or intracranial pressure monitoring. The risk of infection of external ventricular drainage should logically be related to the duration of the drainage, but no proof of this has been given. Elsewhere, the replacement itself of the catheter may implant germs. Overall, infection rate reaches 8 to 10%. Special attention should be given for the insertion in sterile conditions. A sufficient subcutaneous tunnelization of the catheter in the scalp is mandatory to avoid CSF leakage around the catheter issuing and therefore the risk of contamination. Lumbar external drainage, sometimes required after large skull base approaches with high risk of CSF fistulas, is actually replaced by daily lumbar depletive puncture in many cases with a lesser risk of NBM.

Lumbar puncture is exceptionally complicated by infection, in contrast with intrathecal injections (therapeutical or radiological injections).

Head Injury

Both closed and open wound head injuries are associated with a risk of meningitis ranging from 1.4 to 11%. Open wound with dural laceration, particularly penetrating injuries, are exposed to a high risk of meningitis, and therefore require urgent neurosurgical debridement and layers reconstruction (Figure 1).

Closed head injuries may also develop meningitis when there is evidence of skull base fracture from the cribriform plate to the clivus and petrous bones. These skull base fractures are not systematically revealed by CSF leakage from ear or nose, and should be recognized rigorously on thin slices CT-scan and brain MRI. One should keep in mind that head injury remains the most common etiology of recurrent bacterial meningitis. The neurosurgical repair of skull base defects should be precocious, as well as anti-pneumococcal and anti-meningococcal vaccinations should be done.

CLINICAL FINDINGS AND DIAGNOSIS

Clinical Presentation

In the neurosurgical postoperative context, clinical signs of meningitis may be difficult to individualize because of the high incidence of headaches in the absence of infection. Unusual headaches are frequent in NBM (up to 90% of patients), while meningeal irritation signs are absent in 50 % of the infected patients. Fever is frequent but non-specific. A decrease in the level of consciousness and/or the apparition of focal neurological signs in the absence of postoperative hematoma, ischemia or hydrocephalus should alert the clinicians and lead to complementary exams. Globally, fever and consciousness deterioration are very evoking of NBM. The major diagnostic issue concerns sedated or comatose patients. For the specific field of internal shunts, infection signs are not less specific, particularly in children, and may range from intermittent fever, isolated vomiting or diarrhea, and general malaise. Anyway and before lumbar puncture, any clinical anomaly in a neurosurgical postoperative course should prompt an imaging (CT-scan and/or MRI) to clear an expanding mass (hematoma, ischemia, abscess, empyema, hydrocephalus).

Diagnosis Tests

CSF sampling by lumbar puncture (or through the catheter in shunted patients) is mandatory to the accurate diagnosis of NBM. This sampling should include cell counts, Gram's staining, and biochemical tests for glucose and proteins as well as cultures in both aerobic and anaerobic environments. In the neurosurgical postoperative course, interpretation of CSF profile may be difficult because of blood cells are naturally present in the CSF as well as high protein levels secondary to meningeal irritation following cranial or spinal surgeries.

The interpretation of the number of white cells may also be very problematic in patients with associated post-operative subarachnoid hemorrhage. Additional tests have been developed to improve either specificity and sensitivity for the accuracy of CSF analysis in the diagnosis of NBM, such as lactate dosage, C-reactive protein level in CSF and detection of bacterial DNA by polymerase-chain-reaction (PCR) assays. Blood tests are also mandatory and should include white cells count, C-reactive protein level, procalcitonin and blood cultures. NBM should also be differentiated from aseptic meningitis. This latter consists in a postoperative meningeal reaction to surgery, and is thought to result from the presence of blood products in the CSF or toxic substances released by brain tumors during resection. There are no clinical distinctive signs between the two entities. The diagnosis of aseptic meningitis should be retained only if bacterial meningitis has been accurately cleared off and CSF cultures remain sterile at 72 hours.

MANAGEMENT

Despite the advances in therapeutic means, morbidity as well as mortality of NBM is still higher than community-acquired meningitis. After all samples are taken (CSF, blood, wound leakage, scar...), a double bactericide empirical antibiotherapy should be promptly started intravenously. Doses are adapted to renal and liver functions. The choice of first line molecules depends upon pathogenesis of the infection and the ecology of the neurosurgical ward and intensive care unit (Table 3). Usually, a glycopeptide such as vancomycine is used at a dose reaching 40 mg per kg in continuous infusion after a 15 mg per kg bolus (objective is serum concentration of vancomycin between 15 to 20 µg/ml) in association with a large spectrum betalactamine (2 grs every 8 hours of ceftazidim, cefepim or meropenem). For patients allergic to betalactamines, ciprofloxacin (400 mg twice a day) or aztreopam (2 grs every 8 hours) may be proposed. Antibiotherapy is adapted to antibiogram data between day 1 and day 3.

Table 3. First line recommendations for nosocomial bacterial meningitis in neurosurgical practice

MECHANISM	MICROBIOLOGICAL PATTERN	RECOMMENDED EMPIRICAL LARGE-SPECTRUM ANTIBIOTHERAPY	NEUROSURGICAL ADDITIONAL THERAPY
CRANIAL OR SPINAL SURGERY CSF DIVERSION	- Pseudomonas aeruginosa - Other aerobic gram-negative bacilli - Staphylococcus aureus - Coagulase–negative staphylococci (S. epidermidis,…) - Propionibacterium acnes	Vancomycin (15 mg/kg every 8 to 12 hours)* plus ceftazidime** (or cefepime)	Wound debridement, ablation of foreign body (forgotten cotton patties, bone or dural substitutes, spinal material), drainage
PENETRATING HEAD INJURY	- Staphylococcus aureus - Coagulase–negative staphylococci (S. epidermidis,…) - Aerobic gram-negative bacilli (P. aeruginosa)		Wound debridement, abundant washing and layer by layer closure
SKULL BASE FRACTURE	- Streptococcus pneumoniae - Haemophilus influenzae - Group A β-hemolytic streptococci	Vancomycin (15 mg/kg every 8 to 12 hours) plus Ceftriaxone (1 to 4 g/d)	Surgical repair

In cases of allergy to betalactamines, ciprofloxacin may be used 400 mg every 12 hours.
* Doses in adults with normal hepatic and renal functions – Optimal serum level of vancomycin : 15 to 20 µg/ml.
** Ceftazidim 2 grams every 8 hours.

Table 4. Neurosurgical practical recommendations to minimize the risk of nosocomial bacterial meningitis

NEUROSURGICAL RECOMMENDATIONS		
PREOPERATIVE PREPARATION	**IN THE OPERATING THEATRE**	**POSTOPERATIVE COURSE**
- Verification of hole body skin integrity - Showers with antiseptic solution at least the night before and morning of the surgery - Avoid shaving hair - Admission of patients one day before surgery to avoid skin colonization by hospital germs	- No shaving - Shower with iodine solution - Incision preparation with iodine cream - Scalp preparation with iodine solution - Careful draping - Prophylactic intravenous antibiotherapy during the scalp preparation - Minimize tissue injury and blood loss - Double layer of gloves - Change of gloves for each important step (bony approach, dural opening, artificial device implantation, closure) - Abundant irrigation for germ dilution with warm saline - Careful hemostasis to minimize the risk of postoperative hematoma collection - Rigorous layer by layer closure with watertight dural suture - Skin should be sutured correctly while maintaining a good skin perfusion - Drains must be tunneled far from the incision and secured correctly to avoid disconnection	- Sterile dressing should be kept at least 48 hours - Daily showers with antiseptic solution after dressing removal of dressing at day 2 - Avoid bed sores and encourage precocious mobilization from bed

There is no consensus concerning the optimal duration of the treatment, usually between 15 and 21 days. This duration can be prolonged if artificial material is left in place (cranioplasty, plates and other bone fixation devices, dural substitutes, shunt device, catheters). The first-line antibiotherapy should be withdrawn after 72 hours if CSF cultures remain negative.

In rare cases of bacterial ventriculitis associated with meningitis, antibiotherapy can be given directly in the lateral ventricle through an intraventricular catheter related to an external ventricular drainage. Molecules usually used in this case are vancomycin (5 to 20 mg daily), gentamycin (2 to 6 mg daily), amikacin (5 to 20 mg daily) and polymyxin B (5 mg daily in adults).

A special attention should be given to the emergence of new drug-resistant germs, particularly acinetobacter multiresistant.

Common complications of NBM are those of all meningitis including obstructive hydrocephalus (acute or chronic), syringomyelia, vasculitis, cerebral ischemia, brain abscess and pachymeningitis.

Table 5. Proposed algorithm for the management of nosocomial bacterial postoperative meningitis

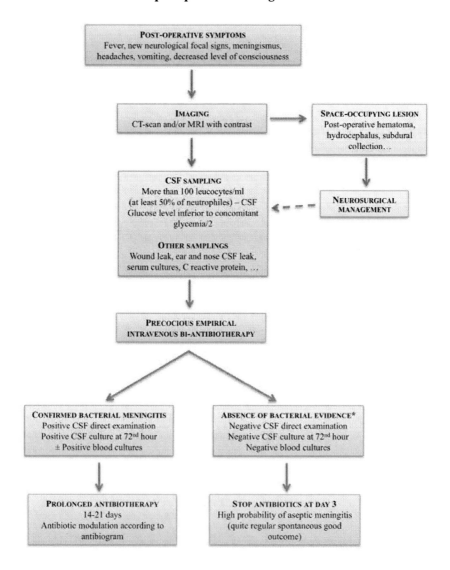

REFERENCES

[1]   Korinek AM, Baugnon T, Golmard JL,van Effenterre R, Coriat P, Puybasset L. Risk factors for adult nosocomial meningitis after craniotomy: role of antibiotic prophylaxis. *Neurosurgery* 2006;59:126-33.

[2]   Lozier AP, Sciacca RR, Romagnoli MF, Connolly ES Jr. Ventriculostomy-related infections: a critical review of the literature. *Neurosurgery* 2008;62:688-700.

[3]   Conen A, Walti LN, Merlo A, FluckigerU, Battegay M, Trampuz A. Characteristics and treatment outcome of cerebrospinal fluid shunt-associated infections in adults: a retrospective analysis over an 11-year period. *Clin. Infect Dis.* 2008;47:73-82.

[4]   Vinchon M, Dhellemmes P. Cerebrospinal fluid shunt infection: risk factors and long-term follow-up. *Childs Nerv. Syst* 2006;22:692-7.

[5]   Kulkarni AV, Drake JM, Lamberti-Pasculli M. Cerebrospinal fluid shunt infection: a prospective study of risk factors. *J. Neurosurg.* 2001;94:195-201.

[6]   Bullock MR, Chesnut R, Ghajar J, et al. Surgical management of depressed cranial fractures. *Neurosurgery* 2006;58: Suppl:S56-S60.

[7]   Sørensen P, Ejlertsen T, Aaen D, Poulsen K. Bacterial contamination of surgeons gloves during shunt insertion: a pilot study. *Br. J. Neurosurg.* 2008;22:675-7.

[8]   McClelland S III, Hall WA. Postoperative central nervous system infection: incidence and associated factors in 2111 neurosurgical procedures. *Clin. Infect Dis.* 2007;45:55-9.

[9]   Wong GK, Poon WS, Wai S, Yu LM, Lyon D, Lam JM. Failure of regular external ventricular drain exchange to reduce cerebrospinal fluid infection: result of a randomised controlled trial. *J. Neurol. Neurosurg. Psychiatry* 2002;73:759-61.

[10] Governale LS, Fein N, Logsdon J, Black PM. Techniques and complications of external lumbar drainage for normal pressure hydrocephalus. *Neurosurgery* 2008;63:Suppl 2:379-84.

[11] Baltas I, Tsoulfa S, Sakellariou P, Vogas V, Fylaktakis M, Kondodimou A. Posttraumatic meningitis: bacteriology, hydrocephalus, and outcome. *Neurosurgery* 1994;35:422-6.

[12] Kestle JRW, Garton HJL, Whitehead WE, et al. Management of shunt infections: a multicenter pilot study. *J. Neurosurg.* 2006;105:Suppl:177-81.

[13] Choi D, Spann R. Traumatic cerebrospinal fluid leakage: risk factors and the use of prophylactic antibiotics. *Br. J. Neurosurg.* 1996;10:571-5.

[14] Adriani KS, van de Beek D, Brouwer MC, Spanjaard L, de Gans J. Community-acquired recurrent bacterial meningitis in adults. *Clin. Infect Dis.* 2007;45:e46-e51.

[15] Baer ET. Post-dural puncture bacterial meningitis. *Anesthesiology* 2006;105:381-93.

[16] Weisfelt M, van de Beek D, Spanjaard L, de Gans J. Nosocomial bacterial meningitis in adults: a prospective series of 50 cases. *J. Hosp. Infect.* 2007;66:71-8.

[17] Mayhall CG, Archer NH, Lamb VA, et al. Ventriculostomy-related infections: a prospective epidemiologic study. *N. Engl. J. Med.* 1984;310:553-9.

[18] Muttaiyah S, Ritchie S, Upton A, Roberts S. Clinical parameters do not predict infection in patients with external ventricular drains: a retrospective observational study of daily cerebrospinal fluid analysis. *J. Med. Microbiol.* 2008;57:207-9.

[19] Schade RP, Schinkel J, Roelandse FW, et al. Lack of value of routine analysis of cerebrospinal fluid for prediction and diagnosis of external drainage-related bacterial meningitis. *J. Neurosurg.* 2006;104: 101-8.

[20] Beer R, Lackner P, Pfausler B, Schmutzhard E. Nosocomial ventriculitis and meningitis in neurocritical care patients. *J. Neurol.* 2008;255:1617-24.

[21] Pfausler B, Beer R, Engelhardt K, Kemmler G, Mohsenipour I, Schmutzhard E. Cell index — a new parameter for the early diagnosis of ventriculostomy (external ventricular drainage)-related ventriculitis in patients with intraventricular hemorrhage? *Acta Neurochir* (Wien) 2004;146:477-81.

[22] Zarrouk V, Vassor I, Bert F, et al. Evaluation of the management of postoperative aseptic meningitis. Clin Infect Dis 2007;44:1555-9.

[23] Leib SL, Boscacci R, Gratzl O, Zimmerli W. Predictive value of cerebrospinal fluid (CSF) lactate level versus CSF/blood glucose ratio for the diagnosis of bacterial meningitis following neurosurgery. *Clin. Infect Dis.* 1999;29:69-74.

[24] Nathan BR, Scheld WM. The potential roles of C-reactive protein and procalcitonin in the serum and cerebrospinal fluid in the diagnosis of bacterial meningitis. *Curr. Clin. Top Infect. Dis.* 2002;22:155-65.

[25] Banks JT, Bharara S, Tubbs RS, et al. Polymerase chain reaction for the rapid detection of cerebrospinal fluid shunt or ventriculostomy infections. *Neurosurgery* 2005;57:1237-43.

[26] Tunkel AR, Hartman BJ, Kaplan SL, et al. Practice guidelines for the management of bacterial meningitis. *Clin. Infect Dis.* 2004;39:1267-84.

[27] Pfausler B, Spiss H, Beer R, et al. Treatment of staphylococcal ventriculitis associated with external cerebrospinal fluid drains: a prospective randomized trial of intravenous compared with intraventricular vancomycin therapy. *J. Neurosurg.* 2003; 98:1040-4.

[28] Kessler AT, Kourtis AP. Treatment of meningitis caused by methicillin-resistant Staphylococcus aureus with linezolid. *Infection* 2007;35:271-4.

[29] Lee DH, Palermo B, Chowdhury M. Successful treatment of methicillin-resistant Staphylococcus aureus meningitis with daptomycin. *Clin. Infect Dis.* 2008;47:588-90.

[30] Beer R, Engelhardt KW, Pfausler B, et al. Pharmacokinetics of intravenous linezolid in cerebrospinal fluid and plasma in neurointensive care patients with staphylococcal ventriculitis associated with external ventricular drains. *Antimicrob. Agents Chemother* 2007;51:379-82.

[31] Tulipan N, Cleves MA. Effect of an intraoperative double-gloving strategy on the incidence of cerebrospinal fluid shunt infection. *J. Neurosurg.* 2006;104:Suppl:S5-S8.

[32] Wen DY, Bottini AG, Hall WA, Haines SJ. The intraventricular use of antibiotics. *Neurosurg Clin. N Am.* 1992;3:343-54.

[33] Ziai WC, Lewin JJ III. Improving the role of intraventricular antimicrobial agents in the management of meningitis. *Curr. Opin. Neurol.* 2009;22:277-82.

[34] Kim BN, Peleg AY, Lodise TP, et al. Management of meningitis due to antibiotic-resistant Acinetobacter species. Lancet Infect Dis 2009;9:245-55.

[35] Rodríguez Guardado A, Blanco A, Asensi V, et al. Multidrug-resistant Acinetobacter meningitis in neurosurgical patients with intraventricular catheters: assessment of different treatments. J Antimicrob Chemother 2008;61:908-13.

[36] Brown EM, Edwards RJ, Pople IK. Conservative management of patients with cerebrospinal shunt infections. Neurosurgery 2006;58:657-65.

[37] Falagas ME, Bliziotis IA, Tam VH. Intraventricular or intrathecal use of polymyxins in patients with gram-negative meningitis: a systematic

review of the available evidence. *Int. J. Antimicrob. Agents* 2007;29:9-25.

[38] Katragkou A, Roilides E. Successful treatment of multidrug-resistant Acinetobacter baumannii central nervous system infections with colistin. *J. Clin. Microbiol.* 2005;43:4916-7.

[39] Schreffler RT, Schreffler AJ, Wittler RR. Treatment of cerebrospinal fluid shunt infections: a decision analysis. *Pediatr. Infect. Dis. J.* 2002;21:632-6.

[40] Yogev R. Cerebrospinal fluid shunt infections: a personal view. *Pediatr. Infect. Dis.* 1985;4:113-8.

In: Meningitis: Causes, Diagnosis and Treatment   ISBN 978-1-62100-833-0
Editors: G. Houllis et al. pp. 255-261   ©2012 Nova Science Publishers, Inc.

Chapter 8

MOLLARET'S MENINGITIS

Poulikakos Panagiotis

ABSTRACT

Mollaret's meningitis is defined as benign recurrent aseptic meningitis characterized by recurrent episodes of fever and signs of meningeal irritation, lasting between 2 and 5 days and is associated with spontaneous recovery. Mollaret's meningitis is seldom seen in clinical practice.

The syndrome was named after Pierre Mollaret, a French neurologist, that in 1944 described recurrent episodes of aseptic meningitis in three patients during a 15 year period. The cerebrospinal fluid (CSF) taken from these patients, 24 hours after the onset of these recurrences, revealed leukocytosis containing many large mononuclear cells, thought to be of endothelial origin (Mollaret cells). After a few days, these cells disappeared. Later immunocytological examination of CSF cells revealed that the so-called Mollaret cells are actually monocytes .

The clinical presentation is indistinguishable from meningitis of other aetiologies, including fever, headache, neck and back pain, myalgias, and neck stiffness. Transient neurologic abnormalities such as epileptic seizures, facial palsy, disequilibrium, speech impairment, syncope and extensor plantar response may be present in 50% of the patients. There is a female to male predominance, approximately 26:15. In general, the episodes tend to reoccur in a period of days to years and the syndrome usually resolves automatically after 3 to 5 years according to some studies.

The aetiology of the syndrome remained obscure for many years. Steel et al. in 1981 were the first to isolate Herpes Simplex Virus type 1 (HSV-1) in the CSF of a patient with diagnosed Mollaret's meningitis, suggesting a viral aetiology of the syndrome. Some researchers followed Steel's hypothesis associating different viruses, such as Herpes Simplex Virus type 2 (HSV-2) or EBV, to the syndrome . However, it was not until the development and the use of the polymerase chain reaction (PCR) technique that the Mollaret's meningitis aetiology became clearer. Since 1991, 69 patients diagnosed with Mollaret's meningitis had their CSF tested with PCR for HSV and were reported in the literature. Remarkably, 56 were positive for HSV-2. Five cases tested negative for HSV. Among them, one was finally attributed to SLE, another to herpesvirus type 6 and only three remained idiopathic.

It has been proposed that the term Mollaret's meningitis should be reserved for recurrent aseptic meningitis where no cause is identified. However, with the existing evidence, recurrent herpetic meningitis is presumably the benign condition that was previously identified as Mollaret's meningitis.

Due to the rarity and the benign course of the disease, there is no definitive treatment recommendation. Intravenous acyclovir may be of value because it has shown to resolve symptoms within 72 h and the majority of patients remain symptom free for many years. However, intermittent or continuous prophylaxis may be considered for frequent episodes.

INTRODUCTION

Mollaret's meningitis is a rare cause of recurrent aseptic meningitis. The term aseptic meningitis refers to patients who have clinical and laboratory evidence of meningeal inflammation with negative routine bacterial cultures. Common aetiologies include viral or other infections, (mycobacteria, fungi, spirochetes), parameningeal infections, medication, and malignancy [1]. However, recurrent meningitis is a clinical entity characterized by recurrent discrete episodes of illness where all symptoms and signs and cerebrospinal fluid parameters of meningeal inflammation resolve completely between the episodes without specific treatment. Recurrent meningitis is most commonly caused by Herpes Simplex Virus type 2 (HSV-2) infection, epidermoid tumor, craniopharygioma, cholesteatoma, Systemic Lupus Erythematosus (SLE), Adamantiadis Behcet syndrome, Vogt Koyannasi Harada syndrome and Mollaret' s meningitis [2] .

Mollaret's meningitis is defined as benign recurrent aseptic meningitis characterized by recurrent episodes of fever and signs of meningeal irritation, lasting between 2 and 5 days and is associated with spontaneous recovery [3].

HISTORY

Pierre Mollaret, a French neurologist, in 1944 described recurrent episodes of aseptic meningitis in three patients during a 15 year period [4]. The cerebrospinal fluid taken from these patients, 24 hours after the onset of these recurrences, revealed leukocytosis containing many large mononuclear cells, thought to be of endothelial origin (Mollaret cells). After a few days, these cells disappeared. Later immunocytological examination of cerebrospinal fluid cells revealed that the so-called Mollaret cells are actually monocytes [5]. The cerebrospinal fluid also initially showed polymorphonuclear cells that changed to predominately lymphocytes, while the other findings (glucose, protein) were consistent with aseptic meningitis [4].

In 1962, Bruyn et al. proposed diagnostic criteria for Mollaret's meningitis [6]. These include attacks separated by symptom-free periods of weeks to months, spontaneous remission of symptoms and signs, recurrent episodes of severe headache, meningismus and fever, cerebrospinal fluid pleocytosis with large 'endothelial' cells, neutrophils, and lymphocytes and no identified causative aetiological agent.

ETIOLOGY

Steel et al. in 1981 were the first to isolate Herpes Simplex Virus type 1 (HSV-1) in the cerebrospinal fluid of a patient with diagnosed Mollaret's meningitis [7], suggesting a viral aetiology of the syndrome. Some researchers followed Steel's hypothesis associating different viruses, such as HSV-2 or EBV, to the syndrome [3]. However, it was not until the development and the use of the polymerase chain reaction (PCR) technique that the Mollaret's meningitis aetiology became clearer. The leading cause appeared to be HSV-2. Among 69 patients diagnosed with Mollaret's meningitis and had their cerebrospinal fluid tested with PCR for HSV since 1991, remarkably, 56 were positive for HSV-2. Five cases tested negative for HSV. Among them, one was finally attributed to SLE, another to herpesvirus type 6 and only three remained idiopathic [8].

After PCR implementation, herpes simplex virus infection is emerging as the cause of neurological diseases that were previously termed as "idiopathic". HSV-1 has been shown to be the most common cause of Bell's palsy [9] and HSV-2 is a well known cause of aseptic meningitis. Additionally, recurrences, though not often, exist in both entities, approximately 7% in patients with Bell's palsy [10] and 20% in patients with herpetic meningitis [11].

It has been proposed that the term Mollaret's meningitis should be reserved for recurrent aseptic meningitis where no cause is identified [12]. However, with the existing evidence, recurrent herpetic meningitis is presumably the benign condition that was previously identified as Mollaret's meningitis in the majority of cases. If herpetic aetiology is excluded in these patients, further investigation should be done to exclude more sinister conditions.

PATHOPHYSIOLOGY

Herpes Simplex Virus type 2 establishes latency in the lumbo-sacral sensory ganglia. Once reactivated, it can cause mucocutaneus disease through peripheral nerve spread. In cases of HSV-2 meningitis, the virus spreads centripetally, from the peripheral activation in the sensory ganglia to the meninges [13].

EPIDEMIOLOGY

Mollaret's meningitis is seldom seen in clinical practice. As mentioned above, since 1991, only 69 patients were reported in the international literature with the diagnosis of mollaret's meningitis after having their cerebrospinal fluid tested with PCR for HSV [8]. There is no age predilection, since the onset of the disease has been observed from 5 to 83 year old [6], with a mean age of 35 years. There is a female to male predominance, approximately 26:15 [3].

PRESENTATION

The medical history of the patient may be indicative for the aetiology of the syndrome. HSV- 2 typically causes genital herpes. Meningitis occurs as often as in 36% of women and in 11% of men during the course of primary genital herpes. Approximately 20% of the patients with an initial episode will have recurrences, while 60% of the patients diagnosed with recurrent meningitis does not mention a history of genital ulcers [11]. Thus, the information of prior HSV-2 infection is invaluable in patients that present with symptoms and signs of meningitis.

The clinical presentation is indistinguishable from meningitis of other aetiologies. Usually there is an abrupt onset of fever, headache, photophobia, neck and back pain, myalgias, and neck stiffness. Signs and symptoms reach maximum intensity within a few hours of onset. Each episode typically lasts 1–3 days, but persistence of symptoms for 3 weeks with subsequent recurrences has been recorded. In general, the episodes reoccur in a period of days to years (median of 3 to 8 episodes) [3] with a tendency to become less common over time and the syndrome usually resolves automatically after 3 to 5 years according to some studies [6]. However, there have been documented as many as 21 recurrent attacks in the same individual, whereas the duration of the syndrome can extend as long as 28 years [14].

Neurologic abnormalities such as hallucinations, epileptic seizures, cranial nerve palsy, disequilibrium, speech impairment, syncope, extensor plantar response or altered levels of consciousness may be present in 50% of the patients. These symptoms are transient and, if they persist, other etiologies should be considered [3].

DIAGNOSIS

The diagnoses of the syndrome is based upon the combination of a typical benign clinical course of recurrent episodes of meningitis with symptoms free intervals without specific treatment and characteristic cerebrospinal fluid findings of aseptic meningitis (increased protein, normal glucose, increased leucocytes with monocyte, lymphocyte or even polymorphonuclear predominance and negative cultures), according to Bruyn's criteria. However, since PCR implementation, the later has been the golden rule for the diagnoses with sensitivity of 95% and specificity of 100% for the detection of HSV-2 in the cerebrospinal fluid.

TREATMENT

Many regimens like steroids, colchicine, antihistamines, and phenylbutazonum have been used for the treatment of Mollaret's meningitis without success [3]. Due to the rarity and the benign course of the disease, no randomized controlled trials are available for the treatment of mollaret's meningitis, so there is no definitive treatment recommendation. Treatment for aseptic HSV-2 meningitis should be individualized according to the number and severity of recurrences. Intravenous acyclovir (5-10mg/kg three times a day) for 7 to 10 days may be of value because it has shown to resolve the symptoms within 72 hours. Alternate agents such as valaciclovir and famciclovir are likely to be equally efficacious. The majority of patients remain symptom-free for many years, suggesting that long-term antiviral prophylaxis may not be appropriate. However, intermittent or continuous prophylaxis may be considered for frequent episodes [11].

REFERENCES

[1]   Connolly KJ, Hammer SM. The acute aseptic meningitis syndrome. *Infect. Dis. Clin. North Am.* 1990;4(4):599-622.
[2]   Koroshetz WJ, Swartz MN. Chronic and Recurrent Meningitis. In: Kasper DL, Braunwald E, Fauci AS, et al., eds. *Harrisson's principles of internal medicine.* 16th ed. New York Q McGraw-Hill, 2005;2491-2493.
[3]   Shalabi M, Whitley RJ. Recurrent benign lymphocytic meningitis. *Clin. Infect. Dis.* 2006; 43:1194-7.
[4]   Mollaret P. La méningite endothélio-leukocytaire multirécurrente bénigne: syndrome nouveau ou maladie nouvelle? *Rev. Neurol.* (Paris) 1944;76:57–76.
[5]   Stoppe G, Stark E, Patzold U. Mollaret's meningitis: CSF-immunocytological examinations. *J. Neurol.* 1987;234:103– 6.
[6]   Bruyn G, Straathof J, Raymakers G. Mollaret's meningitis: differential diagnosis and diagnostic pitfalls. *Neurology* 1962;12:745—53.

[7]   Steel JG, Dix RD, Baringer JR. Isolation of herpes simplex type 1 in recurrent (Mollarets) meningitis. *Trans. Am. Neurol. Assoc.* 1981; 106:37–42.

[8]   Poulikakos PJ, Sergi EE, Margaritis AS, Kioumourtzis AG, Kanellopoulos GD, Mallios PK, Dimitrakis DJ, Poulikakos DJ, Aspiotis AA, Deliousis AD, Flevaris CP, Zacharof AK. A case of recurrent benign lymphocytic (Mollaret's) meningitis and review of the literature. *Journal of Infection and Public Health* (2010) 3, 192—195.

[9]   Gilden DH. Clinical practice. Bell's Palsy. *N. Engl. J. Med.* 2004;351(13):1323-31.

[10] Peitersen E. Bell's palsy: the spontaneous course of 2,500 peripheral facial nerve palsies of different etiologies. *Acta Otolaryngol. Suppl.* 2002;4-30.

[11] Tyler KL. Herpes simplex virus infections of the central nervous system: encephalitis and meningitis, including Mollaret's. *Herpes* 2004;11:57A–64A.

[12] Tedder DG, Ashley R, Tyler KL, Levin MJ. Herpes simplex virus infection as a cause of benign recurrent lymphocytic meningitis. *Ann. Intern. Med.* 1994; 12:334—8.

[13] Kojima Y, Hashiguchi H, Hashimoto T, Tsuji S, Shoji H, Kazuyama Y. Recurrent herpes simplex virus type 2 meningitis: a case report of Mollaret's meningitis. *Jpn. J. Infect. Dis.* 2002; 55:85—8.

[14] Mirakhur B, McKenna M. Recurrent herpes simplex type 2 virus (Mollaret) meningitis. *J. Am. Board Fam. Pract.* 2004;17(4):303-5.

INDEX

I

N

S